Accident and Emergency X-rays Made Easy

This book is dedicated to my Aunts, Margaret, Edith and Betty

'You know my methods ... apply them!'
Sherlock Holmes

Commissioning Editor: Laurence Hunter
Project Development Manager: Janice Urquhart
Project Manager: Frances Affleck
Designer: Erik Bigland
Illustration Manager: Bruce Hogarth
Illustrator: Graeme Chambers

Accident and Emergency X-rays Made Easy

James D. Begg MB BS FRCR

Consultant Radiologist, Royal Victoria Hospital, Dundee;
Honorary Senior Lecturer in Diagnostic Radiology, University of Dundee, Dundee, UK

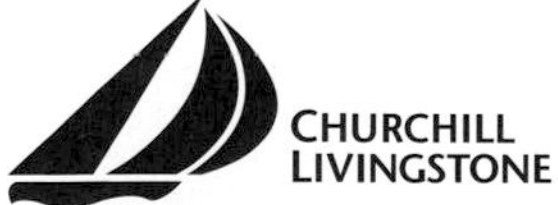

EDINBURGH LONDON NEW YORK OXFORD PHILADELPHIA ST LOUIS SYDNEY TORONTO 2005

CHURCHILL LIVINGSTONE
An imprint of Elsevier Limited

First published 2005

ISBN 0 443 07324 4
International Student Edition ISBN 0 443 07325 2

British Library Cataloguing in Publication Data
A catalogue record for this book is available from the British Library.

Library of Congress Cataloging in Publication Data
A catalog record for this book is available from the Library of Congress.

Notice
Medical knowledge is constantly changing. Standard safety precautions must be followed, but as new research and clinical experience broaden our knowledge, changes in treatment and drug therapy may become necessary or appropriate. Readers are advised to check the most current product information provided by the manufacturer of each drug to be administered to verify the recommended dose, the method and duration of administration and contraindications. It is the responsibility of the practitioner, relying on experience and knowledge of the patient, to determine dosages and the best treatment for each individual patient. Neither the Publisher nor the author assumes any liability for any injury and/or damage to persons or property arising from this publication.

The Publisher

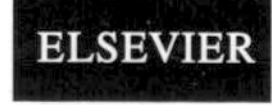

your source for books, journals and multimedia in the health sciences

www.elsevierhealth.com

The Publisher's policy is to use **paper manufactured from sustainable forests**

Printed in China

Preface

The scope for medical error in dealing with Accident and Emergency X-rays is enormous – from misidentifying the patient, to mixing up left and right; from missing fractures which *are* there to 'diagnosing' fractures which are *not* there, all of which has been done thousands of times! A shaky knowledge of anatomy, limited clinical experience and radiological knowledge, combined with the frenetic environment in which such films are often viewed, can combine to form a dangerous cocktail for the junior doctor and his unsuspecting patient, which may lead to disaster. The main object of this book is to help try and prevent that.

When a patient sees a doctor looking at his X-rays, he assumes the diagnosis is straightforward, instantaneous and clear-cut, and that the doctor knows immediately what he is looking at, i.e. 'Yes' he has a fracture, or 'No' he doesn't. Few things could be further from the truth.

Each doctor has a 'duty of care' to every patient and the expectations of the public are rising relentlessly. A small error made in the first few seconds of handling an image e.g. not checking left or right, may go unnoticed by everyone else and rapidly lead to a situation which is irretrievable.

The ever-present threat of litigation hangs constantly in the air, particularly from Accident and Emergency cases. These have littered the Defence Society Annual Reports for years.

A mental glance upward will invariably show the 'legal eagles' circling, flapping their wings, swivelling their eyes and waiting for some lucrative excuse to bare their talons and dive on your head, which can only increase the anxiety of the Accident and Emergency doctor.

The secondary purpose of this book therefore is to help try and prevent 'M'learned friends' from having any excuse to dive on you!

James D. Begg
Dundee
2004

Acknowledgements

There are a great many people to whom I am heavily indebted for their assistance in the production of this book.

Firstly, I must thank Mrs Ann H. Vickers, Senior Radiographer, Royal Victoria Hospital, Dundee, for all her help in the word processing of innumerable drafts and redrafts of the manuscript, and bringing order to what was invariably chaos.

Next I must thank Mrs Alice Harrison and Miss Morag Wilson for their long hours spent with me working on the X-ray images – at times an exacting task.

Many friends and colleagues have kindly contributed X-ray cases, so my thanks go to all of them, even if some of the pictures were not finally used in the present edition.

Among the above I must thank in particular Dr Jason Van der Velde who kindly supplied me with examples of severe trauma and gunshot wounds from South Africa; Dr David Goff and Dr George Aitken, Consultant Radiologists, Raigmore Hospital, Inverness; Dr Ian Kenney, Consultant Paediatric Radiologist, Royal Sussex Hospital for Sick Children, Brighton; Dr Briony Fredericks, Consultant Paediatric Radiologist, Yorkhill Hospital, Glasgow, and Dr Ian Gillespie, Consultant Radiologist, Edinburgh Royal Infirmary, for images of the shoulder and paediatric elbow.

My sincere thanks to Dr Declan Shepherd, recently Consultant Radiologist, Ninewells Hospital, Dundee, Dr David Hardwick, Consultant Radiologist, Borders General Hospital, Melrose, and Dr Robin Sellar, Consultant Neuroradiologist, Western General Hospital, Edinburgh, for images of trauma to the neck. My thanks also to Mr Miles Woodford, Superintendent Radiographer, Spinal Injuries Unit, Salisbury General Hospital, and Mr David Roberts for kind permission to reproduce the neck injury X-rays (Figs 3.9a, b) from Mr Woodford's article in the RAD magazine, of December 2002, pages 21, 22.

My thanks to Senior Staff Nurse Penelope Cunningham, Ninewells Hospital, Dundee for her clever mnemonic regarding the carpus, and Dr Colin Paterson, Reader in Medicine, University of Dundee and Honorary Consultant Physician (Rtd), Ninewells Hospital, Dundee, for images of fractures in infants.

My sincere thanks to Dr Orla Smithwick, Consultant in Accident and Emergency Medicine, University College Hospital, Galway, Ireland for kindly reading and advising on part of the initial draft of the book, and providing many hints and helpful suggestions in regard to the text thereof. The responsibility for any errors of fact or opinions is entirely my own.

I must also thank the Royal College of Radiologists, London, for their kind permission to make reference to their guidelines on the use of X-rays in trauma, particularly in regard to the critical areas of the head and neck which required to be covered in some depth.

Finally I must thank Mrs Janice Urquhart, Project Development Manager and Mr Laurence Hunter for their ongoing support and assistance throughout the work on this project. My thanks also to everyone else at Elsevier, including those overseas who have assisted in the physical production of this book, and not least to the many patients whose X-ray pictures appear here. I feel we owe them a debt of gratitude for enabling us to learn more about the Radiology of Accident and Emergency medicine as a result of their painful and traumatic experiences.

James D. Begg
Dundee

Contents

Chapter 1

The approach to A & E films

Requesting X-rays in A & E: a warning

All X-ray requests in the UK should as far as practicable be in line with the guidance provided in the document *Making The Best Use of a Department of Clinical Radiology*, 5th edn 2003, issued by the Royal College of Radiologists (RCR). In addition to reading the local rules, every doctor who works in A & E should read and be aware of these guidelines in advance of taking up an A & E post, and each department should have a copy of them readily accessible to all medical staff.

Under the IRMER (**I**onizing **R**adiation **M**edical **E**xposure **R**egulations) legislation introduced in 2000, all requests need to be 'justified' by a member of the X-ray staff, which in effect means that each request you make will be vetted and either carried out on its clinical merits, returned for clarification, or refused.

NB Inappropriate exposure of patients to ionizing radiation can now lead to prosecution under UK and European law. Make sure that your request is wholly appropriate as per the guidelines and that you provide full, accurate, relevant and legible demographic and clinical information on every request you write, and always ask yourself this question: 'Could this be defended in court?'. Nevertheless, unforeseen circumstances will sometimes arise which will necessitate that the guidelines be over-ridden, e.g. the CT machine breaks down. This is called 'exercising clinical judgement'.

Another warning!

Look at Figure 1.1. Believe it or not, this patient was sent home by a junior doctor from A & E with a diagnosis of 'no bony injury'. The reasons for such a gross error are not hard to find:

- **Lack of experience** (clinically the fracture was obvious).

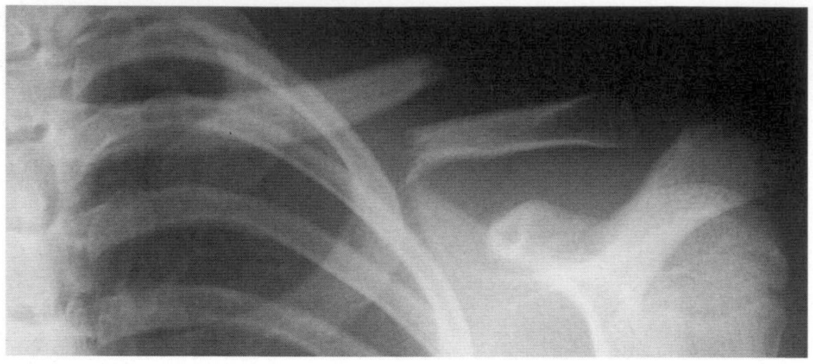

Fig. 1.1 A missed fracture of the clavicle.

- **Lack of knowledge of radiological anatomy** (the clavicle does not have two pieces).
- **Failure to obey the golden rule** of trauma X-rays: **'look right round the edge of every bone'.**
- **Failure to seek a second, more senior opinion,** i.e. not recognizing your own limitations.

Frequently, the least experienced of doctors must try to function in the most stressful of environments, i.e. the Accident & Emergency Department (or Emergency Room), where chaos may frequently reign. With the relentless downgrading of anatomy in UK medical schools, this can only have potentially serious consequences for junior doctors trying to interpret X-rays, particularly of the bones. Very few X-rays have no bony structures on them – so, before you take up that A & E appointment, learn your anatomy!

If you know your anatomy you are already halfway there.

Ways of minimizing X-ray errors and their effects in A & E

Organizational

- *Inception of major trauma centres.* These concentrate resources and expertise in one location but may take longer to reach.

- *24 Hour consultant cover.* Gone are the days when an A & E department was staffed exclusively by junior doctors, with a consultant nominally in charge but physically absent (e.g. in theatre, the orthopaedic clinic or another hospital). Most departments provide close supervision of those in training, so get help early when you need it and never be too self-conscious to seek a second opinion.
- *Major and minor injuries.* Most departments divide their cases into these two important categories so that the most seriously injured patients will automatically come first to the most senior doctors.
- *Red dot system.* This is to alert the inexperienced doctor that the radiographer, who usually has more X-ray experience, has identified (or thinks he has identified) an abnormality. If you cannot see it, go and ask what he is worried about, and if you still cannot see it or disagree, ask a senior clinical colleague or the radiologist. **NB** You must understand that a red dot does *not* mean the patient *definitely* has an abnormality. The responsibility for the interpretation of the film remains yours, being transferred to any senior clinical colleague you show the film to, until such time as it is formally reported by the radiology department.
- *Early review of discharges.* The X-ray films of any patient who is discharged by a junior doctor (e.g. those not returning to the fracture clinic) should be reviewed as soon as possible with senior staff, and preferably with the radiologist, ideally the next morning. All errors, mistakes and 'misses' should be audited and used constructively to teach, and minimize repetition. These may usefully be combined with formal teaching sessions and other relevant teaching films.
- *Timely reporting.* In an ideal world *all* X-rays should be formally reported as quickly as possible, and this applies particularly to A & E films, but staffing limitations can prevent this. Some centres will choose to select the cases which they 'want the radiologist to report'. The radiologist's answer to this is that **he or she wants to see the films which the clinician thinks are normal,** as they may harbour subtle but significant abnormalities. Anyone can see an obvious fracture. It is the subtle secondary signs of trauma with devastating implications (e.g. a small collection of air in the head) which have been overlooked, necessitating the urgent recall of the patient, whereby the radiologist earns his salt. Some centres have 'hot reporting', i.e. as soon as the films are taken, but this is a luxury, and may not be possible due to a lack of staff and non-

availability of previous films for comparison. The acquisition of digital picture archiving and communication systems (PACS) will overcome this.

- *Digital picture and archiving communication systems (PACS).* Centres with image manipulation facilities and immediate access to previous films are at a great advantage. Conversely, radiological errors are known to escalate if reference to previous films is not made. An abnormality may also be highlighted or grossly magnified electronically for closer inspection, or shown not to be of recent origin, by digital and archive retrieval of PFs – previous films.

- *Teleradiology.* Obtaining advice on difficult films from distant regional experts.

Personal

Be utterly ruthless and unrelenting in checking all data relating to X-ray films and images, e.g. the name of the patient, date of birth, current date on films, quality of radiographs, and especially *left* and *right.* Be particularly wary of films already placed on viewing boxes. If someone else asks you to look at one of his cases, check the films as you would your own (for identification, date, left and right, etc.) even if it is the consultant who has asked you. He or she will be glad one day that you spotted the left side was actually the right, before putting a drain in on the wrong side.

That X-ray may look like the perfect Colles' reduction you have just performed, but may in fact be the X-ray done by a colleague on another patient, and yours has not yet come out of the processor.

- Anatomy! Anatomy! Anatomy! (Again!)

- Learn your anatomy, or revise it before coming to A & E.

- Learn about normal variants. This is a huge subject and applies to just about every film you see. Every A & E department should have a copy of *Normal Roentgen Variants that may Simulate Disease* by Theodore E. Keats and Mark W. Anderson (7th edn 2001, Mosby, New York), and if you are actually working in A & E you should both refer to it constantly and study it any time you have a lull.

- Put your own films up on the box. If somebody else does it there is a high probability they will be back to front.

- Be aware of developmental variation. This is included in '*Normal Variants*' but basically relates to skeletal maturation, i.e. the X-ray appearance of the skeleton at different ages. A chart showing the times of appearance and times of fusion of epiphyses should be up on the wall in every department. Refer to it whenever you need to.

- Understand that some X-ray abnormalities are very subtle and hard to see and if you do not even know what you are looking for you certainly won't see it. There is always someone better at looking at X-rays than you, and not all abnormalities with the potential to kill the patient are obvious. Writing 'no gross abnormality' or 'no obvious fracture' in the notes is to avoid responsibility, even if it is understandable.
- **Treat the patient, not the X-ray** (this is an absolutely fundamental principle). Admit that patient with excruciating pain in her hip even if you cannot see a fracture on the initial films!
- Recognize your own limitations and act on them. Seek help early when you need it. That film that you thought was 'normal' at 2 a.m. may look very different in the cold light of day. Hearing that the patient you discharged on the strength of it is now in the mortuary with a ruptured aortic aneurysm is an experience you definitely do not want to have.
- Know what you're looking for. Learn the radiological signs of trauma and pathology and be ready for them when they present. If you have any doubts, go and ask somebody. Never let it be a choice between your pride and the best interests of a patient.
- Do not forget that not all trauma is acute, and remember to be alert to underlying disease. Just because you regard yourself as primarily there to deal with acute injuries, do not forget that your patient may be presenting with a pathological fracture of the humerus due to an underlying malignancy, or osteoporosis with a hip fracture. Do not expect patients to conform to your preconceived notions as to how they should come to medical attention, as 'the patients don't read the textbooks'.
- **Aim for the confidence of absolute knowledge and do not take any chances.**

Chapter 2

The plain skull X-ray in trauma

Background

- There was a time when virtually every patient who received a bump on the head would get a skull X-ray for '? fracture', the anxiety being that 'failure to take an X-ray' would be seized upon as a medicolegal omission in its own right, so that 'defensive medicine' was being practised and 'fear' indeed truly was 'the spur'. Fortunately not every small boy needs a skull X-ray every time he bangs his head on the radiator, even if Mum used to agitate in the past until he got one.
- With the advent of CT, the value of skull X-rays in blunt head trauma has considerably diminished and such films are now often completely circumvented, the argument being that if the patient has sustained sufficiently significant head trauma, a CT is indicated anyway, whether or not the skull films show a fracture.
- The object of the exercise nowadays is to identify those patients who have sustained a *clinically significant brain injury*, and in particular a *neurosurgically removable haematoma*.
- Although CT is poor at demonstrating linear fractures in the same plane as the beam, this does not matter, as the brain is being exquisitely visualized anyway and any associated intracranial trauma can readily be assessed. Nevertheless, it is a stark fact that patients who do have skull fractures are at high-risk for delayed intracranial haemorrhage (around 30 times), especially when such fractures cross the major meningeal vessels. CT is virtually 100% sensitive and specific for fresh intracranial blood, but there is a radiation burden to be borne (e.g. the radiation from one CT corresponds to 1 year's background radiation

(2.0 mSv), which is considerably more than that of three skull films (0.14 mSv)).

- However, patients who do not have skull fractures can still have significant brain injuries (especially children) and the critical factors which dictate appropriate imaging are, as always, the severity of the head or associated injuries, the clinical findings on arrival (i.e. the Glasgow Coma Scale (GCS) score) and any subsequent deterioration in the patient's condition. The GCS uses eye-opening, together with verbal and motor responses, to score neurological status. The maximum score is 15 (fully alert and responding) and the minimum score is 3 (no responses).

- Skull X-ray interpretation is a source of considerable anxiety to the novice. Subtle but potentially life-threatening abnormalities may be present (e.g. a small collection of air inside the head) as well as linear fractures, so **you must know what you are looking for.** Until such time as skull X-rays are completely abandoned we are stuck with the duty of knowing how to interpret them correctly, not only to identify fractures (which is an automatic indication for CT) but to confirm or exclude other critically significant findings. Considerable space is therefore being given here to cover this.

Golden nugget: A patient may suffer a life-threatening injury to the head, without having been knocked out and without having sustained a skull fracture. The lack of such a history or finding should not induce a false sense of security in an inexperienced doctor.

NB You must also, of course, be fully conversant with the *limitations* of a skull X-ray.

Limitations of the skull X-ray

- Crucial fact: skull X-rays provide no direct image of the brain. Look at Figure 2.1 This is the CT equivalent of a skull X-ray which graphically demonstrates this fact.

- X-rays of the skull concern themselves primarily with the cranial vault as such films will not exclude fractures in the base of the skull – hence the frequent format of skull X-ray reports, 'no vault fracture', in recognition of this fact.

- **NB** The actual demonstration of a base of skull fracture is a job for CT, although there are some well-known clinical signs which provide indirect

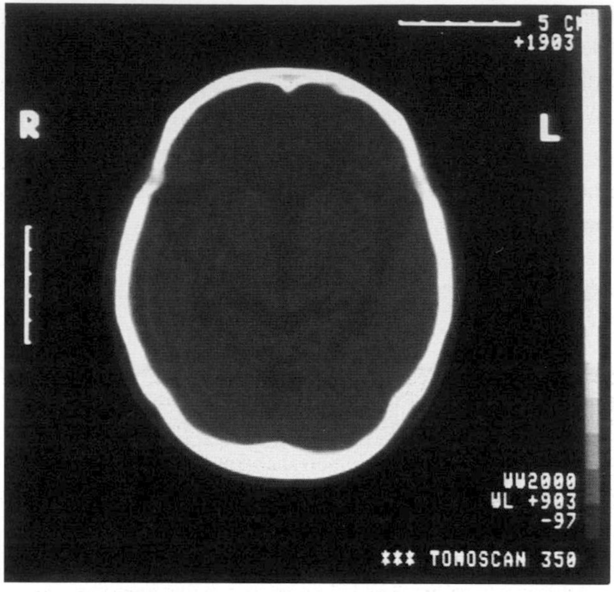

Fig. 2.1 *The CT equivalent of a skull X-ray: a scan set for 'bone windows', rendering the brain invisible. The coronal sutures are just visible.*

evidence of this: CSF pouring out of the nose (rhinorrhoea) or blood pouring out of the ear are dramatic examples. Blood may not actually be leaking out of the ear but accumulating behind the eardrum – a so-called *haemotympanum* which should be sought with an otoscope, as this may also indicate a base of skull fracture. The presence of CSF delays blood clotting.

- Battle's sign. This is the bruising discoloration which may occur over the mastoid area behind the ear after a base of skull fracture and is well worth looking for.
- Racoon eyes. These are the dark blue circles which may be seen around the eyes, indicating a fracture in the floor of the anterior cranial fossa via which blood has tracked out through the orbits.

Some plain X-ray signs may, however, show indirect evidence of a base of skull fracture; for example, a fluid level in the sphenoid sinus or fresh opacification of the mastoid air cells due to bleeding. In this case the differential diagnosis would have to include preceding sinus or mastoid disease, which could be established by immediate access to previous films (say in the middle of the night) – an example of the enormous value of digital archiving systems.

NB Additional views and modified exposures are necessary to demonstrate clearly other parts of the skull (e.g. the facial bones, or soft tissues of the scalp).

Gold medal point: In a viva you could greatly impress an examiner by telling him that a haemotympanum should not be confused with a *congenitally high jugular bulb*, which looks very similar.

Trauma to the head: imaging guidelines and the role of CT scanning

The booklet *Making The Best Use of a Department of Clinical Radiology* (RCR 2003) provides the essential background information and advice on these subjects.

For severe head injury management the ideal set-up is with CT/MRI and neurosurgical facilities on site. Local variations such as CT availability but neurosurgical facilities at a distance will benefit from image transfer software for neurosurgical advice by 'teleradiology' and rapid helicopter or ambulance evacuation to the nearest neurosurgical centre. An essential prerequisite for any centre accepting head injuries is 24 hour availability of CT.

Neurosurgeons, however, look after only 1% of head injuries, leaving considerable decision-making about the remaining 99% to other doctors. The crucial questions that need to be answered on the patient's arrival are:

- Has this patient suffered a clinically significant brain injury?
- Does the patient need an urgent neurosurgical/anaesthetic opinion or transfer now?
- Does the patient need a skull X-ray or a CT scan?
- Are there other significant injuries requiring attention?
- Can the patient be discharged or is admission necessary?

The Canadian Head CT Rule (derived from a study of 3000 cases) identifies focal neurological deficits, post-traumatic seizures, coagulopathy and open or depressed skull fractures as indications for CT. Patients over 64 years of age, or with more than one episode of vomiting, loss of consciousness or retrograde amnesia, must be included, and patients with a GCS score of less than 13 at any time since the injury, or failure to regain a GCS score of 15 within 2 hours of injury, will also require CT scanning. Any suspicion of a high impact injury makes CT a good idea.

NB Similar but slightly modified guidelines exist for children, as they are harder to assess clinically.

So who gets a skull X-ray?

Answer: very few patients compared with times past, and indeed patients who have sustained trivial injury, i.e. were not knocked out and are clinically well, now require no imaging whatsoever.

If the history of trauma is vague (e.g. the patient is drunk), a skull X-ray is a wise precaution. If there is suspected non-accidental injury, a skull X-ray as part of a skeletal survey to document any visible fractures will be required; and if there is a severe head injury, MRI will be the first investigation of choice in order to demonstrate the crucial medicolegal finding of multiple haematomas of different ages.

The object of the skull X-ray is to help predict and prevent those patients with head injuries who have suffered from the visible primary effects of trauma (e.g. a fracture) progressing to and dying from the secondary effects, e.g. an extradural haematoma, raised intracranial pressure, etc. Even so, you do not have to have a fracture to sustain a haematoma. A dural tear could cause it. The interpretation of CT and MRI scans is a problem for the radiologists and neurosurgeons. **Your job as an A & E doctor is the initial interpretation of any skull X-rays you or your colleagues have requested.**

Look at Figure 2.2. This is the CT head scan of a motor cyclist who collided with a truck. You are 36 times more likely to be killed on a motor cycle than you are in a car.

Conclusion: **A CT head scan is therefore mandatory for all suspected clinically significant brain injuries.**

Appropriate consideration also needs to be given to inclusion of the neck at the same examination, and indeed the chest, abdomen and extremities, depending on the presence of coexistent injuries.

NB Skull X-rays will occasionally be taken to find a bullet or trailing fragments in gunshot wounds if there is no exit wound or the patient cannot make it to CT (see Fig. 14.6).

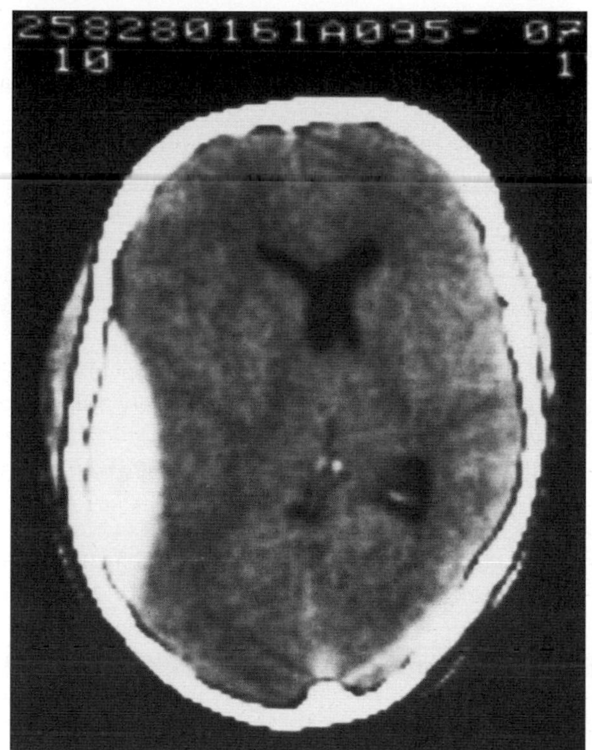

Fig. 2.2 *'The creeping death'. An acute extradural haematoma in a traffic accident victim. Note the compression of the ipsilateral lateral ventricle and shift away of the pineal to the contralateral side. Most CT scans will show calcification in the pineal. Most skull X-rays will not.*

The skull

Radiography

Once the decision has been made to perform a skull X-ray, three basic views are usually taken: the frontal film (AP or PA), the lateral and the Townes' projection, each designed to optimize the view of particular areas of the skull (Figs 2.3–2.6).

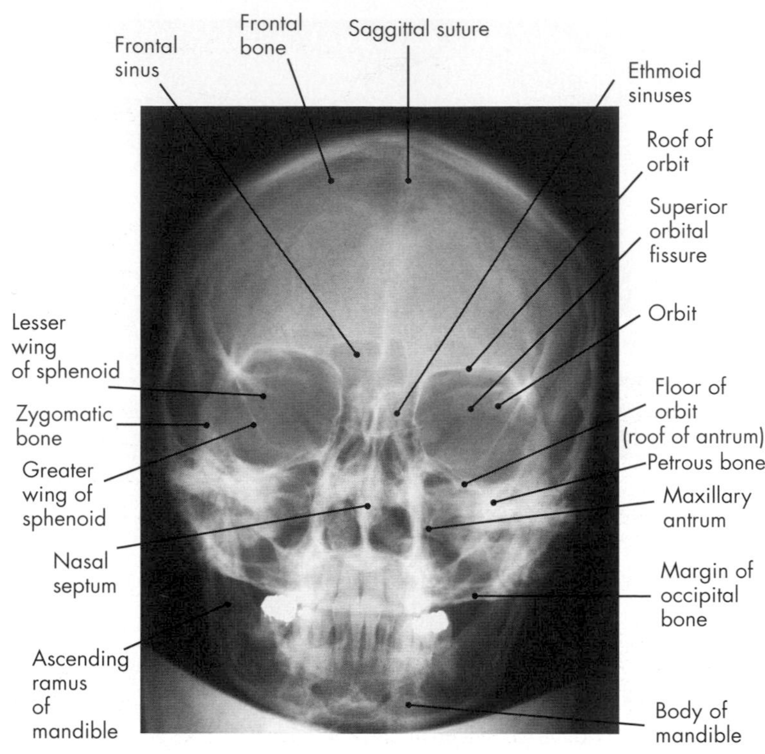

Fig. 2.3 *Normal PA skull X-ray.*

- **NB** It is standard practice following trauma to take lateral skull films with the patient lying on his back, or 'brow up', and the X-ray beam directed horizontally across the table, i.e. parallel to the floor, rather than down from the vertical with the patient on the side (Fig. 2.4); all 'brow up' films should be labelled as such by the radiographer to confirm that this has been done. If, however, the patient was X-rayed erect, this can also usefully be recorded.
- The purpose of this is to optimize the conditions for identifying the presence of air inside the cranial cavity and to generate a fluid level if there has been any bleeding into the sphenoid sinus, neither of which would be so recognizable

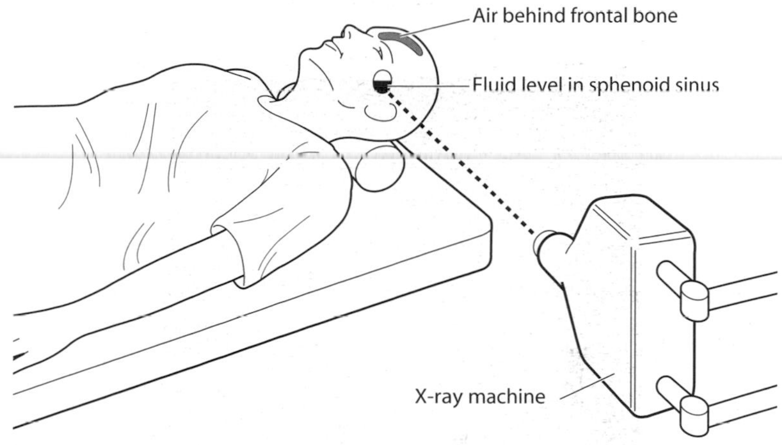

Fig. 2.4 *Horizontal beam technique for demonstration of a fluid level and air in the head.*

without such crucial positioning, as the air will tend to rise to a position directly behind the frontal bone. An astute observer will also be able to identify pockets of air elsewhere in the head (Figs 2.20, 2.21).

- On the lateral film (Fig. 2.5) the traumatized side should lie adjacent to and as close as possible to the X-ray cassette and film or digital detector so that any fracture line is as sharp as possible and therefore as detectable as possible. To understand this principle, hold your index finger above this page then, as you lower it, watch the shadow increase in sharpness as your finger approaches the surface and the penumbra (or surrounding shadow) diminishes. Some centres in the USA use this principle to justify requesting both left and right laterals routinely to optimize the detection of any unilateral fracture line. So, if you suspect a right-sided fracture, request a right lateral. If you do not specify what you want, the radiographer will usually do the job for you.

NB A 'left lateral' means the left side is in contact with the X-ray cassette or detector. A 'right lateral' means the right side is in contact with the X-ray cassette or detector.

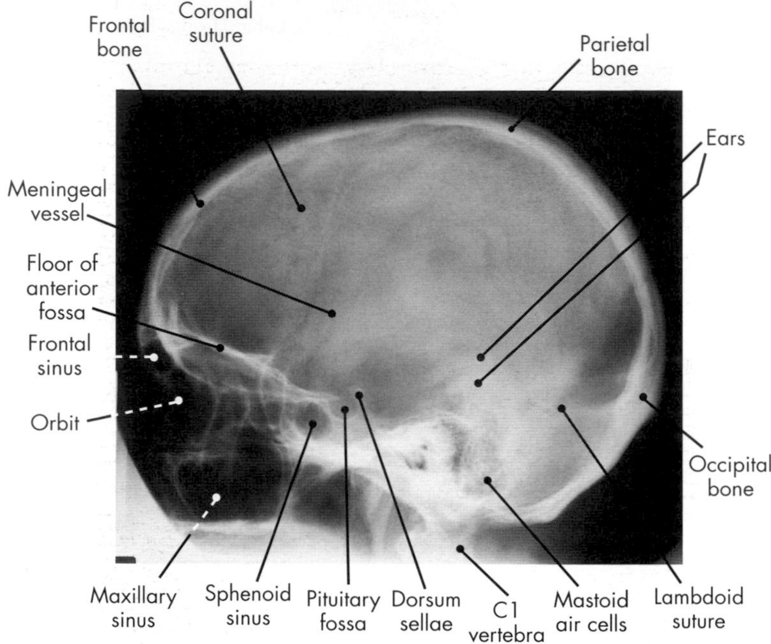

Fig. 2.5 *Normal lateral skull X-ray. Note the branching meningeal vessels and lucency of the frontal, temporal and occipital regions. Study this carefully.*

Each film has a checklist of normal structures that are worth looking for, but first look for the name, date, date of birth, etc. on every film, then consciously identify left and right, then place the films the correct way round on the viewing box. The film above is a left lateral, so you are inspecting it from the left.

Golden rule: Never assume when guided towards a viewing box or workstation and asked to comment on Mr X's films that they are actually the films of Mr X. Always check each one individually for yourself: one day they will belong to someone else!

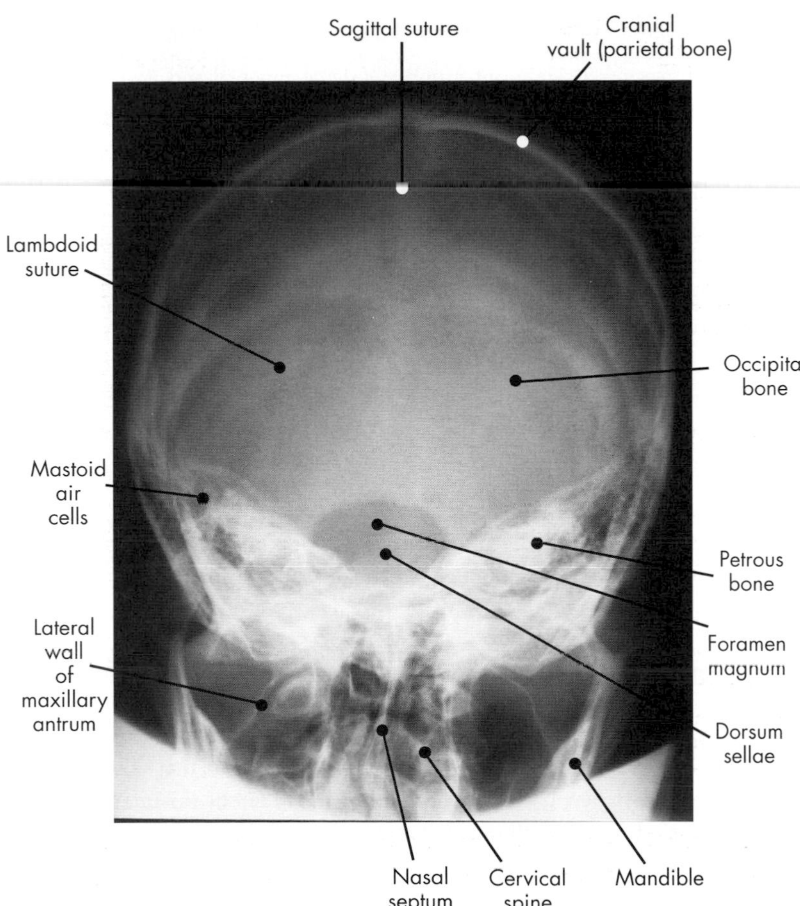

Fig. 2.6 *Normal Townes' view. This is an AP film taken with the patient supine and the X-ray beam angled 30° towards the feet. On a good Townes' view the dorsum sellae will be centred in the foramen magnum.*

Developmental and normal variants

The skull presents a significant number of developmental and normal variants which can easily cause confusion and misdiagnosis, as they simulate fractures and other effects of trauma.

Fontanelles/sutures

- In babies and young children the *anterior* and *posterior fontanelles* may be visible on skull films these being the natural gaps between the frontal/parietal and parietal/occipital bones, respectively. Clinically they should be checked after trauma for tenseness or bulging, and for bulging on the radiographs, which may reflect raised intracranial pressure, but the normal gaps which they present should not be misinterpreted as post-traumatic in themselves. (**NB** These fontanelles allow ultrasonic access to the brain in young infants.)
- The normal sutures are naturally already visible in infants and will often appear significantly wider compared with their adult counterparts. *Accessory sutures* are also very common at this age, and may persist into later life (Fig. 2.7).
- You should be familiar with the normal *coronal, sagittal* and *lambdoid sutures,* which allow the skull to grow.
- *The occipitosphenoid synchondrosis (or suture).* Look at Figure 2.7. This is a sometimes dramatic-looking defect in the base of the skull that exists to permit normal growth here until the late teens. **It should not be misinterpreted as a base of skull fracture, although it looks very much like one**.
- *The metopic suture* (Fig. 2.8). This is a midline vertical suture which divides the frontal bone in a small proportion of normal individuals. It usually has a serrated appearance, thus confirming its anatomical nature, and may remain in adults.
- *Interparietal suture.* This can subdivide the parietal bone when present and may be unilateral or bilateral. When present, it extends from the coronal to the lambdoid sutures.
- *Nasofrontal suture.* This presents as a dark rounded arc above the nasal bones on AP films, and may persist into adult life.

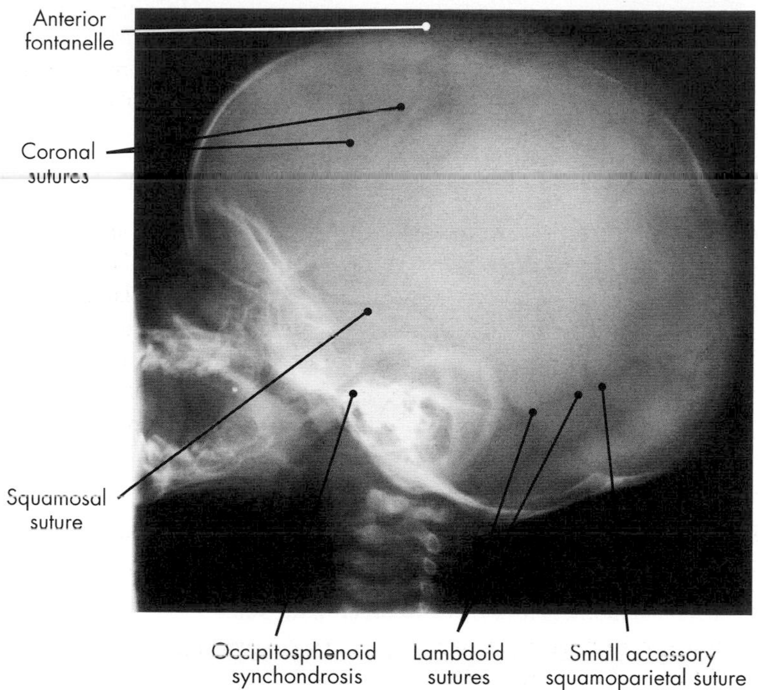

Fig. 2.7 *Normal paediatric skull. Note the many structures simulating fractures. Soft tissue folds in the scalp can also simulate them. The sutures are duplicated due to obliquity.*

- *Occipitomastoid suture.* This can cause trouble posteriorly when present. It is usually seen low down on the Townes' view between the occipital and mastoid bones, sometimes looks linear, and is often more obvious on one side.

- *Sutures containing wormian bones.* These are tiny accessory bones usually seen in the lambdoid sutures and look like crazy paving. They can occur as one or two isolated normal variants or in profusion, but are almost always present in osteogenesis imperfecta – a condition that may easily be confused with the battered baby syndrome. They are not, however, pathognomonic of osteogenesis imperfecta.

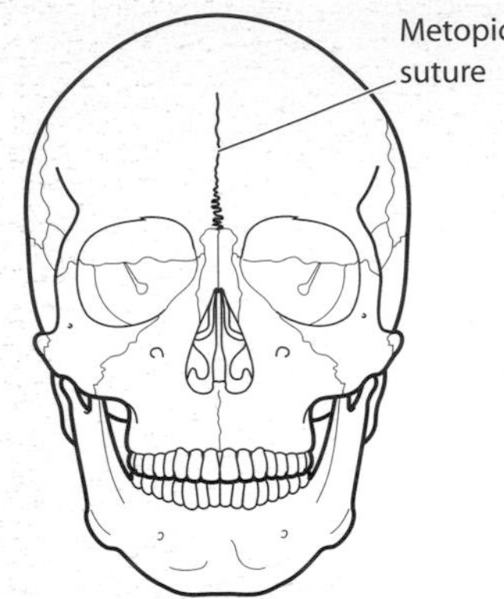

Fig. 2.8 *Metopic suture.*

NB Normal sutures, especially the coronal, can look wider than normal if seen slightly obliquely on an imperfect lateral skull film. A true suture, however, can get 'sprung' or undergo diastasis (separation) in trauma, or – **Gold medal point** – if infiltrated with metastatic disease, especially in children.

Some normal lucent defects that may occur in the vault

- *Parietal foramina.* Usually paired structures best seen on the PA and Townes' views. These may have led at times to incorrect interpretations of 'trephining' or boring holes in ancient skulls of psychiatrically disturbed individuals 'to let the devils out', although genuine trephining is believed to have been done.
- *Venous lakes.* Often clustered in the occipital bone but may occur throughout the skull. Do not go jumping to the conclusion that the patient has multiple myeloma.

Vascular grooves The cranial vault has an inner and outer table and central or diploic space – a bit like Aero (bubbly) chocolate. Apart from the normal meningeal vascular markings, huge and dramatic diploic venous markings can commonly occur, particularly in the parietal bone – variously known as the *parietal spider* (Fig. 2.9) or *parietal star*. A further single large venous channel the sphenoparietal sinus, may also dominate the lateral view, and enlarges down the way (see Keats & Anderson 2001).

NB Unfortunately other vascular grooves may appear just about anywhere in the skull and simulate fractures. 'Persistent strips of membranous bone',

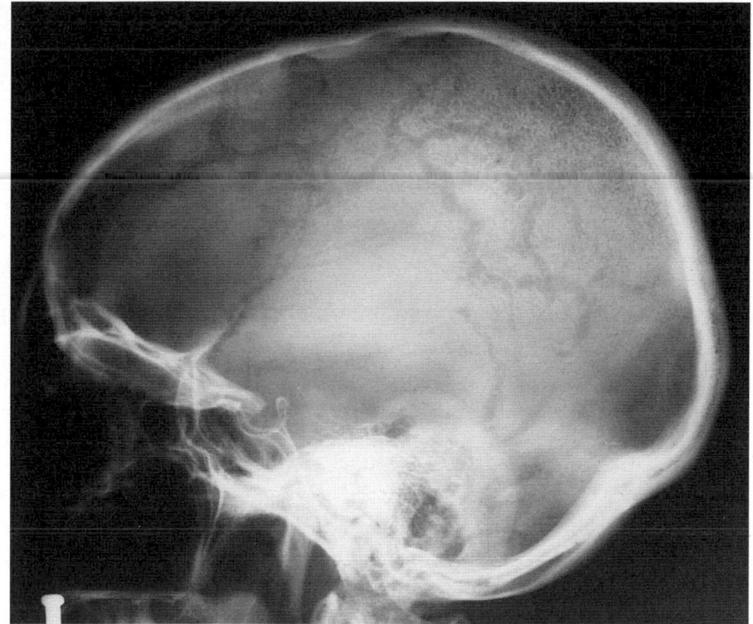

Fig. 2.9 *'Parietal spider'. Could you exclude a fracture amongst all of this?*

which may do the same, are also a diagnostic worry in paediatrics. No-one can always completely exclude a fracture, but the paediatric radiologist is best placed to help you out with children's films – and remember: **always treat the patient not the X-ray.**

Other normal variants (adults)

- *Frontal hyperostosis*. This is irregular dense thickening of the posterior aspect of the frontal bone, usually bilateral. It should not be mistaken for evidence of a depressed fracture. The AP film shows it is invariably bilateral.

Gold medal point: Focal reactive sclerosis in the cranial vault can be a sign of an underlying meningioma (usually unilateral).

- *Bathrocephalic occiput* (Fig. 2.10). This Ancient Greek mouthful (*bathros* = deep, *cephale* = head) refers to the dramatic appearance seen when the occipital bone balloons out backwards or 'deeply', appearing to have sprung out of position and to be overlapping where it articulates with the parietal bone – and it is difficult to believe that it cannot be post-traumatic. Note, however, that it **always occurs where the lambdoid suture reaches the vault posteriorly** and careful inspection of the scalp will (usually) indicate an absence of any swelling over it (i.e. no haematoma). More than one patient has been misdiagnosed with a fracture on the strength of this red herring.

- *Calcified meninges:* Beware of focal calcification in the meninges. For no obvious reason many patients can have plaques of calcification running close to the inner table of the skull. These should not be mistaken for a depressed fracture. Inspection of the film should show that the inner and outer tables are undisturbed above the dural calcification. Sometimes dural calcification can be very extensive.

- *Calcified falx.* (Latin *falx* = sickle; the falx is sickle-shaped.) This is useful when present on AP films as it defines the midline. It can be complete or simply focal and at times remarkably chunky, but is not necessarily age-related.

- *Calcified choroid plexi.* These are sometimes visible as paired faint or slightly more heavily calcified blobs behind the pineal on lateral skulls, but are often asymmetrical. Do not set too much store by them. They are almost always visible on CT scans (Fig. 2.11).

- *Gold medal point*: Very rarely meningiomas and brain tumours will calcify, are usually unilateral, but can straddle the midline.

- *Calcified pineal.* (Useful knowledge for a rare occasion.) Seeking this structure on plain films is much less important than it used to be and is in many senses obsolete; however, it is still worth looking for as an academic exercise as it is sometimes sufficiently calcified to be visible on plain films. If however, **it is not visible on the lateral view it will not be sufficiently calcified to be of diagnostic use on a frontal film. This is the only way plain films will give you direct evidence of an intracranial shift.**

Important fact: In times past, a genuinely displaced pineal as a result of trauma was most likely to be due to an intracranial haematoma; however, the majority of such patients who now receive sufficient trauma to induce a haematoma would

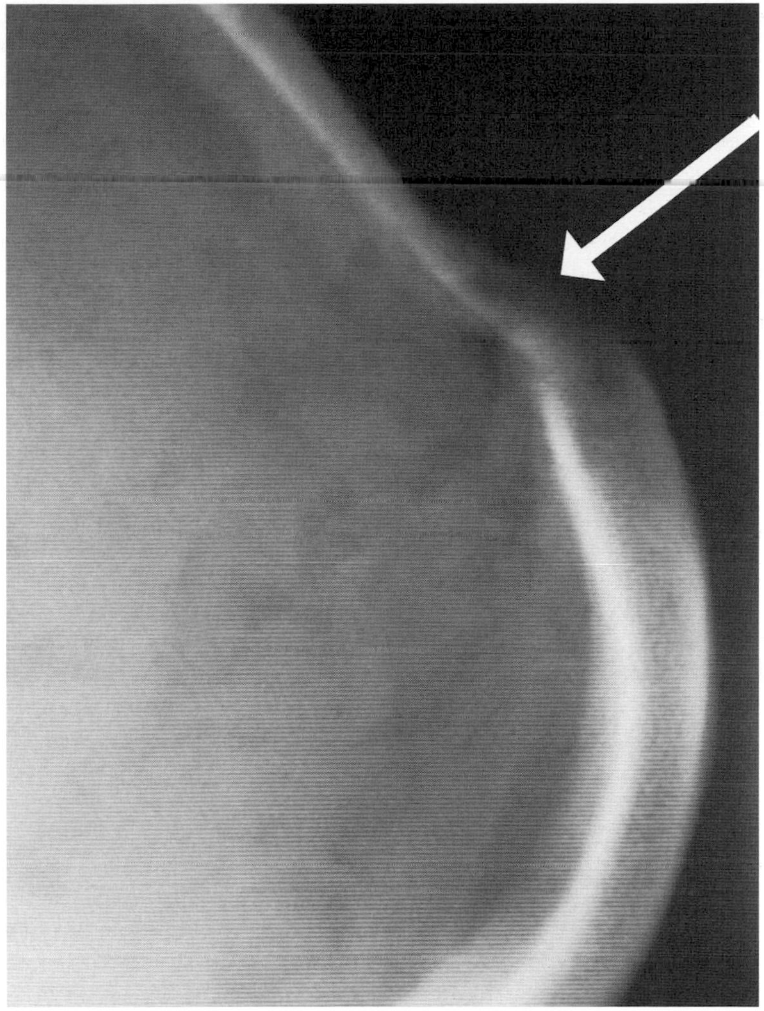

Fig. 2.10 *Bathrocephalic occiput. Alarming but normal! Detail from the skull of a teenage girl without a hard hat who fell off her horse. History from the mother.*

probably go straight to CT, so such skull films with displaced pineals are much less likely to be seen.

Nowadays the assessment of the pineal's position, if it is visible, potentially lies in the misdiagnosis of 'displacement' when displacement is not actually present. Such a conclusion would, however, mandate a CT, which would clarify the situation. Nevertheless, as long as skull X-rays continue to be taken, it is the duty of every doctor who deals with them to know what to look for, as one day it will be the 'real thing' – or you could be working in a developing country where there is no CT, or your CT scanner is out of order.

Effects of obliquity and criteria for diagnosis of displacement of the pineal (Fig. 2.11)

Definition: More than 3 mm off centre from the midline.

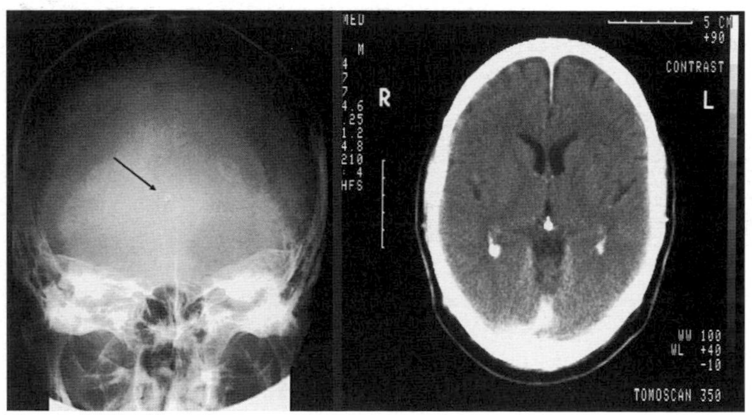

Fig. 2.11 *Spurious displacement of the pineal. Note: the slight positioning of the pineal to the right of the falx on the skull X-ray (arrow) (**A**); The central position in line with the falx on the CT (**B**). Conclusion: slight obliquity of skull X-ray and normally positioned pineal. The two opacities on either side of the pineal are the choroid plexi (where cerebrospinal fluid is formed). Gold medal point: the dense blob at the back of the brain is the torcula herophili or confluence of the venous sinuses 'lighting up' on this enhanced CT scan.*

This sounds easy enough and straightforward to apply but unfortunately it isn't. Displacement of the pineal will be simulated on many AP and Townes' films simply because they are not perfectly straight – something hard to achieve in an injured patient – and sometimes due to objects other than the pineal, like an ivory osteoma in the frontal sinus or gravel in the forehead.

- Check to see if the nasal septum and odontoid (if visible) are in line. If not, the patient is not straight.
- The pineal itself can be eccentrically calcified and you should never assume that what you see of it anatomically is necessarily central in location. This is why there is a 3 mm leeway in its interpretation (Fig. 2.12).

Hint: Learn the CT anatomy of the head. This will help you to understand skull X-rays better.

Importance of checking the scalp on skull X-rays

Look at Figure 2.13. The initial assessment of this AP film showed what looked like a pineal displaced to the right. The detailed lateral view of the frontal region of the skull at the standard exposure showed nothing abnormal. The opacity on

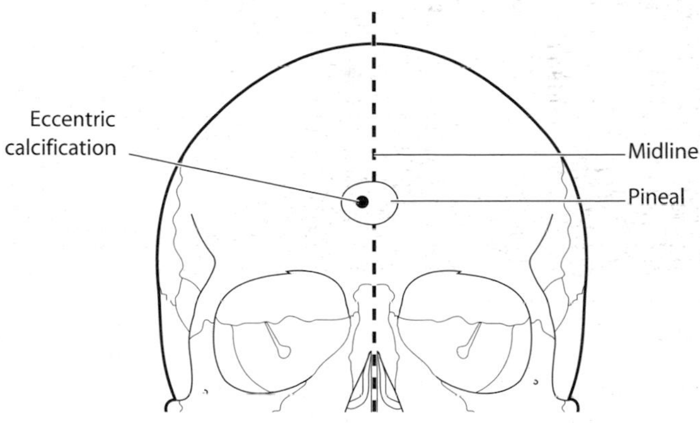

Fig. 2.12 *Concept of eccentric calcification in a central pineal simulating displacement, even when the skull is straight.*

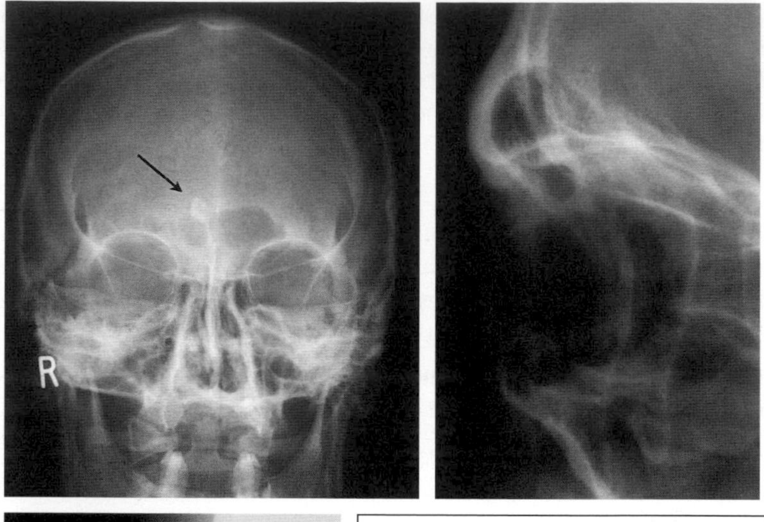

A

B

C

Fig. 2.13 A–C *Gravel in forehead (arrow) simulating displacement of the pineal. History: fell off a bicycle – no helmet.*

the AP film, however, was considered to be too low down for the pineal. Another film set for soft tissue exposure showed opaque foreign material in the scalp (gravel) – and a broken nasal bone! This was causing a spurious appearance of displacement of the pineal. (The gravel and nasal fracture were, however, visible on 'bright-lighting' the original film.)

Moral: Do not get caught out by something like this. Always put a bright light behind the scalp and look right round it on every skull film, or bring it up electronically on your workstation. Before the advent of CT, this patient might have been subjected to burr holes or carotid arteriography to look for a left-sided intracranial haematoma displacing the 'pineal'. The main reason for inspecting the scalp nowadays is to check for haematomas and to exclude air and foreign material, which can predispose to infection. **NB** A haematoma over a suspect line in the vault makes it more likely to be a fracture, and the absence of a haematoma makes it less so. **Always tell the radiologist where the swellings are clinically. The scalp can bleed very profusely.**

Hairstyle artefacts

Dense linear strands on skull X-rays from clotted blood in the hair alert the radiologist to the fact that the patient has probably sustained a laceration of the scalp, but cosmetic hair gels can have a similar effect. Multiple round densities from short curly hair are the corresponding finding in Afrocaribbean patients.

A look at some fractures and how to tell what is a fracture and what isn't. (Figs 2.14, 2.15, 2.16)

Linear fractures

- Fractures tend to be either jagged, like lightning, or straight cracks; vessels are usually meandering or describing gentler radii of curvature.
- Fractures have sharp edges.
- Fractures tend to look darker than vessels and the bigger they are the darker they tend to be, although the latter is also true for vessels.
- Fractures may cross anatomical landmarks.
- Fractures are unilateral and asymmetric, with different sharpness on left and right lateral films. Anatomical structures will be duplicated, e.g. the coronal

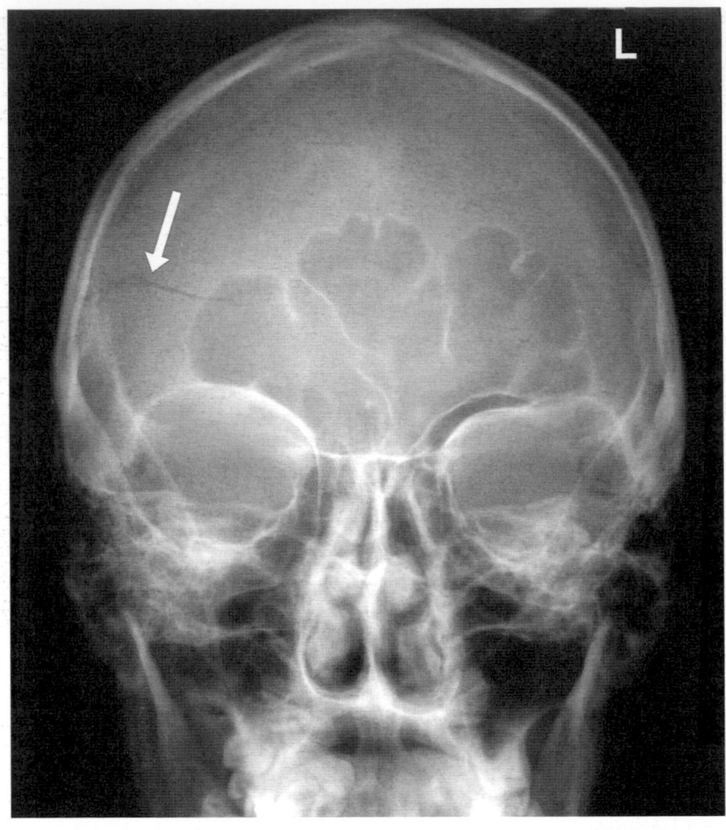

Fig. 2.14 *A fracture (arrow) of the right cranial vault. Relatively dark and straight. Note: fractures tend to be dark because they involve the full thickness of the skull; vessels only groove the inner or outer surfaces (check this on any dried skull). Note the huge frontal sinuses (see p. 45).*

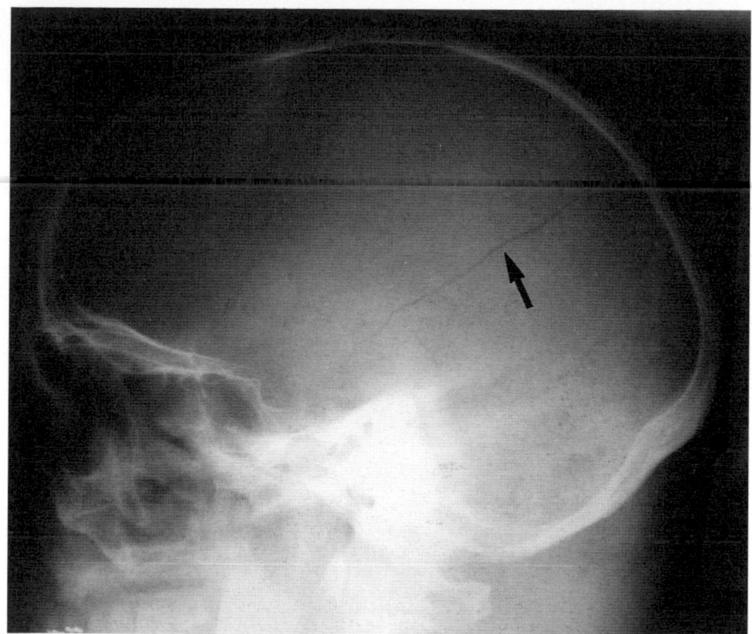

Fig. 2.15 *Crack fracture (arrow) of parietal and temporal bones. History: fell off a skateboard – no helmet. Again dark, sharp and relatively straight. This is crossing the 'danger area' of the branches of the middle meningeal artery, causing 30 times the risk of an extradural haematoma.*

and lambdoid sutures – but obviously not the sagittal which is a solitary and midline structure, or a unilateral accessory fissure.

- Fractures often have an overlying haematoma.
- Crack fractures are just black lines. Vessels and sutures tend to have sclerotic margins.

Vessels

- The main vessels have known locations, e.g. the middle meningeals.
- Vessels change calibre: arteries taper distally, and veins enlarge proximally.

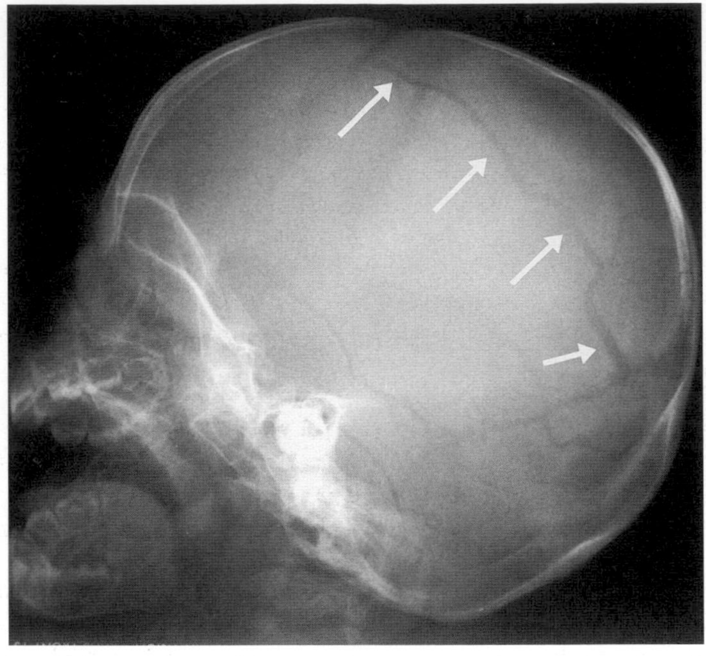

Fig. 2.16 *Fractured parietal bone in non-accidental injury of an infant.*

- The middle meningeal arteries curve alongside the coronal sutures (Fig. 2.5). Their posterior branches cross the squamous temporal bone and are at high risk in the presence of a fracture.
- Vessels tend to have unsharp edges.
- Vessels tend to show organized branching.

Golden rule: If you are truly in doubt about something, ask someone senior what he or she thinks; if you are on your own, regard it as a fracture.

What about sutures?

The main sutures, the sagittal, coronal and lambdoid, have well known positions, but learn where to look for the accessory ones as well (see Keats & Anderson

2001). Sutures take a very tightly tortuous path within their general linear direction. Remember Lennon and McCartneys *Long and Winding Road*? – that's sutures. They are also usually bilateral and symmetrical, e.g. lambdoid, coronal and occipitomastoid. Note, however, that they fuse in the elderly and can undergo premature fusion in some infants, causing craniostenosis – forming 'turret heads', etc. A few of your patients will have congenital abnormalities as well as trauma. Sutures, especially the lambdoid, may show a 'crazy paving' effect if wormian bones are present. Sutures also tend to have sclerotic margins – a startling feature in some older patients when this contrasts with the background osteoporosis, causing 'perisutural sclerosis'. Both sides of the coronal and lambdoid sutures are often visible as a result of slight obliquity on lateral films.

Depressed fractures

These occur when part of the cranial vault has fractured, causing either a part of it to be driven in, for example by a hammer, or a plate of bone which has broken round the edges to be tilted relative to the remains of the vault.

NB The appearance of the same focally depressed fracture looks very different depending on the angle from which it is viewed (Fig. 2.17).

Most of these patients will, however, need to go on to CT for assessment of the underlying brain for haematomas, air, etc., and a decision about the necessity for surgical elevation. Greater than 50% depression or 0.5 cm displacement usually requires elevation. Sometimes the skull simply crumples and collapses with cracks within a circular fracture line, a so-called 'wagon-wheel fracture', a little like the earth crumpling and sinking when a nuclear test explosion is detonated underneath it.

Hint: Sometimes the glare from a viewing box coming through a conventional film makes it impossible to see the thin rim of the soft tissue on the outer aspect of the skull, which constitutes the scalp, preventing a successful hunt for air, glass or other potentially infectious foreign bodies within it. An easy way to deal with this is to make a fist with your hand and move it to a position in front of the X-ray where it just corresponds to the size of the intracranial cavity, to occlude the glare (e.g. on the AP view) (Fig. 2.18). Then, at just the correct position, the scalp should suddenly appear like the corona at the instant when the moon blots out the sun's disc in a solar eclipse. Selective shielding can also be carried out around the circumference of the vault with the edge of the hand. However, occasionally the film will still be too overpenetrated for you to see the scalp at all, but opaque objects may be just visible in the darkness.

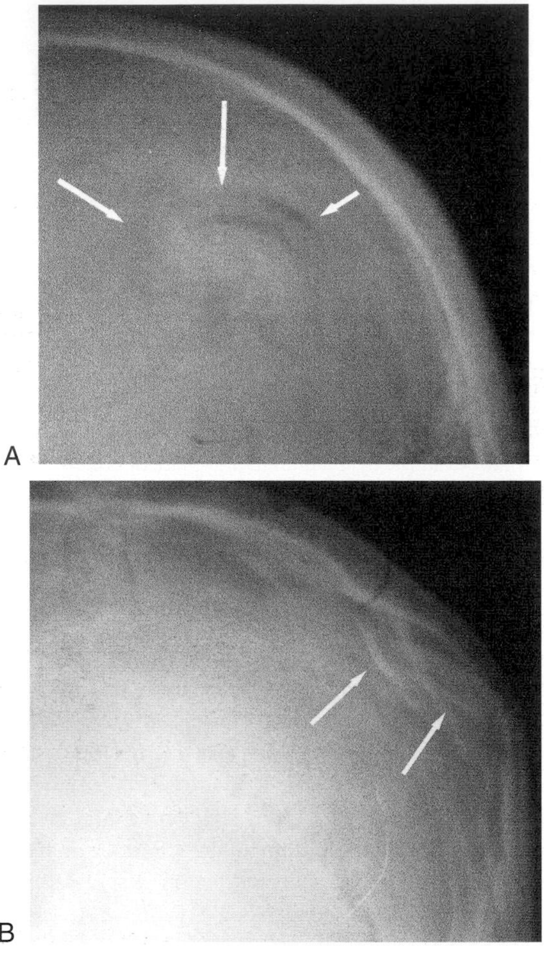

Fig. 2.17 *This patient was kicked in the left side of the head by the hooves of a zebra at a zoo and knocked out for a while. A large boggy haematoma remained and these details from the skull were obtained. Note:* ***A*** *The lateral view shows concentric dark fracture lines (like a usual 'crack' fracture where the X-ray beam is in the same axis as the depression); and* ***B*** *the AP view shows curved dense depressed splinters 'inboard' of the vault where the X-ray beam is tangential to the depression. Learn to recognize these different appearances of the same thing.*

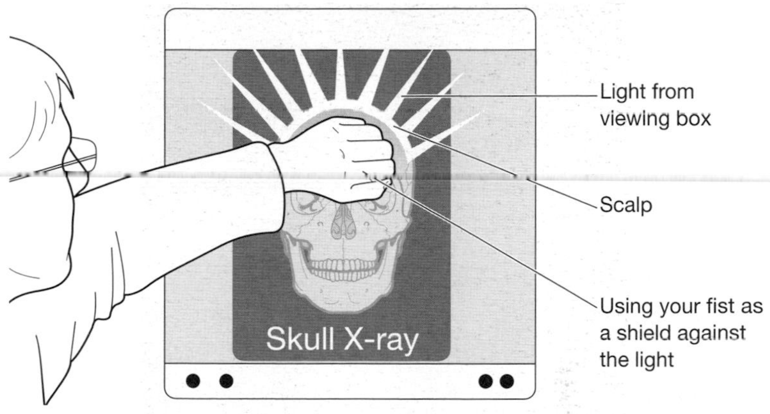

Fig. 2.18 *The doctor should use his fist as a shield against the light.*

Radiological signs not to miss

Fluid in the sphenoid sinus

Question: What shall we do with the drunken sailor?
Answer: Whatever you do, do not assume his state of unconsciousness is all due to drink; and check the blood glucose while you're at it.

Look at Figure 2.19. This is the view of a brow-up lateral skull X-ray taken as part of an initial trauma survey (including the chest, pelvis, etc.) on a sailor who had been involved in a drunken brawl after his ship docked in port. On arrival at hospital he smelt strongly of alcohol and was almost unrousable.

Look at the sphenoid sinus:

- Remember this X-ray has been taken with the patient lying on his back, and the beam directed horizontally across the table.

- Note the razor-sharp interface contrasting with the air in the posterior part of the sphenoid sinus. This is a fluid level in the sinus due to a crack fracture in its wall which has extended down from the vault, leading to bleeding, and indicates a **base of skull fracture,** and therefore increased severity of injury. **NB** This is a rare radiological sign but it is one of the main reasons the lateral

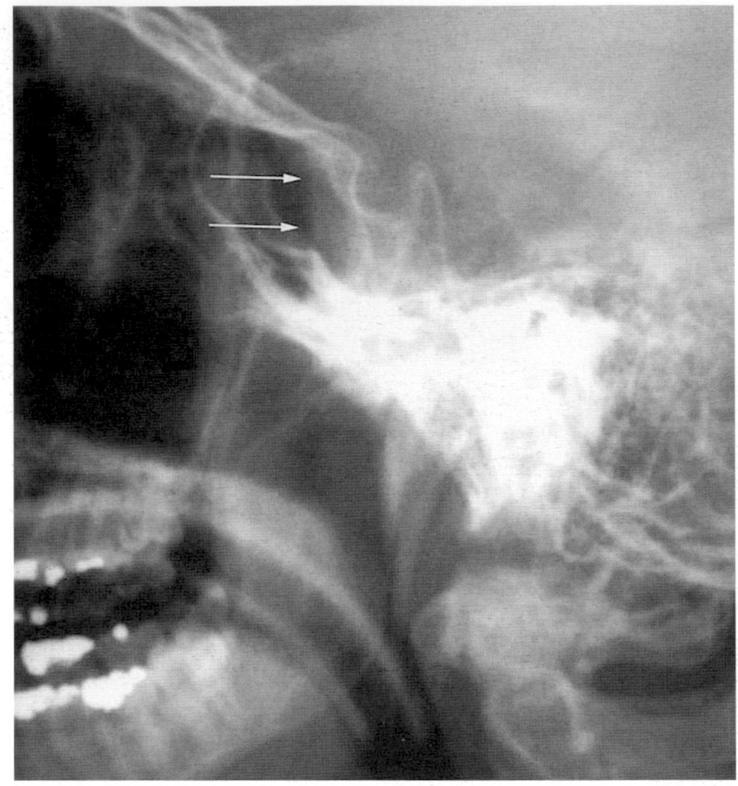

Fig. 2.19 *'Brow-up' lateral skull X-ray showing a fluid level (horizontal arrows) in the sphenoid sinus. Remember the patient is lying on his back for this view. Note the endotracheal tube in situ.*

skull is taken 'brow up', and **you must train yourself to look for it on every lateral film.**

Diagnostic pitfall The sphenoid sinus is just an opaque bone in early life. It then begins to form a central enlarging air cavity, a process called pneumatization. In some adults this is incomplete and a proportion of the back of the sinus remains opaque with bone, the anterior cortex of which can resemble a fluid level;

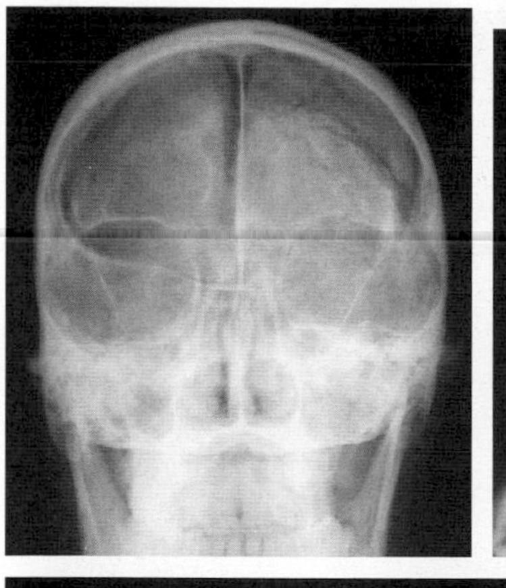

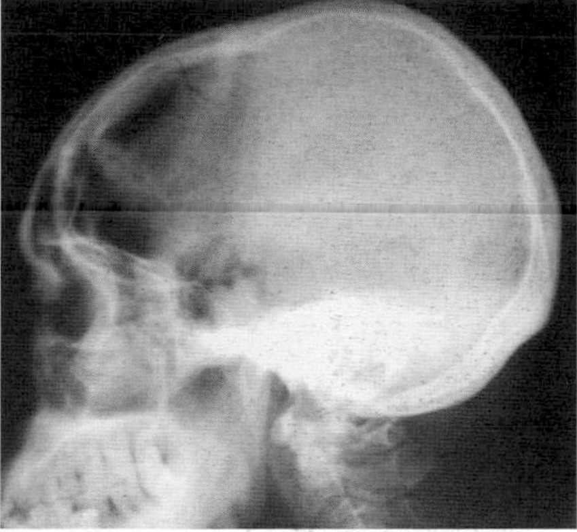

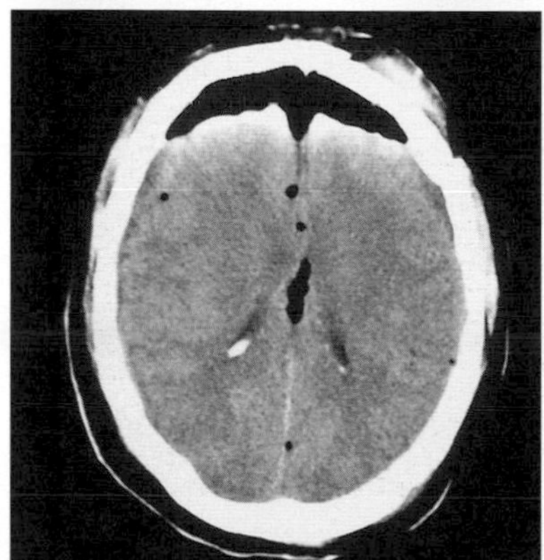

Fig. 2.20 *Victim of assault. Air in the head. Note the sharp outlining of the frontal lobes of both cerebral hemispheres of the brain on the AP skull film (**A**), the marked anterior radiolucency on the lateral view (**B**), and the unequivocal confirmation of air in the head on the CT scan (**C**).*

however, this is often slightly curved and sclerotic, with clear anterior and posterior cortical margins.

Intracranial air (Figs 2.20, 2.21)

What does it look like? Dark!

Traumatic pneumocephalus Air inside the head is extremely bad news, and **is a disaster that has already happened.** It means a pathway for bacteria has been opened up by a dural tear, with all the attendant risks of intracranial infection –

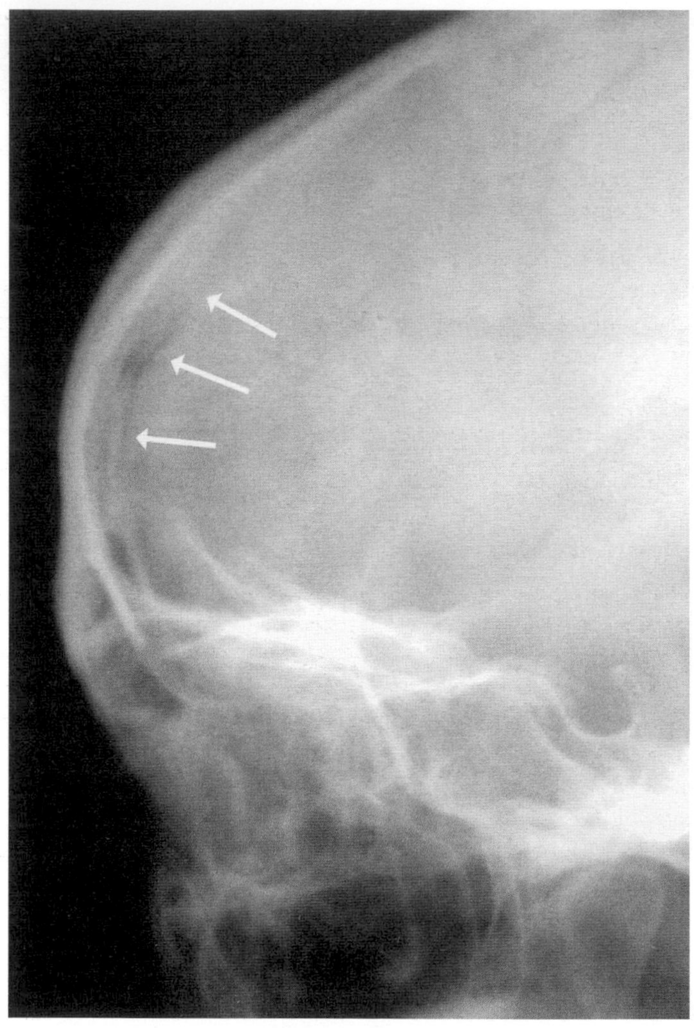

Fig. 2.21 *A more likely scenario – a life-saving observation of air in the head. Detail from a brow-up lateral film of the victim of a road traffic accident.*

meningitis, cerebral abscess, etc. **The presence of air within the head should therefore be conscientiously sought on the films of every patient who has sustained blunt trauma,** which, remember, is the other main reason for doing the lateral 'brow-up'. Following any form of penetrating injury to the head the automatic introduction of bacteria is assumed and appropriate antibiotic prophylaxis must therefore be given.

Gold medal points:

- Rarely in some patients a *tension pneumocephalus* may develop, analogous to a pneumothorax in the chest, and cause backward compression of the brain. Patients with air in the head should be told to avoid blowing the nose, which may exacerbate the situation, and to try and avoid coughing or sneezing.
- A scalp avulsion (e.g. from long hair caught in machinery) can cause a big and dramatic lucent defect. Scalp tissue is fibrous and contributes greatly to the apparent density of the skull – do not mistake such a defect for air in the head.

Important points

The whole clinical approach to head injuries is designed to pre-empt rare events which, in most patients, never happen. Similarly, a displaced pineal, air in the head and fluid in the sphenoid sinus are rare plain film findings, but with potentially devastating consequences if missed. The corollary of this is that if you do not look for these signs, there is little to be gained from taking any films in the first place, apart, of course, from looking for fractures, which are first and foremost what is being sought. The life of a patient with a rare radiological finding will then well and truly lie in the alertness of the doctor to that radiological sign, which in turn presupposes knowledge of it. Or, to put it another way – you see what you look for!

Remember: Always check for air in the head.

And finally: Sometimes in the elderly, the frontal, temporal or occipital bones can be very thin and strikingly radiolucent. This phenomenon should not be mistaken for collections of intracranial air. Look how lucent these areas are even on the normal lateral skull film (Fig. 2.5, p. 14).

Summary of analysis of skull films

In the light of the clinical findings ask yourself: **What am I looking for?**

Frontal film: checklist

- Confirm patient's name, today's date, date of birth, etc. (this applies to all films).
- AP or PA? An AP will probably have been taken supine. Is the patient straight or rotated?
- Look for any gross abnormality that strikes you immediately.
- Find the L/R marker. Make sure you put the films up the right way round.
- Check for linear fractures, i.e. straight or jagged edges that are darker than vessels and which may be crossing anatomical boundaries.
- Check for depressed fractures – crumpling of tables of the skull; either lucent or focal area of increased density.
- Check the scalp for haematomas and foreign bodies, e.g. air, gravel, glass, and their relationships to suspected underlying fractures.
- Check for accessory sutures especially in children.
- Look at the maxillary sinus region. Despite the underlying petrous bones, opacification on one side may still be seen. If so, get formal facial views.
- Look for air in the head due to penetrating injury or surgical emphysema in the scalp.
- Check the pineal for midline displacement (often not visible). Check for obliquity if you think the pineal is not central. Do not mistake other things for the pineal.

Lateral film: checklist

- Confirm patient's name, today's date, date of birth, etc.
- Any gross abnormality?
- Radiographic data? Is this a left or a right lateral? Find the marker. Is the film marked 'brow up' or 'shoot through'? If not, find out why or get the radiographer to confirm how it was taken.
- Any obvious major fractures? Look for linear and depressed fractures.
- Scalp (bright light or digital interrogation). Check for foreign bodies as above (e.g. if the patient went through a car windscreen or was hit over the head with a bottle).

- Cranial vault – status of frontal, parietal, occipital, temporal bones.
- Identify suture lines/vascular channels, especially middle meningeals. Be aware of profuse venous channels which may occur as normal variants, e.g. parietal star/spider (Fig. 2.9).
- Check fontanelles and presence of any accessory sutures in children.
- Any extra jagged lines crossing anatomical boundaries?
- Check directly behind frontal bone for air inside head and for fluid in the sphenoid sinus.
- Cervical spine – look at the upper neck anatomy and check for evidence of trauma at the occipitoatlantal and at the atlantoaxial joints and bones of the upper neck. Any prevertebral swelling? (see Ch. 3)
- Pineal – calcified? If not, it will not be visible on AP film.

Townes' view: checklist

- Confirm patient's name, today's date, date of birth, etc.
- Radiographic data, e.g. 'patient restless' written on film, or back of request card?
- Is dorsum sellae visible in the foramen magnum? (The definition of a good Townes' view.) Sometimes it won't be, e.g. if the patient is drunk.
- Which is left and right? (Often difficult to see.) You will probably have to peer into the darkness beyond the skull to find the marker, especially on a Townes' view.
- Make sure you put the film up correctly having checked left and right.
- Is all of the arc of the vault visible? May require bright light/interrogation to see the top properly.
- Identify lambdoid suture. Any wormian bones? (Useful in osteogenesis imperfecta.)
- Any evidence of fractures?
- Any accessory fissures especially in children?
- Any scalp haematomas/foreign bodies/air in soft tissues?

- Mastoid air cells – clear/opaque? (Opacification may indicate base of skull fracture in petrous bone.)
- Look at neck and sinus anatomy, if visible on films, and zygomatic arches.

And finally: Anything I cannot explain? Anything I am unhappy with? Do I need to seek help now? If so – go and get it!

NB These concepts and level of self-interrogation must be applied generally: looking at X-rays is an active not a passive process, and should be applied to all X-ray images that you see.

The orbits

Background

Emergency imaging of the orbits usually involves either *blunt trauma* for a suspected blow-out fracture, or *penetrating injury* by an opaque object, often a small metal particle, or penetration by a some other kind of object or material such as plastic, e.g. a knitting needle or a chopstick. Patients who arrive in A & E with spontaneously swollen infected orbits are another group, but would normally always go straight to CT.

Radiography

Plain film frontal views usually suffice for initial suspected radio-opaque foreign bodies and trauma.

Anatomy

The orbits consist of conical cavities which hold and support the globes of the eyes. Any injury is always therefore a potential threat to sight and they have crucial anatomical relationships with the brain above, the ethmoid sinuses and nasal cavities medially and maxillary antra below.

Blow-out fracture of the orbit ('BOF')

A failed catch

Look at Figure 2.22. This is an X-ray of a pitcher who was hit over the left eye by a baseball when he missed the catch. He had limitation of upward gaze. This is presumptive evidence of a blow-out fracture of the orbit. Note:

- The increased opacification of the left orbit due to overlying swelling. Such swelling can at times be so severe as to completely obscure the underlying anatomy.

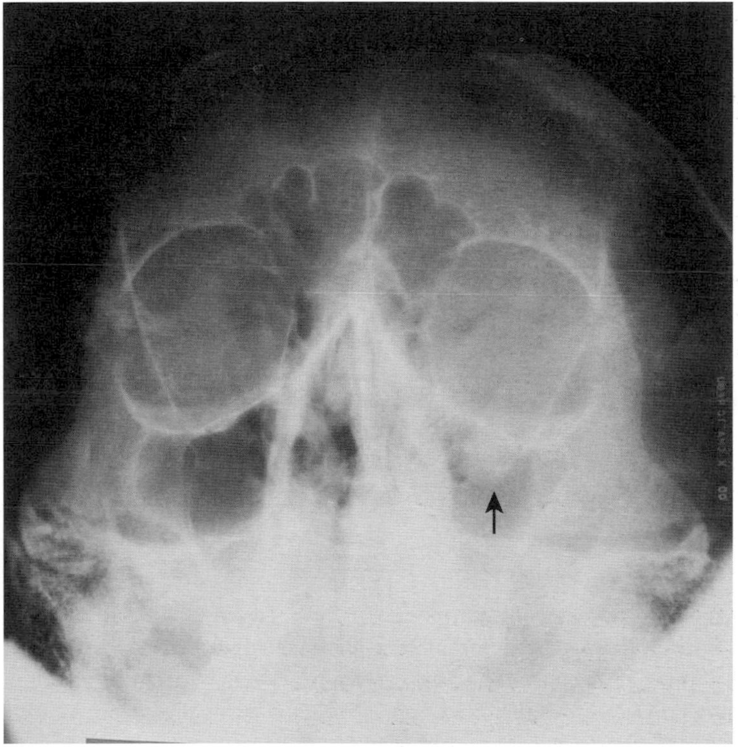

Fig. 2.22 *A failed catch! Erect facial film showing blow-out fracture of the left orbit.*

- The downward angulation and partial collapse of the left orbital floor/ maxillary antral roof.
- The rounded soft tissue density contrasting with the air in the maxillary antrum.

NB This is radiological confirmation of a blow-out fracture of the orbit. The momentum of the speeding ball has been transferred to the bony orbit, causing it to fracture at its weakest point. This allows the inferior oblique eye muscle (which contributes to upward gaze) and orbital fat to herniate downwards into the antrum. Sometimes this is hard to see on plain X-rays due to overlying swelling. Direct coronal slices on CT will confirm or exclude the diagnosis.

These cases will sometimes require surgical release of the herniated orbital contents. Interestingly, however, some of them are managed conservatively and reduce spontaneously.

Gold medal points: Other orbital injuries include a medial blow-out into the ethmoids, and fracture of the lateral orbital wall from a direct blow known as a pistol-whip type injury. A blow-out fracture of the orbital *floor* should still show an intact inferior orbital *rim*. The collapsed floor is further back.

The 'black eyebrow sign'

Following trauma to the face, e.g. from an assault, X-rays may show no apparent immediate abnormality to the casual observer. Meticulous scrutiny of such films is, however, necessary in these situations as a subtle radiological sign may be present, which, if missed, may have serious consequences.

Look at Figure 2.23. Note:

- The opacification over the lateral and inferior aspects of the left maxillary antrum caused by the overlying soft tissue swelling.
- The dark crescent in the upper left orbit. **NB** This is intraorbital emphysema or *air in the orbit*. This means that the ethmoid air cells have blown out, allowing air to enter around the eyeball, which also means bacteria can now get in. Once established, intraorbital sepsis may rapidly progress to intracranial infection and, if untreated, quickly kill the patient – a high price to pay because you have missed the air. This crescent of air is known as the *black eyebrow sign*.

NB Fainter dark crescents can sometimes be seen in non-injured patients. These constitute *normal intraorbital fat*, usually symmetrical on both sides and of equal radiolucency when present.

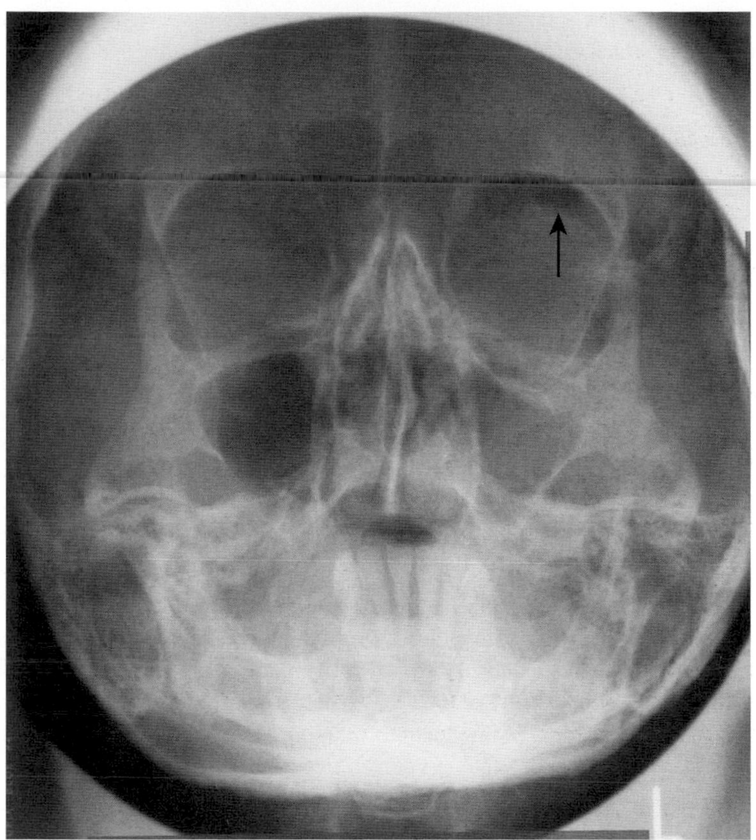

Fig. 2.23 *Air in the roof of the left orbital cavity. This policeman tried to intervene in a fight and received a vicious punch to the left side of his face. Note: the blow you receive when trying to separate two combatants is one of the most dangerous you can get.*

Sometimes air can be caught in the conjunctival sac when blinking, simulating orbital emphysema. A repeat film might be necessary to resolve it.

Foreign bodies in the eye (Fig. 2.24)

The classic injury is that of a metal particle from a lathe entering the eye of someone who should have been wearing protective goggles. These show up on X-ray as tiny metallic opacities over the orbit. Unfortunately, most normal X-ray cassettes contain minute 'screen marks' from dust particles inside the cassettes which block the X-rays, producing an identical appearance. (Now that you know they exist, have a look for them on conventional X-rays – before you go digital; there are often half a dozen or more on one film such as a chest X-ray). The solution is to take one film of the orbits, e.g. with the eyes looking up. A metallic foreign body will show up on the film, in which case a second film should be taken, marked 'down', and the foreign body will change position with the moving eyeball (this excludes a screen mark), and its location can be assessed from the relative motion. If no foreign body is seen on the first film, a second is not necessary. Further ways of assessing a foreign body include with a slit-lamp (i.e. clinical examination), ultrasound for the anterior chamber of the eye, and CT of the orbit (to look both for foreign bodies and for secondary signs of sepsis). An appropriate method of removal can then be planned.

Crucial point: An MRI scan is absolutely contraindicated if there is a suspected ferrous metallic foreign body in the eye, as it is liable to take off like a bullet, so do not make a fool of yourself by asking for one.

Facial bones

Background

Facial injuries due to motor vehicle accidents, assaults, sports injuries, etc. are extremely common. They may occur in isolation or in association with head, neck and multiple injuries, but even when present on their own may threaten life due to severe blood loss or obstruction to the upper airways. Facial disfigurement is also a potential and rightly feared long-term sequel.

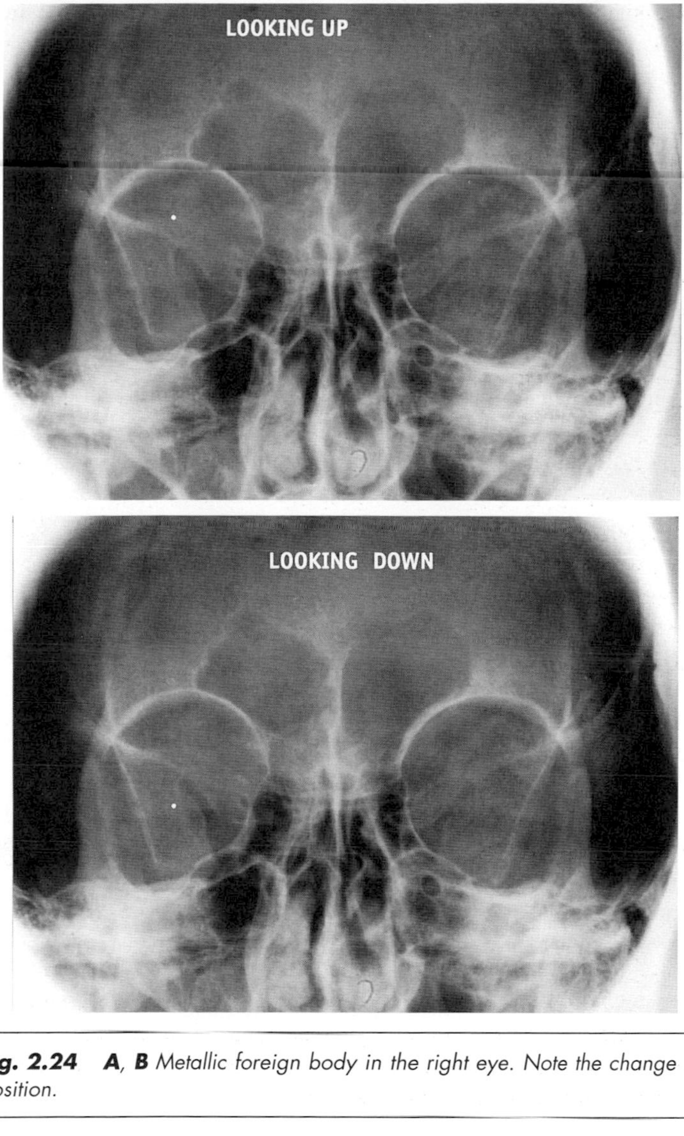

LOOKING UP

A

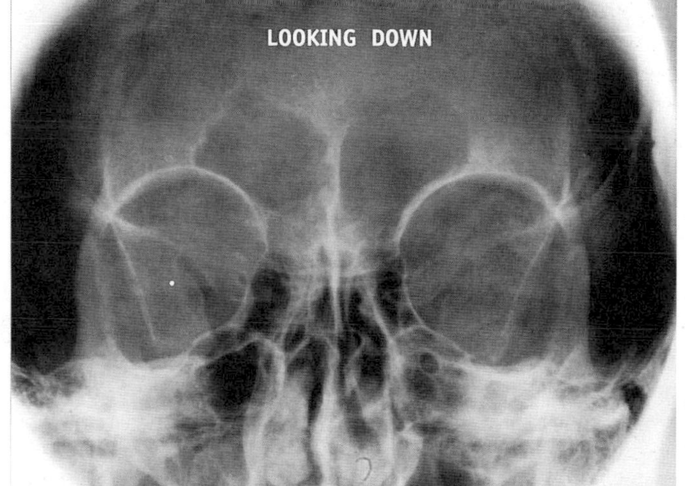

Fig. 2.24 ***A*, *B*** *Metallic foreign body in the right eye. Note the change in position.*

The bad news Gross soft tissue swelling may combine both to inhibit adequate clinical examination and further cloud the bony structures and radiographic anatomy on X-rays of the face.

The good news Evolving guidelines now tend to recommend both early involvement of maxillofacial surgeons with all but the simplest of facial injuries and a low threshold for proceeding to low-dose CT. Clearly, if the face is badly damaged from the outset, or the patient either head-injured or multiply injured, the entire diagnostic exercise may be conducted exclusively by CT, and plain films circumvented. The CT examination will nowadays usually include three-dimensional (3D) reconstruction for optimum evaluation of the injuries to enable the maxillofacial surgeon to plan the surgical reconstruction of the face.

Crucial point: If necessary, surgical intervention in severe facial injury may be delayed for several days until the swelling has subsided, so it may also be possible to delay imaging for that period if required (unlike imaging of the brain).

Radiography

The ideal view is an erect PA film (occipitomental) (Fig. 2.26, p. 46) with the patient facing the cassette and the head tilted back, to optimize the view of the facial anatomy with the *petrous temporal bones projected down out of the way*. This position will maximize clarity and allow any fluid levels in the maxillary or frontal sinuses to become manifest.

NB Always look to see where the petrous bones are so that you know what, if anything, is being obscured.

Important fact: It is incredibly helpful to have films of the facial bones labelled **'erect'** or **'supine'** (as AP chest films are labelled) because a fluid-filled antrum cannot be distinguished from mucosal thickening on a supine film, but it can on an erect view if a fluid level is seen. It may be obvious to another radiographer how such a film was taken but certainly not necessarily to the A & E doctor, who can really benefit from this information.

NB Severely injured patients who obviously cannot sit up will have to be examined supine and AP but the radiographer can carry out reverse angulation to generate the necessary positioning.

NB In addition to the petrous bones dropping as the head goes further back, more of the zygomatic arches open out as your viewpoint drops beneath them. Sometimes films have to be a compromise, with intermediate degrees of

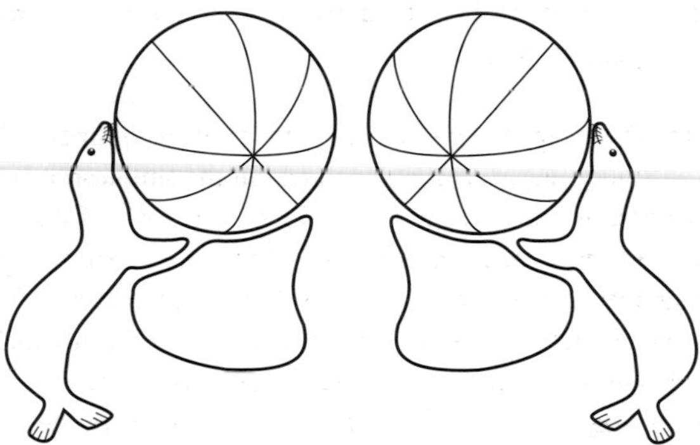

Fig. 2.25 *The zygomatic sea lions with their beach balls.*

angulation, but now you can assess what is going on. The decision to go for CT first if necessary should already have been made by this time.

Hint: The zygomatic arches are usually visible on Townes' views but you may require bright lights to see them (Fig. 2.25).

Anatomy (Fig. 2.26)

This needs to be learnt or properly revised. The relevant structures comprise the *middle third of the face,* which effectively means everything from just above the superior orbital rims to the sockets of the teeth in the maxilla. The key to understanding the facial anatomy is first to identify the maxillary sinuses and orbital cavities. The thin plates of bone between them form both the roofs of the antra and the floors of the orbits. Above the orbits lie the scalloped margins of the frontal sinuses. Sometimes these are so large and overdeveloped that neurosurgical approaches have to be rerouted around them (Fig. 2.14, p. 26). The ethmoid air cells lie medial to the orbits and the nasal cavities between the antra.

Look at the frontal occipitomental view of the facial bones (Fig. 2.26). This is taken with the head tilted back so that the chin is against the cassette. Note the resemblance to the 'Man in the Moon' and the low position of the petrous bone below the inferior angles of the maxillary antra. Next time you look at the full moon think of the facial bones.

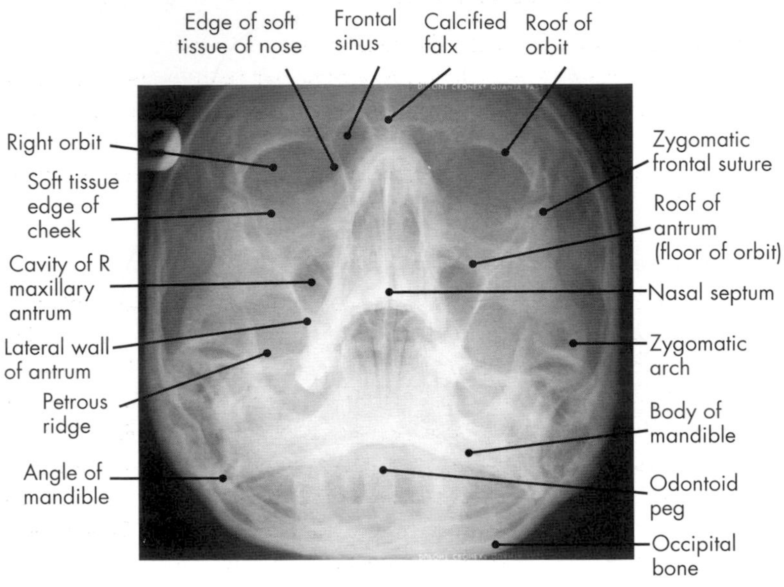

Fig. 2.26 *Normal facial bones. Occipitomental view.*

The maxillary and other sinuses are usually symmetrically 'clear', i.e. dark because they are empty, but blood or mucosal thickening will render them opaque. The zygomatic arches are placed like a pair of flying buttresses, or the bodies of 'rampant' sea lions in heraldic posture blending with the frontal bones at the zygomaticofrontal sutures and anterolateral walls of the antra with their noses and front flippers respectively. Talking of noses – note the Norman arch style sweep of the nasal bones and the central nasal septum.

Normal variant

Sometimes there may be an accessory suture in the arch called the zygomaticotemporal suture which looks like fracture but will not be displaced.

Radiological signs of facial trauma

The X-Ray paradox: The effects of trauma to the facial bones are quite unlike those to long bones such as the humerus or femur, where the observer is simply looking primarily for breaks in bony continuity. Certainly the bones break in facial fractures, but the combination of overlying oedema, bleeding and escape of air provide evidence of, while simultaneously obscuring, the underlying trauma.

NB Face 'just a mess' – go straight to CT.

Le Fort fractures

Mention may be made of the French surgeon Le Fort, who, in the early part of the 20th century conducted some violently macabre experiments with dead bodies. He smashed the faces with a sledgehammer and from the dissected remnants he traced out the pattern of common fracture lines which led to his eponymous classification of facial injuries. These relate to arcs of increasing radii, first across the lower maxilla (I), then up through the medial orbital floors and over the vault of the nasal bone (II), and finally through the zygomaticofrontal sutures and backs of the orbits (III). The Le Fort III fracture renders the maxilla loose and essentially separates the facial skeleton from the rest of the skull.

However, not all facial injuries fall into the Le Fort classification, nor can the full Le Fort status of an injury necessarily be established from plain films. Nowadays such patients need to go to CT. The likely types of facial injuries which the A & E doctor may encounter therefore fall into several groups:

- Orbits.
- Isolated fracture of the zygomatic arch.
- Depressed fracture of the zygomatic bone ('tripod fracture').
- More complex and mixed fractures of the facial skeleton, of incremental severity.

Some examples of trauma

Look at Figure 2.27 (patient punched in the right side of the face). Note:

- The fluid level in the right maxillary antrum. The facial bones are otherwise intact.
- The low position of the petrous bones just crossing the lower antra.

Comment: One can deduce that this film was taken erect (fluid level present). This is presumptive evidence of a crack fracture in the wall of the right antrum with bleeding into it, and therefore of an *open* fracture with the risk of *infection* getting in.

Caveat: The differential includes *preceding sinus disease* (with an effusion) or a recent *antral wash-out* – so make sure you get a proper history.

NB Fluid levels may also be seen in the frontal sinus.

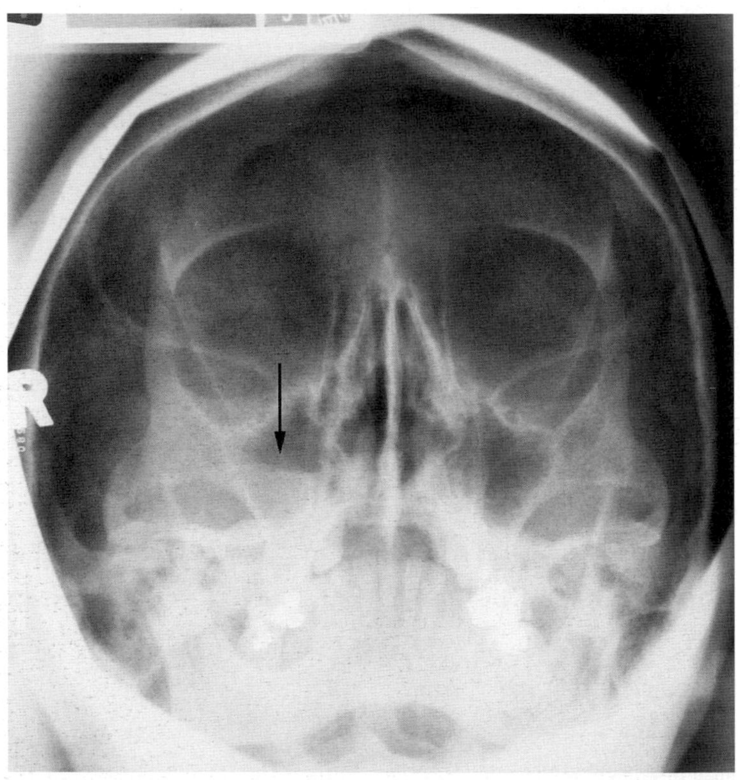

Fig. 2.27 *Erect view of the facial bones showing fluid level (arrow) in right maxillary sinus.*

Look at Figure 2.28 (patient hit in the face with a cricket bat). This is a 3-point or 'tripod' depressed fracture of the right zygomatic bone. Note:

- The opacification of the right maxillary antrum.
- No fluid level; ? supine/erect – does not say.
- The disruption of the lateral wall of the right maxillary antrum and the right zygomatic arch.

NB

- Look to see if the films are labelled erect/supine, or are unlabelled. (If you have seen the patient you should have a good idea which one is likely.)
- If you see a fluid level in an antrum or frontal sinus, obviously the film was done erect. If just a clouded antrum and unlabelled it could be fluid in the antrum in the supine position or mucosal thickening due to submucosal haemorrhage or preceding sinus disease. If you are still unsure, ask the radiographer how he or she took the films (and mark them for future reference).

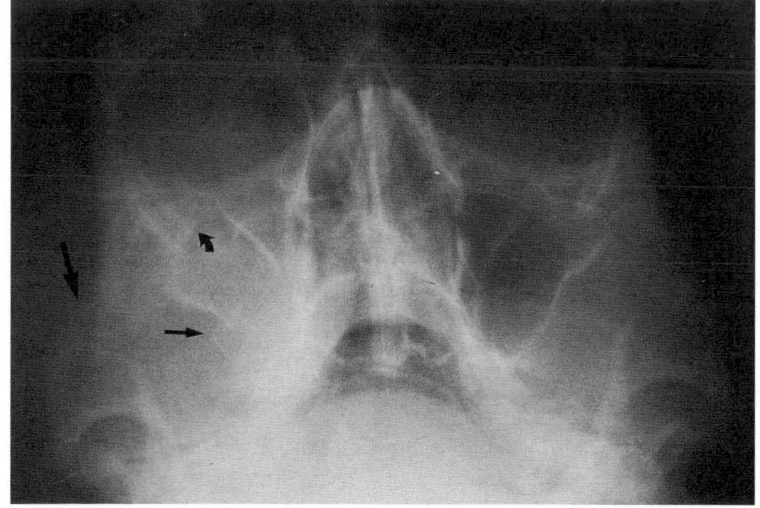

Fig. 2.28 *'Tripod fracture' of right zygomatic bone (arrows).*

- If one side of the face is swollen and ballooned up clinically, expect a marked increase in density over that side of the face on the X-ray films and a corresponding increased difficulty in seeing the underlying bones, which may look underexposed (too pale). This may also cause misinterpretation of perceived but spurious clouding of the antrum.

Summary of assessment of facial bones

As always check, name, date, etc. After locating the position of the petrous bones and any immediately obvious abnormalities start at the top and work down, looking for:

- Opacification of or fluid levels in the frontal sinuses or disruption of their bony margins.
- Roofs of the orbits – ?symmetrical lucent crescents (= normal fat); ?asymmetrical lucent crescents (= ?air in orbit); the 'dark eyebrow sign'.
- Zygomaticofrontal sutures – often asymmetric due to obliquity, which can make one look wider than the other; often fused in the elderly. Smooth margins when anatomical.
- Look right round the edge of every bone, including the inner and outer bony margins of the orbits, and follow the latter downwards. They blend with the zygomatic arches.
- Look for asymmetry/unilateral depression of, or cracks in, the zygomatic arch on the affected side.
- Check the integrity of the lateral walls of the antra, and if both of these are broken you are dealing with some kind of Le Fort fracture, as this is a bilateral injury. The face is likely to be unstable.
- Check for specific evidence of a blow-out fracture (BOF) of the floor of the orbit into the upper part of the antrum (Fig. 2.22, p. 39).

Remember that the basic radiographic responses to trauma consist of:

- *Interruption of normally placed bony margins*, with comminution or gross displacement depending on the degree of impact.
- *Bleeding into cavities* (i.e. sinuses), rendering them partially or wholly opaque.
- *Escape of air* from sinuses into adjacent cavities (i.e. orbits).

And that:

- It is the mixture of fluid/air and gravity which produces fluid levels, plus of course the appropriate radiographic projection – preferably erect.
- Escaped air or 'surgical emphysema' can cause extensive irregular dark mottling and confusing shadows, greatly hindering plain film interpretation. The air itself can dissect up around the head or down into the neck, sometimes right down into the chest to cause a pneumomediastinum, which may (1) mimic non-existent chest trauma, and (2) allow bacteria to cause mediastinitis – a dangerous and unwelcome complication.

If there is extensive damage, call the radiologists and maxillofacial surgeons and get a facial CT. You cannot fully evaluate the Le Fort status from plain films. If the maxilla is mobile clinically and the face has clearly become disconnected from the skull there is obviously a serious problem.

Pause to:

- Take a look into the hinterland of the skull just to see what's going on. Occasionally a fracture line will be visible in the vault, an unsupected calcified mass or cranial vault lucency necessitating full skull films. (The corollary of requesting facial views after spotting an opaque antrum on a skull X-ray.) Ask the patient first whether there is a history of neurosurgical procedures, e.g. burr holes. That is good practice.
- Look at the jaws and upper neck for incidental trauma. These are often just about a white-out and the uncritical observer fails even to bother looking at them. **Remember! You are responsible for any abnormality on the film.**
- Look for surgical emphysema, and do not confuse it with normal fat lines.

NB Radiologists help to justify their existence by picking up things on the edge of visibility – all it takes is a little thought and the time to take a determined look to find some missing teeth or a break at the angle of the mandible. The Odontoid process may also be sitting there centrally, like a crocus. Have a look at this as well. (**Moral**: Seek and ye shall find.)

Some tiresome normal variants

- Air caught in the conjunctival sacs simulating gas in the orbits.
- Thin lucent lines crossing the orbits – air between the eyelids in the palpebral

fissure if shut at the moment of exposure. If unilateral – patient winking at radiographer?!

- Small maxillary sinuses (either underdeveloped due to age or congenitally hypoplastic) will tend to look more opaque than normal, mimicking trauma, and the bony edges are harder to find.
- Soft tissue crescentic edges over the maxillary sinuses, e.g. due to edge of the upper lip – follow it across from right to left. The margins of the nostrils may also simulate submucosal swelling or haemorrhage. Remember it is not just bones that appear on X-rays – soft tissues do as well.
- Overdeveloped ethmoid/sphenoid air cells may mimic gas pockets projected over the orbits and maxillary sinuses.
- The intense osteoporosis of the very elderly, making the facial bones look ghost-like and difficult to see.
- The infantile facial skeleton. Go and see the paediatric radiologist (unless you've done a special study module (SSM) on the subject as a student).
- Small cortical 'breaks' in the lateral antral walls. Normal 'posterior superior alveolar canals'.

What about the nose?

Background

The nose is frequently subject to injury in facial trauma because (1) it sticks out anatomically, and (2) it is frequently inserted uninvited into other peoples' business!

Radiographic anatomy

The bones of the nose are actually present in the fields of AP and lateral skull and facial films, but are usually 'burnt out' on the lateral views because of the energy needed to demonstrate the cranial vault, etc. In the past, special views at reduced penetration were frequently taken to demonstrate fractures of the nasal bone itself and the nasal spine of the maxilla – the latter often being associated with severe soft tissue swelling of the upper lip following a blow to the mouth.

Radiology

A lucent line is often discernible at the base of the nasal bone – the nasofrontal suture. Any line that crosses the crest of the nasal bone further down the slope on the lateral view can be regarded as a fracture.

NB The nasociliary vessels and nerves often generate normal markings on the nasal bones, but these do not cross the upper edge.

NB The routine X-ray of most nasal injuries has fallen from favour. Nowadays it is likely to be left to the discretion of an ENT surgeon, mainly in the context of nasal obstruction, and CT will better assess any comminution, septal displacement or soft tissue swelling than will plain films. **Find out what your own local rules are**.

Important fact: A non-central nasal septum is not necessarily post-traumatic in origin.

The mandible

Background

John Wayne and the traditional Western movie (e.g. *The Sheriff of Fractured Jaw*) with all those flying fists have a lot to answer for in regard to the apparent indestructability of the human mandible! Rarely would a concession be made to what could really happen: you must regard the mandible as a rather delicate object.

Teeth also appear to be highly resistant to flying fists in the movies. Meanwhile, back in the real world where so many assaults and motor vehicle accidents occur these days, mandibular fractures are common, either in isolation or associated with facial or multiple injuries.

Radiography (Figs. 2.29, 2.30, 2.31)

Views employed here are the straight PA (to get the bone detail as close to the film as possible), rather than the AP, and oblique views of both sides, which are essential because mandibular fractures have a tendency to be bilateral, and a suitably exposed Townes' view, which may show the regions of the temporomandibular joints and upper rami well. Best of all, however, is an orthopantomogram (OPT, p. 57), which 'unwraps' the mandible and allows it to be viewed without the inevitable bony overlap seen on lateral and oblique projections. Oblique views of the mandible can be confusing, and the OPT is easier to understand and interpret.

Crucial point: An OPT requires a cooperative patient in the upright position, but it may not always do justice to the temporomandibular joints at the extremities of the film. Recent developments in OPT technique allow specific parts only of the mandible to be shown with appropriate shielding.

In serious cases CT scanning should be used to sort out complex injuries. CT may well reveal fractures undetectable on plain films, or further fracture components not apparent on conventional X-rays, and does of course offer a 3D reconstruction facility. Basically, the harder you look the more you find.

Dental injuries These are a special case and may require referral to a dental surgeon, who in turn may ask for specific dental films of the affected teeth.

Anatomy (Figs 2.29, 2.30)

The mandible has a body, two horizontal and two vertical rami. It then divides on either side like a catapult – the posterior component forming the condylar process and the anterior component the coronoid process. The alveolar fossae accommodate the teeth.

Trauma

History: This patient (Fig. 2.31) said she had stood on a rake which 'came up and hit me'. Fifty minutes later her husband came to A & E with fractured 4th and 5th metacarpals. Note:

- The crack and split fractures of the angle and posterior aspect of the ascending ramus of the left side of the mandible.
- The second break at the base of the mandibular condyle on the opposite side.
- The loss of many of the teeth (long-standing), with consequent atrophy of the horizontal rami.
- The dark **air column of the pharynx crossing over the mandibular angles, especially on the left**.

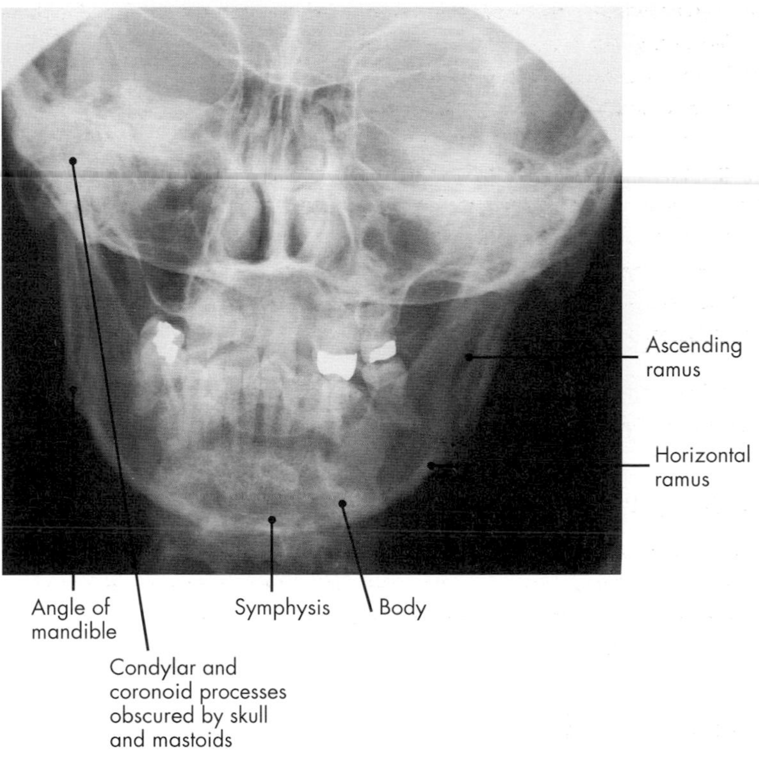

Fig. 2.29 *Normal AP view of mandible. Note the obscuration of the condylar and coronoid processes.*

The weakest points of the mandible are in the body at the mandibular foramen and at the angle of the mandible beside the 3rd molar. Fractures are therefore common here but can occur anywhere, so all of the above must be carefully inspected, especially on the opposite side from the main injury, as the mandible is effectively a ring.

A big mistake not to make: Do not mistake the air in the pharynx contrasting with the dorsum of the tongue on conventional lateral or oblique views of the

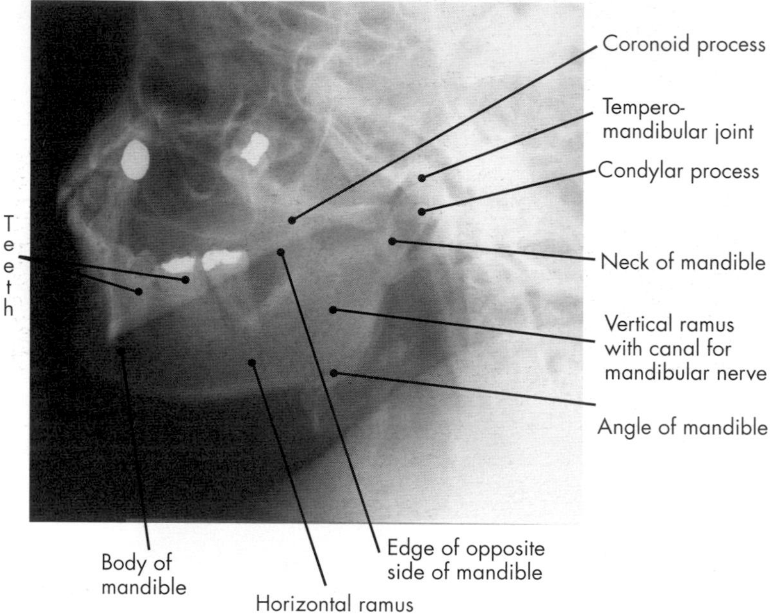

Fig. 2.30 *Oblique view of mandible showing the horizontal and vertical rami isolated on one side. A second view is required for the opposite side.*

mandible for a fracture. Get used to identifying the back of the tongue on lateral skull films, which you'll probably see more often.

Golden rule: Always look inside the mouth (if possible) to assess mandibular trauma **in case you are dealing with an open fracture** which has split the jaw, loosened an adjacent tooth or ripped the buccal mucosa. Conversely, fracture fragments may already be jutting out through the skin, revealing glistening white bone.

Fractures that do not communicate with the surface are regarded as 'simple' and usually involve the rami or condyles. Fractures at the body of the mandible may be difficult to see on plain films because the plane of the fracture lies obliquely to the beam, but will usually show up well on CT.

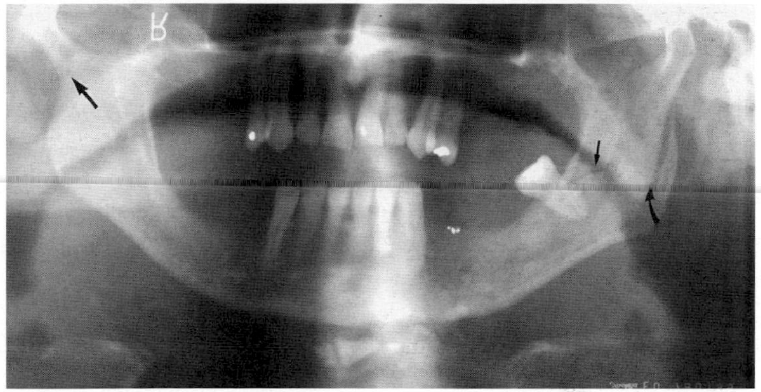

Fig. 2.31 *Orthopantomogram showing bilateral fractures of the mandible.*

Danger of death

A severely bilaterally fractured mandible adjacent to the symphysis may allow the tongue to float back and occlude the airway, as important muscles of the tongue are attached here (the *swallowed tongue syndrome*), or the whole bone may be driven back, (remember John Wayne?) necessitating a tracheostomy or traction suture to hold the tongue forward.

What about the temporomandibular joints?

These are the joints involved in dislocation of the jaw – usually due to trauma or an excessively big yawn.

Experiment: Place an index finger in your ear with the pulp pointing forwards. Then move your jaw. What you feel moving anteriorly is the head of the mandible in its glenoid fossa (yes, the same name as the socket for the shoulder).

Important fact: On X-rays in the 'open' and 'closed' positions these structures move right out of their sockets, downwards and forwards. This is known as physiological subluxation. A dislocated jaw is usually stuck in this position, but do not mistake the normal degree of excursion for a dislocation. When the mandibular condyle is anterior to the glenoid tubercle (which is just in front of the socket) in the closed position, or the patient is unable to close the mouth when the condyle remains forward, the jaw is definitely 'out'. **NB** Such films are hard to interpret and you should get help early with them if you have any doubts about what you are looking at.

Films of painful non-traumatized temporomandibular joints will normally be marked 'open' and 'closed' for you by the radiographer, so that you know exactly what you should be seeing on each view.

Hint: Do not get mixed up with 'left' and 'right' and 'open' and 'closed' – you'll have four films to inspect and be feeling the strain. It's easily done!

Chapter 3

The neck

Background

- **In multiple trauma a very high index of suspicion must be maintained for neck injuries because of the potentially devastating consequences of missing such lesions at the outset**; whatever other findings dominate the clinical picture, the presence of a lesion must invariably be assumed in the first instance.

- In practice this boils down to immediate immobilization of all suspect necks at the scene, which is how they will usually present in A & E, and **the support must remain in place until the patient is stabilized and all appropriate clinical and imaging evaluations are completed.**

  Crucial X-ray fact: Following some neck injuries, the position of the bones and joints at the moment of impact may be totally different from that at which they are later seen at the instant the X-ray is taken, due to temporary traumatic dislocation which damages the cord but then spontaneously reduces.

- Conventional X-rays to show the current alignment on arrival in A & E, however, including a 'shoot-through', or horizontal beam lateral are mandatory and may provide the necessary initial radiological information. If not, early progression to CT or MRI will be necessary to **'clear the neck'** before the green light can be given to remove any immobilization device, **the order for which should come only from a senior doctor.**

- Road traffic accidents, accidents at work, at home or during sports activities form the bulk of the injuries. Trampolines, diving into impossibly shallow pools or being thrown from a horse are other potent causes. Unfortunately, irreparable damage is sometimes done by subsequent mishandling of casualties after the initial injury has been inflicted. (**Moral:** Don't mess about with necks!)

Point of interest: It is said a significant number of fatalities occurred among those who jumped from the *Titanic* because their necks were thrown back and snapped by their buoyant life-jackets when they hit the sea.

A look at the guidelines in neck injuries

As with head injuries and the brain, the RCR guidelines are designed to optimize the pick-up rate of injuries, in this case to the cord, to minimize any chance of damage to an uninjured cord in the presence of an unstable neck, and indeed to prevent a partially transected cord being turned into a completely transected one by inappropriate handling or premature movement.

In common with the brain, the spinal cord is completely invisible on plain X-rays. So too are the ligaments that maintain the neck's stability. Any deductions from conventional films are therefore made indirectly.

Clinical reasons why the diagnosis may get overlooked

- A lack of knowledge by the doctor of the mechanism and severity of injury.
- Patient unconscious on arrival due to head injury or other condition causing a fall (e.g. stroke).
- Multiple injuries, e.g. a 'red blanket' or emergency case, such as a sky-diver or crashed pilot with flail chest, vascular injury or massive haematuria, causing distraction and dominating the clinical picture.
- Minimal neurological signs giving a false sense of security – but an unstable neck. A disaster waiting to happen.

So who gets what imaging?

Because there is so much at stake, the imaging requirements of patients with various categories of neck injury merit close attention to detail. The RCR guidelines identify the following groups.

1. Conscious patients with apparent head and/or facial injury only

These patients do not need any X-rays routinely, but still need to be checked to exclude evidence of cervical injuries. The necessary criteria to exempt them from X-ray examinations are that they:

- Are fully alert and not intoxicated by alcohol or drugs.
- Show no neurological deficit.
- Have no midline posterior cervical tenderness.
- Have no other major, more painful injuries (patients may just complain about what hurts most), distracting attention from the neck.

2. Unconscious patients with head injury (or suspected head injury)

NB No one must manipulate the neck at this stage. These cases require high quality X-rays of the entire cervical spine from the odontoid to T1/T2, but these may not be achievable in muscular or obese individuals despite traction/oblique views, etc. Advice? Go directly to CT or MRI. If multiply-injured, the entire head, neck, chest and abdomen assessments may best be accomplished at the same time by CT anyway. If MRI is available this may be preferable for the spinal cord but restlessness may compromise both modalities. Anaesthetic assistance with light sedation may be invaluable.

3. Neck injury with pain

These patients warrant cervical spine films in the first instance. If the X-rays are problematical or the findings not straightforward, go and discuss them with your seniors and the radiologists regarding possible CT/MRI for further evaluation. **A painful neck will usually have a cause.**

4. Neck injury with neurological deficit

These warrant urgent orthopaedic or neurosurgical assessment and plain X-rays of diagnostic quality as a baseline. However, if necessary, go directly to MRI to assess:

- The cord itself.
- Extrinsic cord compression.
- Soft tissue injuries (ligaments).
- Fractures at multiple levels.

Or CT myelography if MRI is not available.

5. Neck injury with pain and suspect ligamentous injury (e.g. self-reduced subluxation from moment of impact)

These require X-ray assessment in flexion and extension, if necessary with screening (i.e. real-time X-rays) to show any latent instability. A doctor must be in attendance (preferably the one who requested the examination) and any movements should only be initiated by the patient and not forced. The patient should be warned to stop if he or she experiences excess pain or paraesthesiae down the arms.

Radiography

The objective is to demonstrate all the relevant anatomy, which may be much easier said than done in a thick-set severely injured and unconscious patient.

Standard views include:

- A lateral film which shows all the vertebrae in the cervical spine, from C1 to the top of T1 in the thoracic spine (Fig. 3.1). This may be the only plain film taken in severe trauma.
- The AP view (Fig. 3.4).
- An open-mouth view of the C1/C2 vertebrae (atlas and axis), also known as a 'peroral' or 'peg' view (Fig. 3.5, p. 69).

NB In well-built or obese individuals the shoulders may completely obscure much of the cervical spine, from as high as C3 down in some cases, but generally the problem is of the view being cut off at around C7/T1.

Crucial fact: The implications of this are that, if using conventional films, you must consciously check to see if all the relevant anatomy has been included. Unless you can tell at a glance that the view gets well down into the thoracic spine, **you must count the number of vertebrae from C1 down**, and the films as a minimum must demonstrate the upper end-plate of T1 (or preferably all of it). If using digital radiography you should be able to bring up the relevant anatomy purely by image manipulation.

What should be done if this cannot be achieved with conventional films? Traditionally the radiographer has several options:

- *Films of increased penetration.* These may solve the problem but tend to come out very dark and be hard to interpret, even with a bright light.

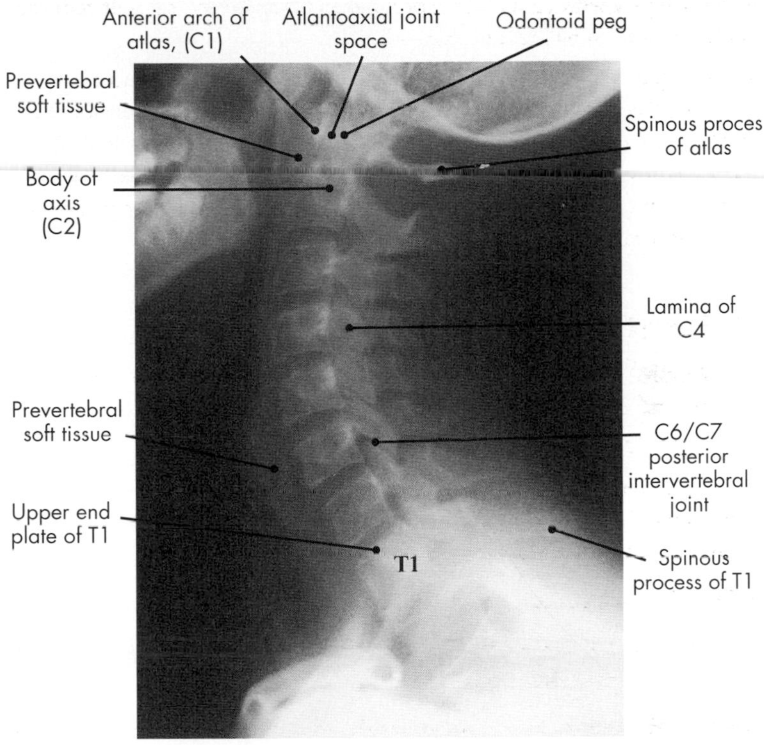

Fig. 3.1 *X-ray heaven! Excellent lateral view of neck showing vertebrae down to T1 and beyond.*

- *Films with arm traction gently pulling the shoulders down* out the way (traction views) (Fig. 3.9, p. 75).
- *'Swimmers' views'* (taken with one arm up and one arm down) (Fig. 3.2), but this may not be possible, e.g. with fractured shoulder girdles.
- *'Trauma obliques'*. By angulation these project the shoulders out of the way, and the view is no longer lateral; but may be sufficient to confirm normal alignment and integrity of the vertebral bodies.

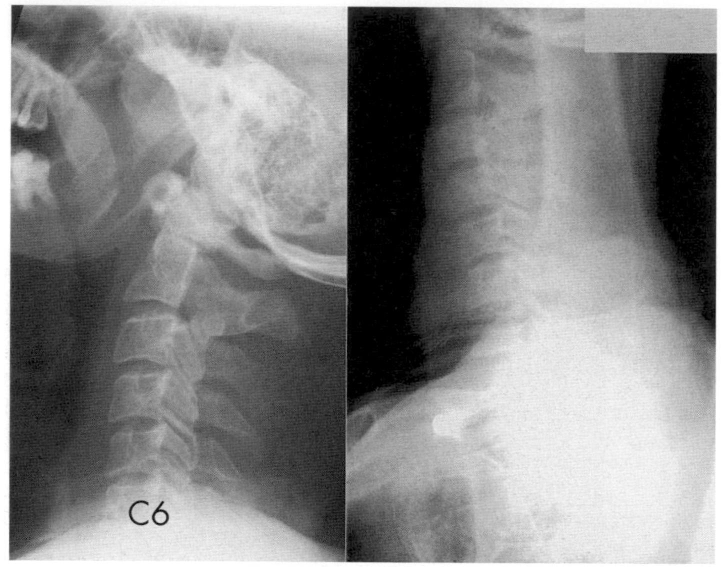

Fig. 3.2 **A** *Attempted lateral showing only down to C6.* **B** *'Swimmer's view' with slight obliquity and arm elevated in a 'Hail Caesar!' Roman salute showing down to T1 upper end-plate.*

All these views should be attainable without moving the patient as a whole.

Question: Why all this fuss about the cervicodorsal junction?

Answer: Because this is where the curve of the spine reverses and is particularly susceptible to trauma. Many injuries have been overlooked here in the past, with subsequently devastating consequences for the patient **(because somebody did not bother to count the vertebrae)**.

Anatomy

Look at Figure 3.3:

- This shows the lateral view of a normal neck.
- A normal neck in 'neutral' (i.e. relaxed) position describes a gentle forward curve convex anteriorly, which constitutes the cervical lordosis. This curve

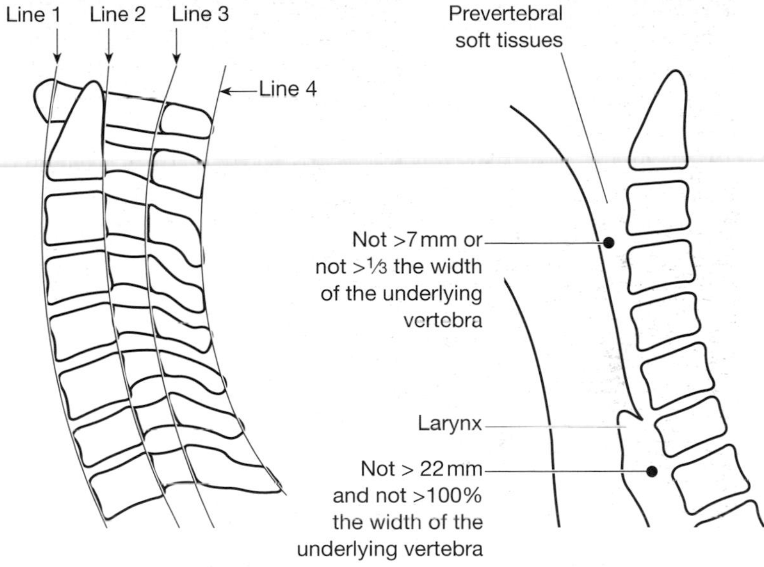

Fig. 3.3 *Lateral view of the neck showing normal alignment lines to be checked.*

may be lost or reversed in trauma due to spasm, or chronically with degenerative disease.

- Lines drawn connecting the anterior and posterior aspects of the vertebral bodies and anterior aspects of the bases of the spinous processes will run parallel to each other. Interruption of these lines is used in the assessment of traumatic displacements. Sometimes line 3 bypasses C2 by a whisker.
- The first two lines anteriorly correspond to the ligaments holding the bones together, i.e. the anterior and posterior longitudinal ligaments.
- Because of overlying mastoids and earlobes, the craniocervical junction (or occipitoatlantal joint) is not clearly discernible on the lateral view, but the gap between the anterior arch of the atlas and the odontoid process or dens is visible (Greek *odous, odontos* = tooth, Latin *dens* = tooth from its tooth-like shape). The dens is anatomically part of C2 but functions as the body of C1.

In an adult this should not exceed 3 mm. In a child it should not exceed 5 mm.

- Note how the shoulder partially opacifies the level of T1 and the area behind it on the lateral X-ray (Fig. 3.2).

NB Physiological subluxations can occur on children's X-rays, simulating dislocations, particularly of C2 on C3 and C3 on C4 on forward flexion. In such circumstances there may be steps in lines 1 and 2 but line 3 will remain intact. All three lines are out of alignment with a real subluxation.

Prevertebral soft tissues

Look at the prevertebral soft tissues in front of the spine contrasting sharply with the dark air in the pharynx and below the larynx in the trachea. Between the base of the skull and the odontoid these form a gentle anterior concave margin but may become convex here in adenoidal enlargement. They are normally convex over the anterior tubercle of the atlas, then concave immediately below it. Where these retropharyngeal and retrotracheal soft tissues normally run almost parallel to the spine, e.g. between C2 and C4 and C5 to C7, they should not exceed around 7 mm and 22 mm in width, respectively, as a rough guide.

Swelling of these tissues may occur in trauma **but an absence of such swelling does not exclude significant trauma.** Other causes for swelling include infected impacted foreign bodies, spontaneous retropharyngeal abscess, tonsillitis, osteophytes and malignant disease.

NB False swelling may appear to be present on shoot-through laterals due to pooling of blood and saliva in unconscious patients but will have a sharp anterior margin due to this fluid level or flexion of the neck in children.

Look at Figure 3.4:

- This is an AP view of the neck. Its clear segmental form is apparent with the body of each bony vertebra being separated by a radiolucent intervertebral disc, in vertical alignment. The diverging beam is angled slightly up about 15–20° to get through as many of the discs as possible but increasing obliquity will blur their margins.
- The spinous processes, some of which are often bifid (or forked), define the midline, as does the overlying air column of the trachea, which is therefore a sensitive indicator of rotation. When the trachea does *not* overlie the spinous

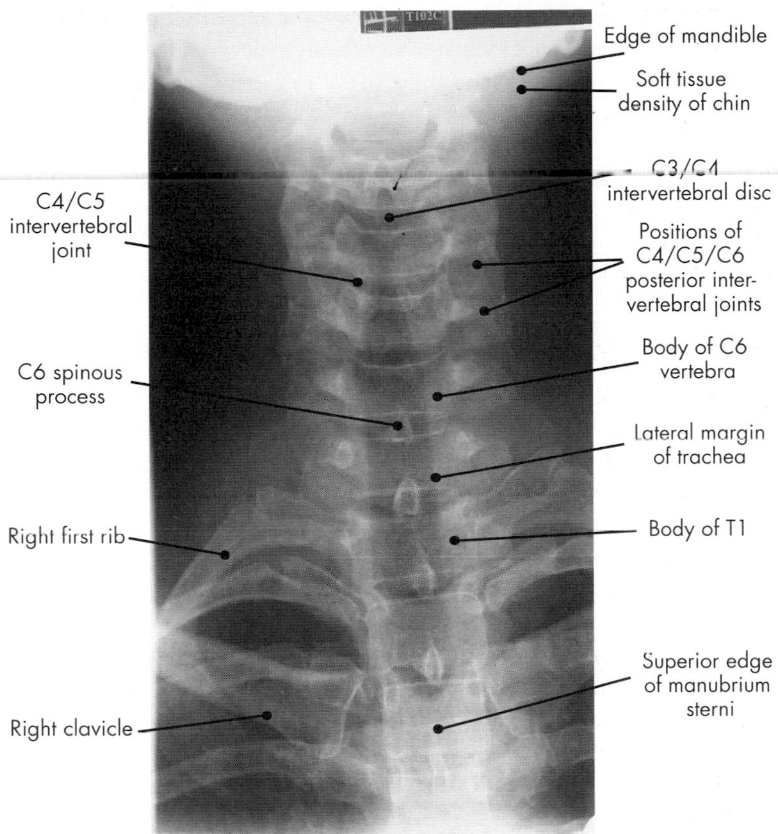

Fig. 3.4 *AP view of the neck (there is slight rotation to the right).*

processes, this may also be due to anatomical rotation, pathological displacement of the trachea or malalignment of a vertebral body (scoliosis). In older patients the lower trachea will deviate naturally to the right to negotiate an unfolded aorta.

- The Luschka joints and their uncinate processes (Latin *uncus* = hook) are usually clearly visible over several levels at and adjacent to the central X-ray beam, but become progressively distorted and less sharp due to obliquity.

Normal variants

- The joints between the lateral masses are out of alignment with the beam in this projection so do not show up. Note the steep downward directions of the posterior intervertebral joints on the lateral view (Fig. 3.1). Steep downward angulated views running parallel to these axes can be taken (i.e. 'pillar view') to demonstrate occult lateral mass fractures if required.

This illustrates a fundamental principle worth knowing: **the best view of a disc or joint space will come from a beam centred on and parallel to its axis** – and the same of course is true of a fracture line.

The atlantoaxial joint

Looking is not the same as seeing in radiology and you must learn to 'see' the anterior atlantoaxial joint space on the lateral view (Fig. 3.1) and be able to resolve it in your 'mind's eye', as Shakespeare called it. The joint space should not exceed 3 mm in an adult or 5 mm in a child. It usually increases minimally in flexion compared with extension, more so in children.

Look at Figure 3.5. This shows the frontal anatomy of the adult odontoid, which looks like a meditating Norman knight in armour with huge shoulder pads, and the appearance of the lateral atlantoaxial joints. The spinous processes look like steepled fingers resting on his sword.

Important fact: The odontoid peg is bedevilled by a number of dark bands and edges which cross over it, simulating fractures, including the top of the tongue and the dark edge along the margin of the shadow of the occiput – a so-called Mach band effect. The margins of teeth will also sometimes produce such an edge but should be fairly obvious. Apart from these, the main anatomical and artefactual edges can usually be traced well beyond either side of the odontoid.

Radiographic hint: Asking the patient to say 'Aahhh!' at the instant of filming will lower the tongue and help to remove at least one confusing edge from the odontoid.

Normal variants

Paediatric patients

An important variant is the normal synchondrosis, which is present in very young children, causing a genuine lucent (but cartilaginous) defect at the base of the odontoid. This may also be discernible on the lateral film and very rarely will

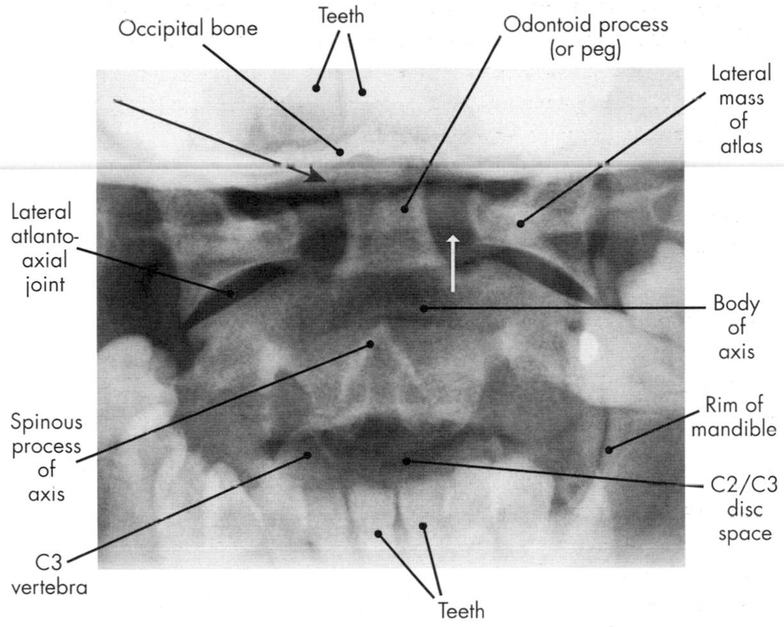

Fig. 3.5 *'Open mouth' view of the odontoid. Black arrow indicates soft tissue fold at the back of neck; white arrow indicates dorsum of tongue.*

persist as a sclerotic-margined remnant in the adult. Odontoid peg views are, of course, very difficult to obtain in infants.

Elderly patients

Degenerative changes in a sense are physiological, giving rise to disc space narrowing, sclerosis and osteophyte formation, the classic signs of osteoarthritis of the spine (cervical spondylosis). In addition, however, particles of bone can appear on the anteroinferior aspects of such vertebral bodies and anterior disc spaces and may be confused with 'teardrop' fractures (a manifestation of hyperflexion injury). These are due to incompletely fused epiphyseal ring remnants. In addition, severe hypertrophic degenerative disease in the posterior intervertebral joints can cause one vertebra to move gradually forward relative to another, producing a *subluxation of degenerative origin* (Fig. 3.6), which may be impossible to prove as non-acute unless there are previous films.

Breaking your neck

This sounds dramatic – and it is, although technically speaking both a small chip fracture and a complete fracture dislocation constitute a 'broken neck', a

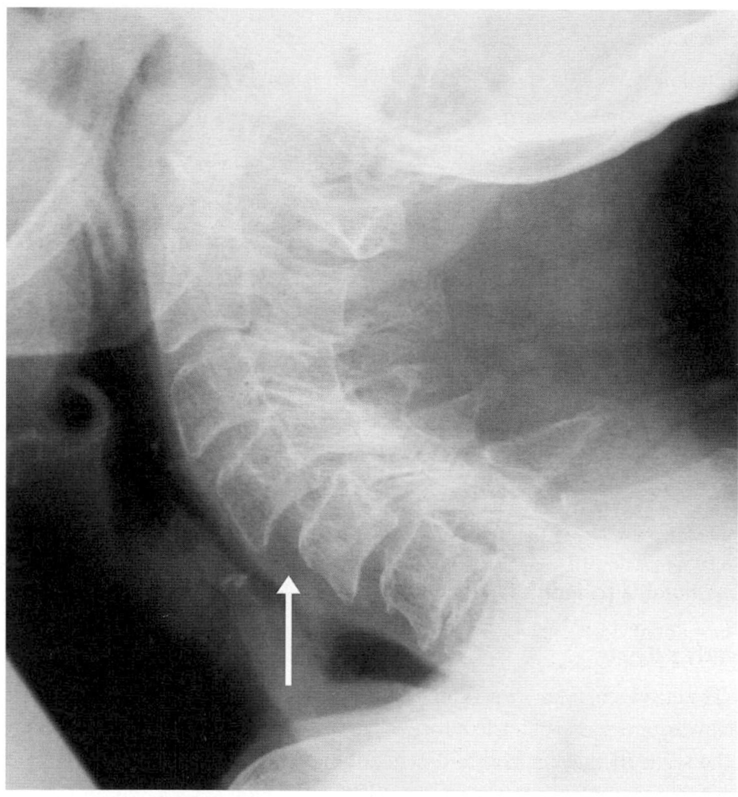

Fig. 3.6 *Degenerative subluxations of C4 on C5 (arrow) and C5 on C6. Note the posterior disk space narrowing and posterior intervertebral joint sclerosis due to osteoarthritis. There was no history of trauma.*

distinction often lost on some newspapers. Active lives can, however, be over in an instant, sometimes due to thoughtlessness, like letting your tractor roll over, or driving too fast on an icy road, which delivers your spinning car into a tree. All your tomorrows pass down through that narrow space that is the cervical spinal canal, so just bear it in mind the next time you decide to go skydiving, and jump out of a fully serviceable aeroplane.

With regard to neck injuries, there are four basic mechanisms:

- flexion
- extension
- rotation
- compression

but combinations of these will often contribute to the injury.

Flexion injuries

Flexion injuries are the commonest type of trauma to affect the neck, particularly at its lower end, and the most frequent components of these include:

- Simple wedge fractures.
- Posterior ligamentous tears.
- Facet joint dislocations.
- Combined fracture/dislocations of vertebral bodies.

However, look at Figure 3.7.

A memorable patient: a flexion dislocation of the head

This patient lost control of his vehicle at high speed. Note the massive prevertebral swelling.

The head can dislocate completely backwards or forwards given sufficient extension or flexion forces at the occipitoatlantal joint. Many of these patients die at the scene. If they survive, the injury is unstable, but with modern intensive care techniques some of them do survive.

Simple wedge fractures

These are due to downward compression of the superior end-plate of a vertebra at its anterior aspect, giving this injury its 'wedge' shape and its name. It may be

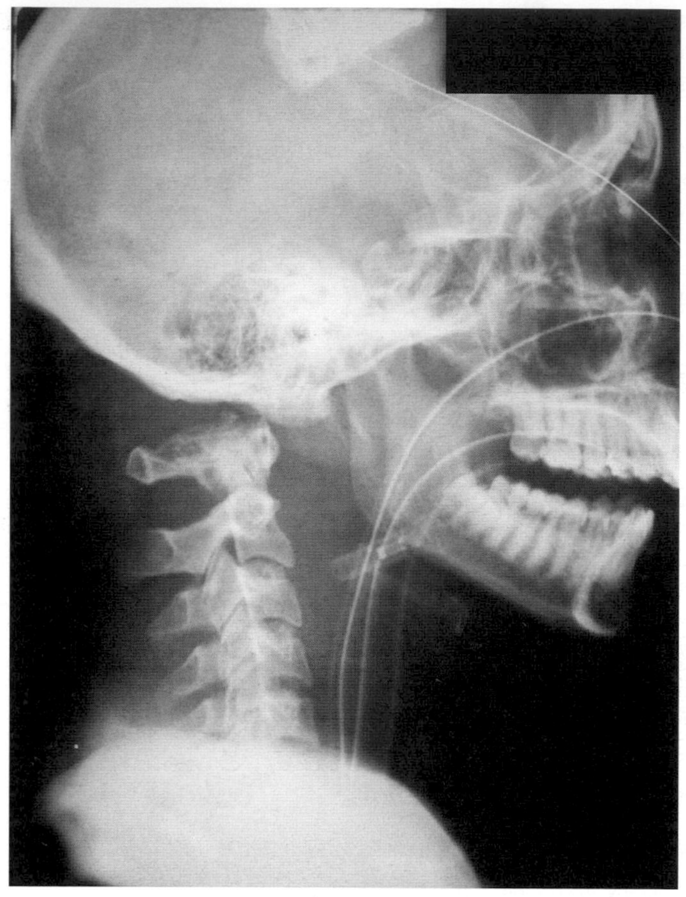

Fig. 3.7 *A dislocation of the head. The odontoid is now behind the mastoid process instead of adjacent to it. Just about as bad as it gets.*

associated with buckling of the upper anterior wall cortex creating a small step (look at Figure 3.8, p. 74).

NB The inferior end-plate and posterior vertebral body cortex are intact. If the degree of compression is less than 25%, the traumatic force applied is unlikely to have been sufficiently severe for ligamentous rupture to occur and the supraspinous ligament will hold, rendering this injury stable. Beyond 25% of **compression, ligamentous rupture and instability should be assumed.**

Important normal variant Some cervical vertebrae are already anatomically wedge-shaped. Look for prevertebral swelling and cortical breaks as further evidence of suspect trauma.

A nasty dose of reality

Look at Figure 3.9A. This is the film of a patient whose car ran into the back of a stationary vehicle. This shows a 'normal' neck with no fractures and good alignment. Unfortunately, if you count the number of vertebrae there are only **six**. A second lateral X-ray was then performed with arm traction. Look now at Figure 3.9B. This now shows **seven** vertebrae with a burst fracture of C7.

Moral: In practice, the aim must be to ensure that all the relevant anatomy is demonstrated radiographically, from C1 to the top of T1. Horrendous fracture/dislocations have been missed here in the past, with permanent damage to the cord when patients with inadequate films were discharged and started to move their necks. With CT and MRI available there is no longer any excuse for failing to achieve an adequate demonstration of the neck. Not for nothing has this area been called 'the A & E doctor's graveyard!', although it's actually the patient who may end up in the graveyard, not the doctor!

Ligamentous ruptures

In some patients sudden severe flexion will tear the interspinous and supraspinous ligaments, rendering the neck unstable. The neck may look normal in the neutral position. Any flexion allowed at this point would, however, cause the spinous processes to separate from each other ('fanning') and may lead to permanent cord damage. In the longer term, if the ligaments do not heal, this can lead to delayed instability.

Facet joint dislocations

Bilateral unstable 'jumped facets' An element of rotation associated with a flexion injury can cause the facet joint capsules to rupture and the facet joints to sublux or dislocate. These are unstable. Look at Figure 3.10. Note:

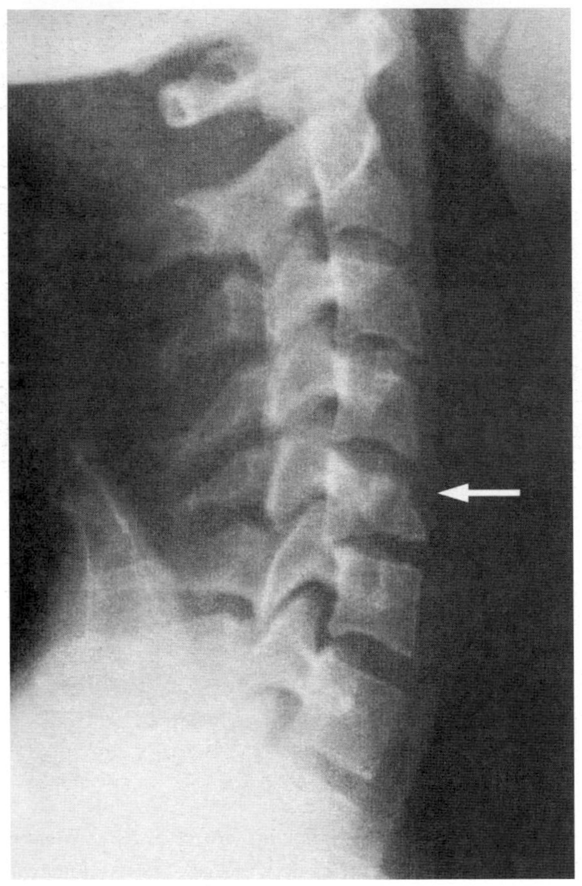

Fig. 3.8 *Wedge fracture of C5.*

- The considerable anterior positioning of C5 upon C6, with interruption of the anterior and posterior longitudinal lines. (The apparent forward positioning is exacerbated by the big osteophyte on C5.)
- The anterior positioning of the C5 facets relative to C6 – the arrow points to the position where they should be articulating with the C6 facets behind.

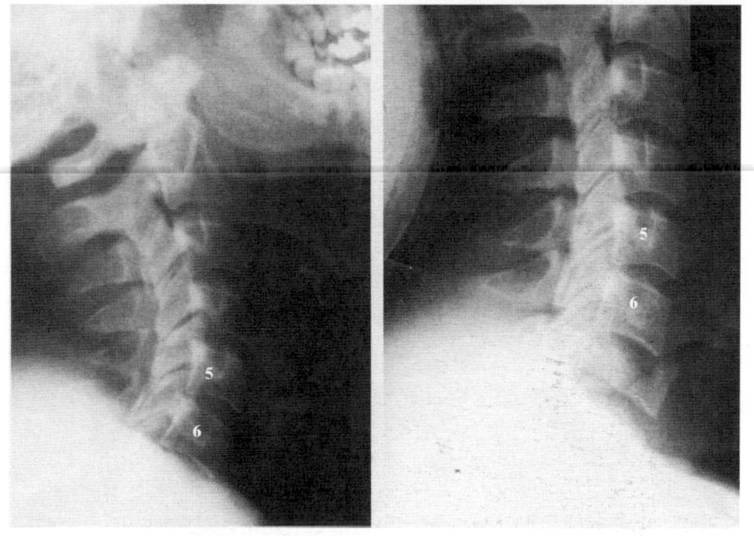

Fig. 3.9 ***A*** *Lateral view of neck showing only down to C6.* ***B*** *Same patient with arm traction revealing down to C7 where there is a burst fracture.*

- This is a *bilateral facet joint dislocation*. All the ligaments of the spine are ruptured in this condition and there is a high risk of cord injury.

NB If both facets have completely 'jumped' there will be no rotational element but up to a 50% or more anterior over-riding.

The appearance of facet joints on lateral films is a source of endless angst and difficulty, usually due to anatomical variations, slight degrees of flexion and obliquity, and occasional reversal of the cervical lordosis which makes facets 'ride up' on the ones beneath them. If, however, there is ongoing concern about facet joint injuries, 45° oblique films can be used to confirm or exclude the normal relationships.

Unilateral facet dislocation (stable) (Figs 3.11, 3.12) This is a more subtle injury than the bilateral version but, again, it will not usually occur without some visible forward movement of the affected vertebra on the one below. Such movement

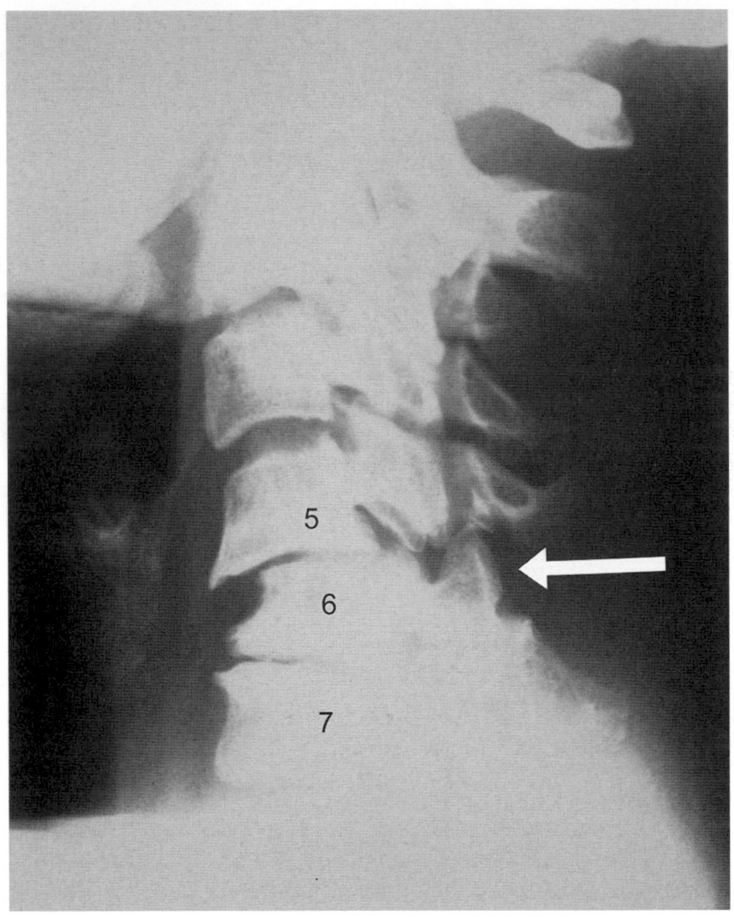

Fig. 3.10 *A C5/C6 dislocation with jumped facets (arrow). The patient hit a brick wall on his motorcycle. These are unstable with up to 50% over-ride.*

can, however, be minimal or masked by obliquity, and difficult to appreciate (but not >25%). If only one facet has 'jumped', the affected vertebra should also show:

- Some rotation of its spinous process to the opposite side on the AP view.
- Increased clarity of the affected lateral mass posterior to the intervertebral joint due to altered positioning.

Imagine a ship coming straight at you – it then turns to starboard (the ship's right, your left). The prow then moves off to your left and the stern begins to stick out to the right. Similarly, the spinous processes will come out of alignment in a unilateral facet dislocation and move to the dislocated side.

Perched facets (the 'in-betweenies') An in-between condition can occur, between normality and established dislocation, when the facet joints become 'perched' upon each other with point to point contact.

NB Although associated with degrees of displacement and occasional root symptoms, facet dislocations are not usually associated with neurological deficits and are treatable by traction and manipulative reduction.

Fracture dislocations

When flexion violence is sufficiently severe to cause a fracture and dislocation, cord compromise with quadriplegia is likely. The initial films will give likely warning of the severity of the injury and cord damage will be both clinically apparent and anatomically demonstrable by MRI.

Odontoid peg fractures

These are usually divided into three types (Fig. 3.13):

1. Through the upper peg – stable.
2. Through the base of the peg – unstable.
3. Through the base of the peg and into the body of the axis – stable.

These fractures are very painful and the patient may think his head is 'going to fall off'. Unfortunately it is easy to miss them, or misdiagnose their presence when absent. The radiographer will assist you by taking an open-mouthed AP view if possible – the problem is one of interpretation.

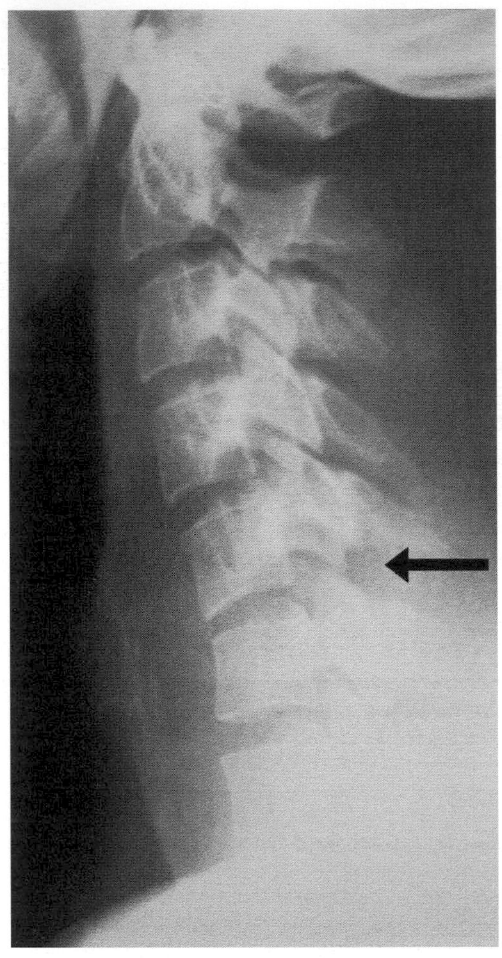

Fig. 3.11 *Unilateral facet dislocation. Sudden forced flexion of the neck in a rugby scrum. Note the prevertebral swelling. This is stable.*

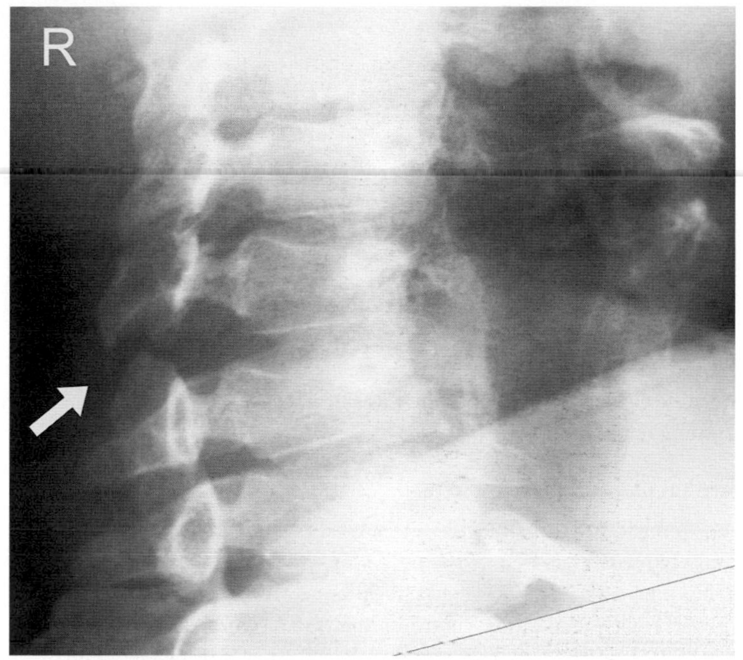

Fig. 3.12 *Oblique view of same patient as in Fig. 3.11, showing the dislocated C5/6 facet. This is stable.*

Important mnemonic: Scarlet and Black!

There are many red herrings that can cause black lines to cross the odontoid and simulate a fracture, such dark bands often accompanying the white edges of bony structures, known as the *Mach effect*, which has already been demonstrated (Fig. 3.5).

NB Whilst mainly a flexion injury, which causes the top of the peg to move forwards, an extension injury as here (Fig. 3.14) may cause it to go posteriorly.

An interesting congenital abnormality

Look at Figure 3.15. The tip of the odontoid is separate from its lower part. This is a congenital non-fusion of the odontoid (Os odontoideum), with no history of

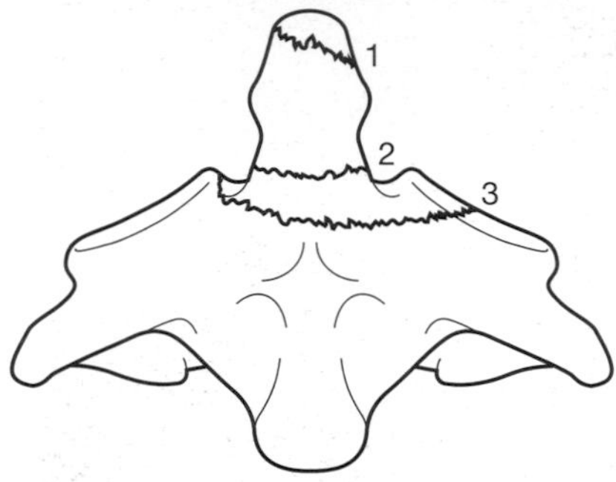

Fig. 3.13 *Odontoid peg fractures (see text).*

trauma. Real fractures can look like this but note the smooth sclerotic margins, indicating that it is not acute.

Clay shoveller's fracture (Fig. 3.16, p. 83)

This is a fracture of a spinous process caused by sudden severe flexion stress or a direct blow. The AP view of the neck may show what looks like two adjacent spinous processes – 'the ghost sign'. Its differential diagnosis includes non-fusion of an accessory ossification centre at the spinous process (so the history is important) or normal variant anatomical calcification in the ligamentum nuchae. Its name is supposed to have arisen from clay miners in Australia, and a high incidence of it was recorded in Germany during the construction of the autobahns – using shovels without crossbars.

'Teardrop' fracture (flexion injury of lower cervical spine) (Fig. 3.17B)

Despite its quaint name, **this is the most vicious and unstable injury to the cervical spine,** as 'everything goes': all the ligaments rupture and there will often be one or more fractures in the anterior and posterior parts of the affected vertebra, leading to paraplegia.

Some patients may suffer an incomplete *anterior cord syndrome*: loss of pain and temperature sense due to involvement of the spinothalamic tracts, but preservation of proprioception due to sparing of the dorsal columns.

Time to revisit some anatomy: two important lookalikes

- A normal cervical vertebra will often have a small corticated chin reminiscent of the little goatee beard of King Charles I of England (Fig. 3.17A). The

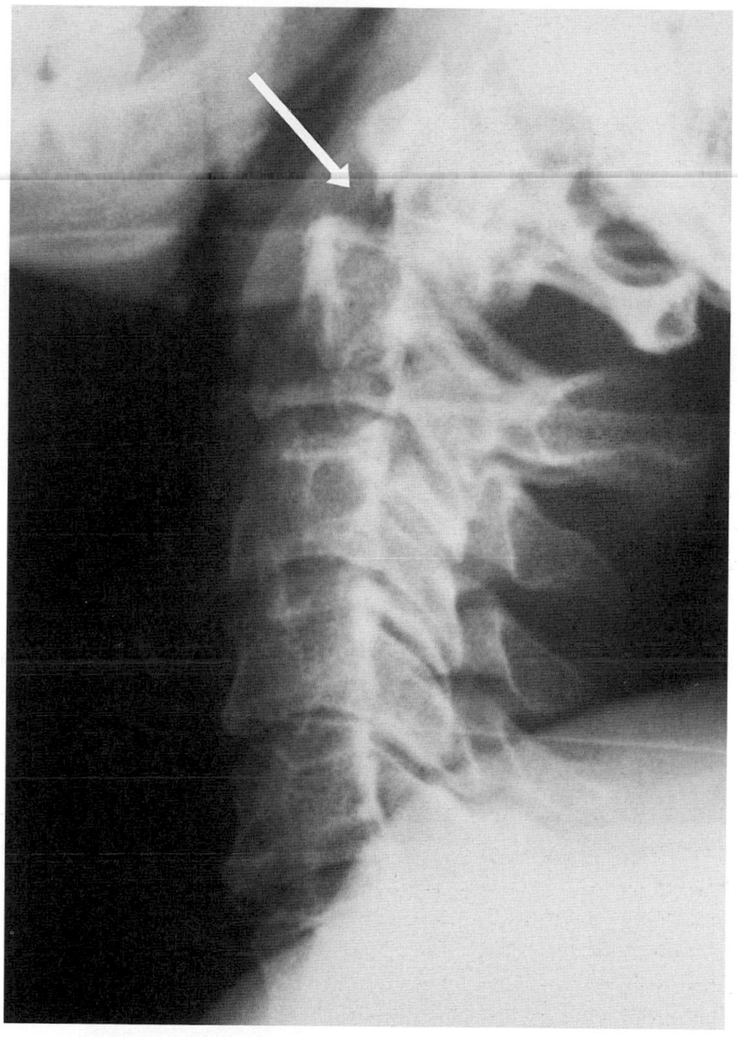

Fig. 3.14 *Fractured odontoid with backward displacement (the arrow points to where the odontoid should be).*

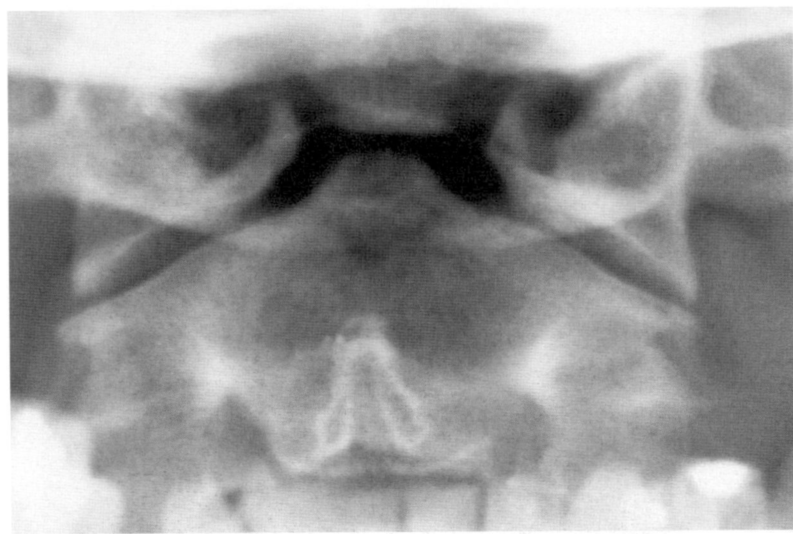

A

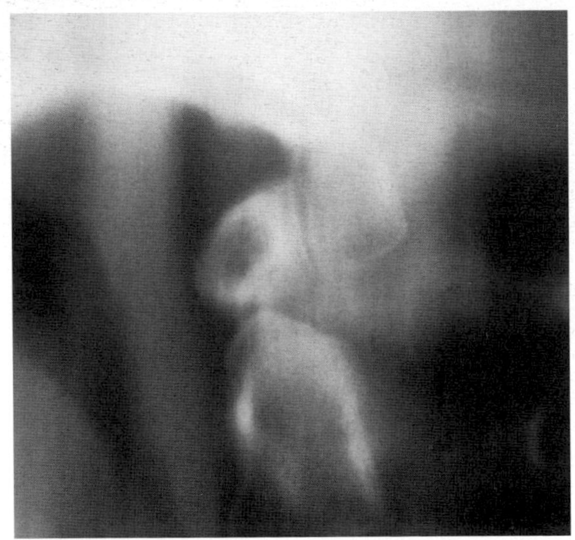

B

Fig. 3.15 *Congenital non-fusion of the odontoid.* ***A*** *AP;* ***B*** *lateral tomogram – a vertical 'slice' through the atlantoaxial joint area.*

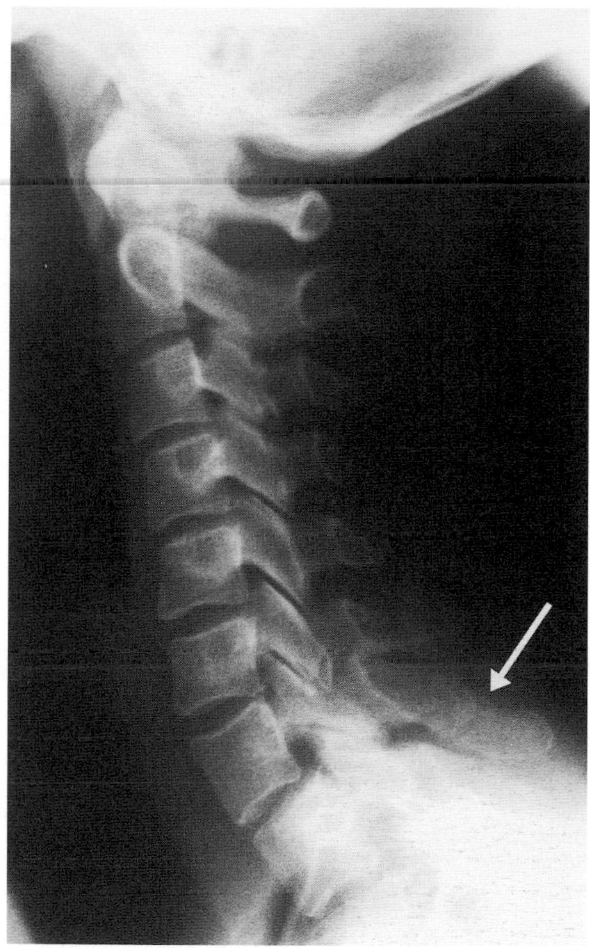

Fig. 3.16 *Clay shoveller's fracture.*

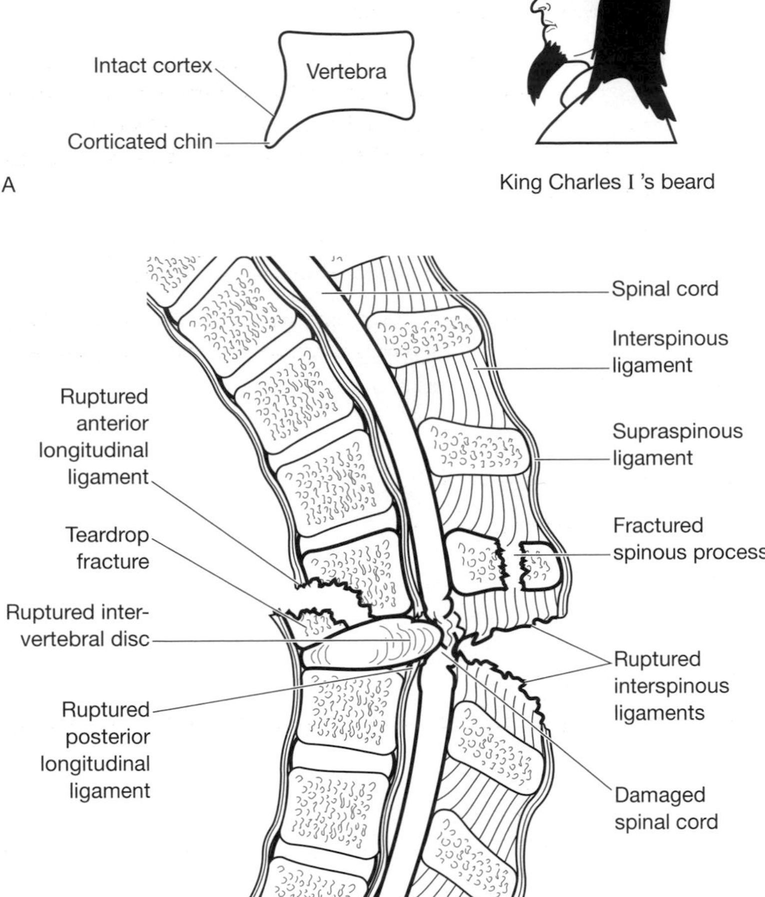

Fig. 3.17 ***A*** *Vertebra with 'corticated chin'.* ***B*** *Flexion teardrop fracture and associated injuries.*

anomaly (Fig. 3.17a) becomes more prominent with age, and sometimes undergoes osteophytic enlargement in osteoarthritis. Little detached bony fragments also often present in front of the disc spaces as a result of incompletely fused epiphyseal remnants.

- When looking for a teardrop fracture (Fig. 3.17B), check for an incompletely corticated chin and corresponding defect on the adjacent vertebral body. A further fracture and variable backward dislocation of the vertebra above will also be present with interruption of the 'spinal lines', depending on the severity of the injury.

Extension injuries

These are commonest in the upper cervical spine and usually less devastating than flexion injuries, but they can still be very serious and will occasionally lead to death. They include:

- Odontoid fracture.
- Fracture of the posterior arch of C1.
- Hyperextension fracture dislocation.
- Hangman's fracture.
- Extension teardrop fracture.

Odontoid fractures (as above).

If due to flexion, the peg may go forwards. If due to extension, the peg may go back.

Fracture of the posterior arch of C1

Careful inspection of this difficult area may show a fracture line or cortical discontinuity. This injury is stable.

Important normal variant Sometimes there are congenital defects in the posterior arch of the atlas. See also the Jefferson fracture (pp 88, 90).

Hyperextension fracture dislocation

Sufficient hyperextension trauma can cause a severe fracture dislocation with backward displacement of the superior components. If it has occurred, it should be apparent on the initial film taken on the patient's arrival.

Two special cases

- *Prolapsed intervertebral disc.* Sometimes when a fracture is found the clinical signs may be out of proportion to the visible radiographic abnormality. An MRI scan may then show that a *simultaneous disc protrusion* has occurred which has severely damaged the cord.
- *The geriatric neck.* Because an elderly patient's rigid neck will inevitably harbour extensive degenerative changes, consisting of osteophytic lipping and ligamentous thickening, an abrupt extension injury can wrinkle the posterior longitudinal ligament (attached to the posterior aspect of the vertebral body) and compress the anterior spinal artery, leading to cord damage. This causes the *anterior spinal artery syndrome*, which will weaken the arms but spare the legs.

The hangman's fracture (fracture dislocation of C2 on C3) (Fig. 3.18)

It is relevant for the A & E doctor to understand the distinction between 'hanging' causing death by protracted strangulation, a ghastly fate suffered by countless thousands over the ages, and even those today who commit suicide, and the judicial execution called 'hanging' due to a drop, which, if carried out 'efficiently', would lead to virtually instantaneous death. Emergency cases will still sometimes present at A & E half-strangled, having just been found and cut down in time. These patients may have suffered a fractured larynx, damaged trachea, etc., and may exhibit extensive surgical emphysema.

Traditionally the hangman would visit the condemned man before the execution to obtain the height, weight and assess the thickness of the neck. A specific drop could then be calculated from tables, plus any further nuances and adjustments based on past experience. At the end of the drop, the knot placed under the left side of the mandible on top of the hood would throw the head back, distract the neck and inflict the fatal injury. With too much or too little drop, a 'hanging' could cause decapitation or strangulation.

What is today called a *hangman's fracture* or *traumatic spondylolisthesis* is a fracture through the pars interarticularis of C2. This may present as an isolated crack (type I) or continue down into the intervertebral disc (type II) and in severe cases go on to a complete fracture dislocation (type III). Needless to say, these days it is usually caused by a road traffic accident in which the head strikes the

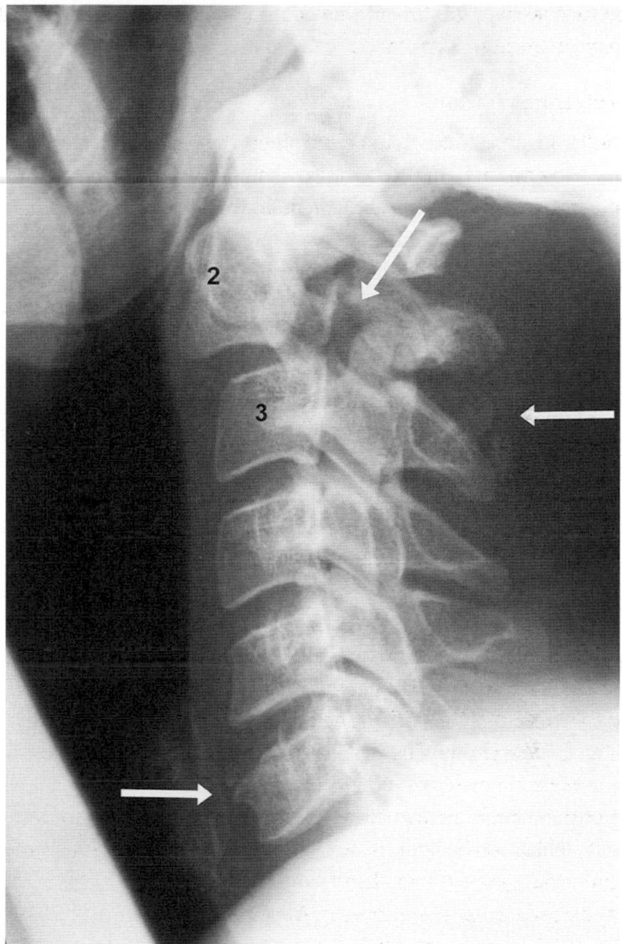

Fig. 3.18 *Hangman's fracture. Note the crack in the posterior lamina and forward dislocation of C2 on C3 (top arrow). Note also the gap between the spinous processes of C2 and C3 ('fanning', middle arrow) and also the previous trauma to C6 (bottom arrow).*

windscreen, so perhaps it is time it was called a 'windscreen fracture'. This injury is unstable.

Extension teardrop fracture

This is similar in appearance to its 'big brother' the flexion teardrop fracture, but much less serious. It is due to an extension injury with avulsion of a small fragment or fragments of bone, but there is no subluxation and this injury is stable. It usually occurs around C2 or C3 and there is likely to be prevertebral swelling of more than 7 mm with this injury.

The atlantoaxial joint

On the lateral view of the neck the anterior arch of the atlas normally sits 2–3 mm in front of the odontoid peg, forming the anterior atlantoaxial joint space. Following trauma, the surrounding ligaments may rupture, leading to atlanto-axial subluxation, i.e. a gap forming here of more than 3 mm in an adult and more than 5 mm in a young child (a child's neck normally being more mobile).

NB The atlantoaxial joint may also destabilize laterally, although such lateral displacements can be simulated by lateral head flexion and obliquity of positioning, but when positional there will be no offset (see below).

Important point: Many pre-existing diseases may lead to atlantoaxial subluxation, the most important of which is rheumatoid arthritis. Often the films look normal in the neutral position but a subluxation is unmasked by forward flexion (Fig. 3.19), and rarely by extension or lateral flexion. The most important application of this knowledge (other than when sitting examinations) lies in the checking of rheumatoid necks before excessive hyperextension for intubation in anaesthesia, which can be fatal.

Compression injuries

It does not take too much imagination to realize what may happen if a patient falls from a height on to the top of his head or a concrete block falls and hits it. Exactly the right spot needs to be struck to transmit a truly vertical force and most impacts will cause sudden severe flexion or extension to occur. Such vertical forces may, however, break and disturb the ring of the atlas, causing a *Jefferson fracture* (Fig. 3.20). This is identified by inferolateral displacement of both lateral components beyond the articular margins of the axis on the AP view of the upper neck. This plain film finding is known as a *bilateral offset*. If identified, or even suspected, further evaluation by CT is warranted. Alternatively, a 'burst fracture' of a vertebral body may occur at a lower level, causing comminution (i.e. shattering). A CT scan will demonstrate any spicules of bone extending into the spinal canal (Fig. 5.4, p. 112).

Hard to spot, but requiring a high index of suspicion too, is a fracture of the occipital condyles, so do not switch off that CT machine just yet.

Question: Is it true a patient with a congenital defect in the posterior arch of C1 can have a bilateral offset without trauma?

Answer: Yes.

Rotational injuries

The more one understands about neck injuries, the more it becomes apparent that multiple forces are at work necessitating extending the concept of injury

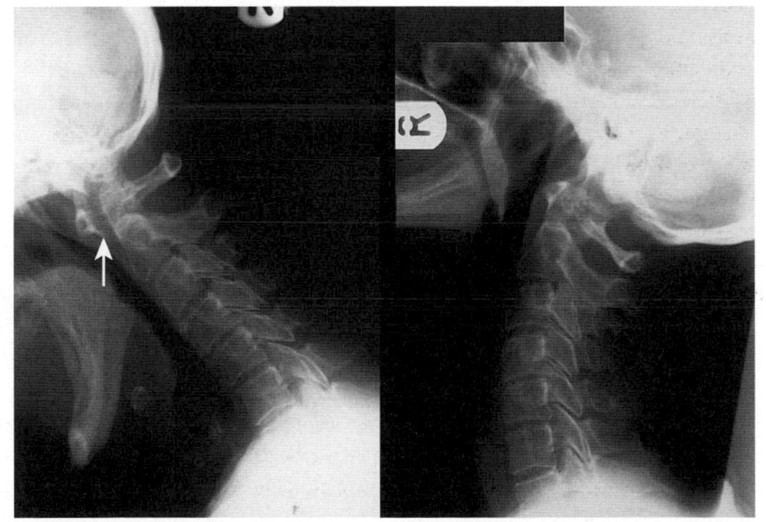

Fig. 3.19 ***A*** *Flexion and* ***B*** *extension views of neck showing atlantoaxial subluxation (arrow) on full forward flexion and reduction in full extension.*

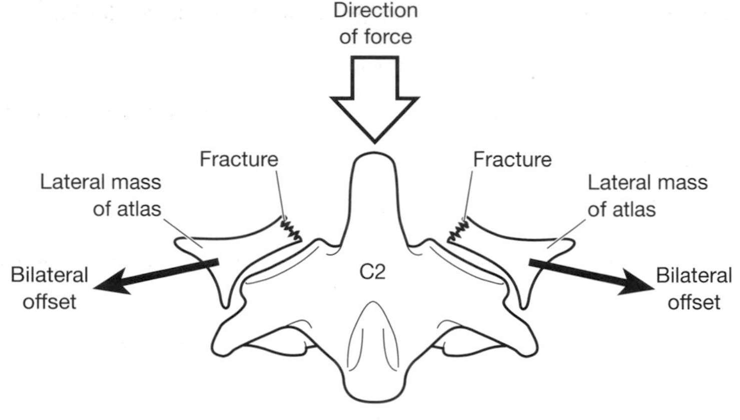

Fig. 3.20 *A Jefferson fracture.*

from simple flexion and extension events. Rotational forces contribute to dislocations at the craniocervical junction, 'rotary dislocations' at C1/C2 and unilateral facet joint dislocations at a lower level. Even more complex shearing and distraction forces may cause lateral mass and transverse process fractures, as well as disc space narrowing or even widening with hyperextension. Confirmation of the esoteric signs of such findings is a job for the radiographer to demonstrate, radiologist to interpret and the orthopaedic or neurosurgeons to treat.

Whiplash injury

This is a combined flexion/extension injury caused at the moment of a collision ahead or shunt from behind, the second movement being a recoil from the first. The headrests in modern vehicles are designed to cushion the extension impact but in older vehicles only the chin on the chest limits forward movement, but now hopefully our quick-acting airbags will inflate spontaneously in our faces.

The severity or speed of the impact will determine whether or not ligamentous or neurological damage is sustained.

Summary of normal variants that may cause diagnostic confusion

- Congenital non-fusion of the odontoid.
- Dark bands from overlying bony and soft tissue structures (tongue, tonsils).
- Congenital defects in the arch of the atlas.
- Block vertebrae with failure of segmentation.
- Small developmentally detached fragments of bone at the lower anterior margin of a vertebral body (limbus vertebra).
- Persistent developmental wedge-shape of a vertebra (most vertebrae from C3 to C7 look the same).
- Increased mobility of the neck in children, causing 'pseudosubluxations'.
- Extensive gaps between spinous processes simulating 'fanning'. Interpret this apparent finding with caution and compare against any previous films.
- Ring apophyses causing bony spicules on developing vertebral bodies (children).
- Sagittal chunks of calcification in the ligamentum nuchae.
- Accessory ossification centres at spinous processes (simulating clay shoveller's fractures).
- Normal upward riding of facet joints on forward flexion and reversal of normal lordosis in, for example, 'the military position' (chin on chest).
- Wide prevertebral soft tissues in children (see p. 190).

Check Keats & Anderson (2001) for more examples.

Non-traumatic neck pain

Patients will frequently arrive in A & E with a sore neck. The vast majority will have degenerative osteoarthritis. A few will have rheumatoid arthritis and a very few will be presenting with a metastasis. Think also about retropharyngeal infection, plus very rarely a cord tumour.

Some general principles in dealing with necks

- Maintain a high index of suspicion for neck trauma in all patients but particularly in those with head and facial injuries.
- Try and establish the mechanism of injury from the patient, relatives, police or paramedics.
- Consider every injured neck unstable until proved otherwise.
- Do a thorough neurological examination.
- Get senior help early with severe neck injuries – if such patients have not already been commandeered as departmental policy.
- Ensure a thorough X-ray examination is done, or the optimum possible.
- Remember to move rapidly to CT/MRI if conventional films do not give the answer. Plain films have their limitations.
- Remember the false fullness of prevertebral tissues in children due to expiration, flexion, crying and swallowing.
- In every injury think: **What has happened to the ligaments?**
- Always look for more than one injury: 8% of patients will have another one.
- Forget Kia-Ora, the drink, and think about SCIWORA (Spinal Cord Injury Without Radiographic Abnormality). In this entity you can have a severe neurological injury with a normal X-ray. The patient's best chance then lies with you (1) doing a thorough neurological examination, and (2) having the nous to treat the patient not the X-ray.
- Remember the concept of delayed instability – early spasm and pain can mask it. Do flexion/extension views at 14 days if the patient is still in pain, if not contraindicated, and **make sure the patient stays in a collar in the meantime.**

Summary of approach to radiographic analysis of trauma neck X-rays

- Confirm the patient's name, date of birth and date of X-ray prior to any assessment of each film. Do not forget to ask the $64 000 question: **Who's neck is it anyway?** It's too easy in the excitement of a major incident to overlook this. Remember you may have six neck injuries in A & E simultaneously after a train crash – and three 'unknowns'.
- Check the radiographic quality and confirm you have lateral views from C1 to the top of the T1 vertebra. If not, the radiographer will already have attempted a swimmer's view or trauma obliques. Getting down to C7/T1 may show up 90% of relevant injuries if other circumstances are favourable.
- Check left and right.
- Consider the need for CT/MRI .
- In the light of the known or likely mechanism of injury, check for any immediately apparent gross abnormality – some will hit you right between the eyes – e.g. a complete 2 cm anterior separation of C3 upon C4, which will be obvious.
- If there is no immediately obvious abnormality, carry out a systematic analysis of the films, but do it afterwards anyway, and do not stop looking just because you have found one abnormality.
- Check the four main 'magic lines' for smooth continuity or steps (Fig. 3.3).
- Check the prevertebral soft tissues for swelling.
- Check for evidence of preceding disease, especially severe rheumatoid arthritis or osteoarthritis. These may be associated with degenerative or rheumatoid subluxations and separate bony particles anterior to the spine (to be distinguished from teardrop fractures and narrowing of the disks).
- Check the atlantoaxial joints for widening on the lateral views and asymmetry on the AP view.
- Check the atlantoaxial joints for bilateral offset, indicating Jefferson fractures.
- Check the odontoid and follow all the dark lines crossing it to make sure that they go all the way beyond it before diagnosing a fracture.

- Look through the bones and do not just give up because the anatomy looks complex.
- Put a bright light on the dark areas if necessary (e.g. spinous processes), or make optimum use of image manipulation at your workstation.
- If there is bony overlap of vertebral bodies assess its degree and look for facet dislocation or locking. Up to 25% = unilateral; >50% = bilateral. Bony overlap of >3.5 mm with a fracture indicates instability.
- Look for 'fanning' of the spinous processes: suspect it if more than 12 mm separation is visible, which may indicate instability, but remember that even wider separation can be a normal variant. Check against previous films and remember flexion will accentuate it. >10% of angulation between vertebrae = instability.
- Check the AP film for malalignment of the spinous processes. They should be in line and equidistant.
- Check for disc narrowing and widening or air in the discs (distraction/chronic degeneration).
- Look around and through the films at the skull base and cranial cavity (lateral and AP) and do not miss something gross like a dislocation of the head. (p. 72).
- Ask yourself again: **Do I need more views now? Do I need CT/MRI urgently? Should I contact the neuro- or orthopaedic surgeons?**

Chapter 4

The thoracic spine

Background

The guidelines here rest on a history of trauma and the presence or absence of pain or neurological deficit. If the patient is alert and without pain, no films are required. If there is pain, the painful area should be X-rayed plus or minus CT/MRI. If there is pain and neurological deficit, CT/MRI are definitely required.

- Sufficient violence can always disrupt any part of the human frame, for example the avalanche of disintegrating metal that constitutes an air crash. Of those who survive their trauma, however, the spectrum of injuries in the thoracic spine is different from elsewhere, mainly due to its relatively narrow spinal canal and reduced mobility.
- As with the neck, flexion, extension, compression and shearing forces can be applied, occasionally in isolation but usually in combination. Specific differences are, however, notable; for example, for a given force, facet joint dislocations are less likely to occur.
- If the violence is sufficient to disrupt these joints it will usually be sufficiently disruptive to inflict severe damage on the bones, the displacement of which, or fracture fragments from which, will be sufficient to traumatize the cord and render the patient paraplegic. **Identifiable trauma to the thoracic spine therefore tends to be obvious and serious.** Falls, road traffic accidents, plunging masonry, etc. all take their toll but the thoracic spine is also a huge source of human misery from spontaneous excruciating fractures due to osteoporosis in the elderly and destructive metastatic disease.

Gold medal point: Osteoporosis may be the only manifestation of *multiple myeloma*.

Radiography

Standard films are the AP and lateral views, which sound straightforward enough. Unfortunately, the thoracic spine is a long curved structure and, because each X-ray exposure consists of a diverging beam, often only the central and adjacent rays will give an undistorted image (Fig. 4.1).

Important point: Usually this does not matter, e.g. with a long bone like the femur, but with a structure like the thoracic spine, built up like a pile of small

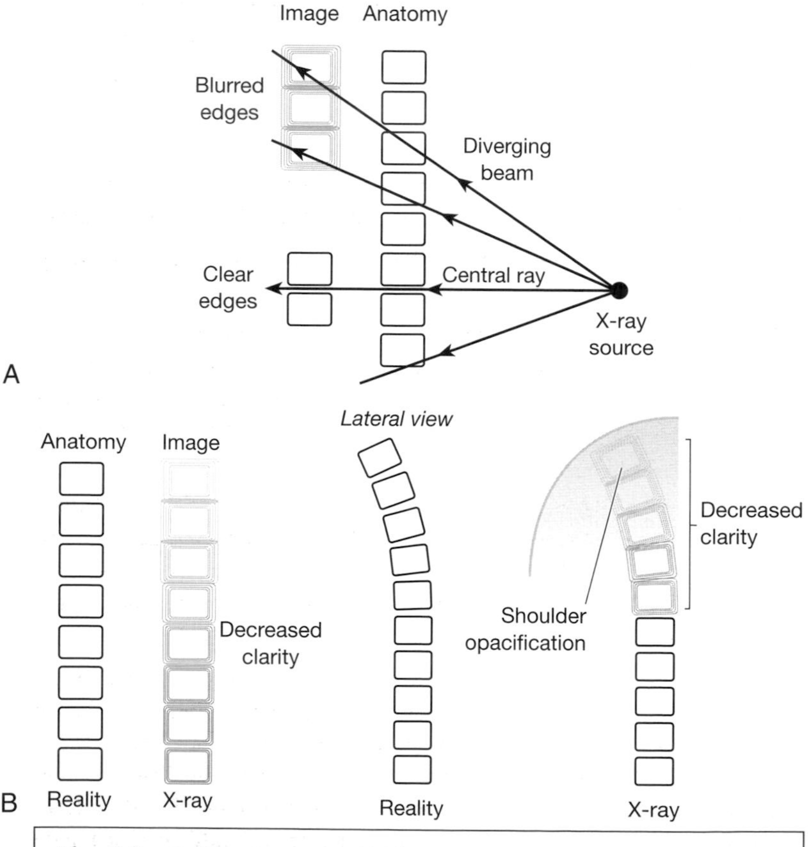

Fig. 4.1 ***A** Diverging beam. **B** AP view.*

bricks each with each edge parallel to the other, it can be important. Sometimes the effects of distortion on a lateral view can simulate pathology, due to a lack of clarity of the end-plates superiorly or inferiorly, depending on the precise position of the centring point. Erroneous diagnoses of vertebral body collapses and even metastatic disease have frequently been made in the past.

On the AP film, however, the thoracic kyphosis can compensate for the diverging beam to some degree but, again for example with a low centring point, ultimately the upper end-plates may tend to look blurred (Fig. 4.2).

NB As with the neck, the shoulders usually obscure the uppermost thoracic vertebrae on the lateral projections, making this a blind spot. Obliques (or swimmer's) views, and if indicated CT or MRI scanning, may be required to elucidate this area.

Some important anatomy (Fig. 4.3)

- Look in particular at the *paraspinal line* where the pleural surface is reflected off the spine (horizontal arrows). This normally runs parallel to the spinal column.
- Another paraspinal line may on occasion be visible on the right but is usually less obvious here.
- **NB** The left paraspinal line needs to be consciously identified and distinguished from the lateral margin of the descending thoracic aorta (oblique arrows), which will start further out and approach the spine at an oblique angle (especially in the elderly where the aorta may be very ectatic and incredibly tortuous).
- In obese individuals, the paraspinal lines will tend to stand off more laterally, but remain parallel to the spine, if normal. When abnormal, a paraspinal line is convex laterally, and in serious pathology biconvex paraspinal masses may frequently be visible. These take a characteristic spindle shape around the relevant abnormality (Fig. 4.4).

Crucial fact: Displaced paraspinal lines are a sensitive index of spinal pathology and are among the most crucial radiological signs in trauma, indeed in clinical medicine. They will usually represent a haematoma following injury with a spinal fracture, or an expanding metastasis in malignant disease. They are often just on the edge of visibility on pale chest films or even completely hidden from you, and this is why it is so crucial that **all chest X-rays should be of adequate penetration** (p. 200).

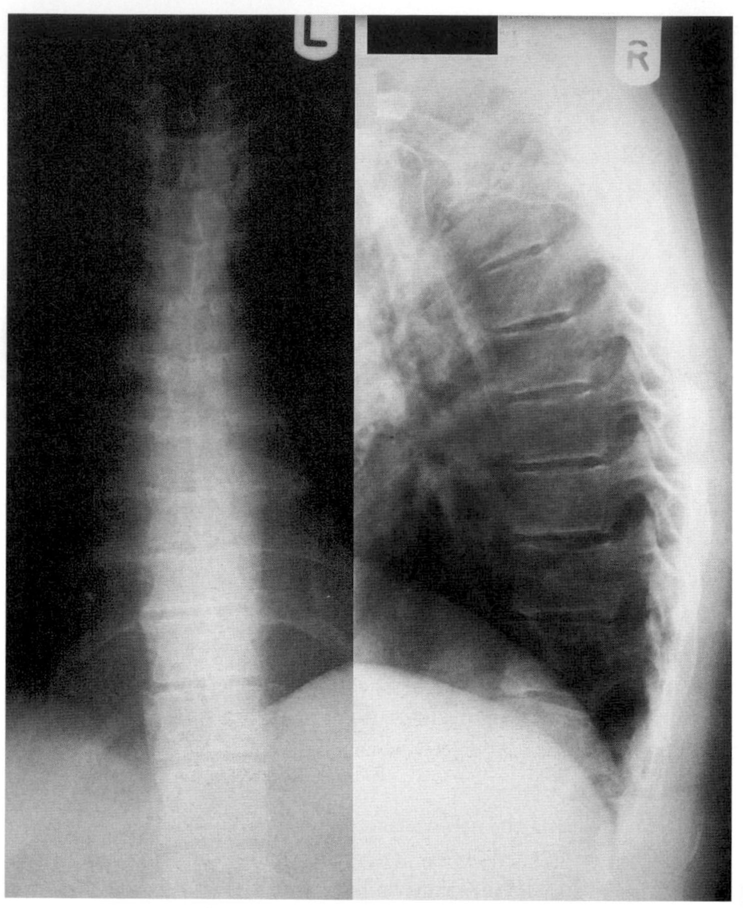

Fig. 4.2 ***A** AP and **B** lateral views of the normal thoracic spine.*

Definition: A well-penetrated chest X-ray is one where you can see the lower thoracic intervertebral disc spaces without undue effort.

And finally: watch out for osteophytes. These can also displace the paraspinal lines, but are totally benign.

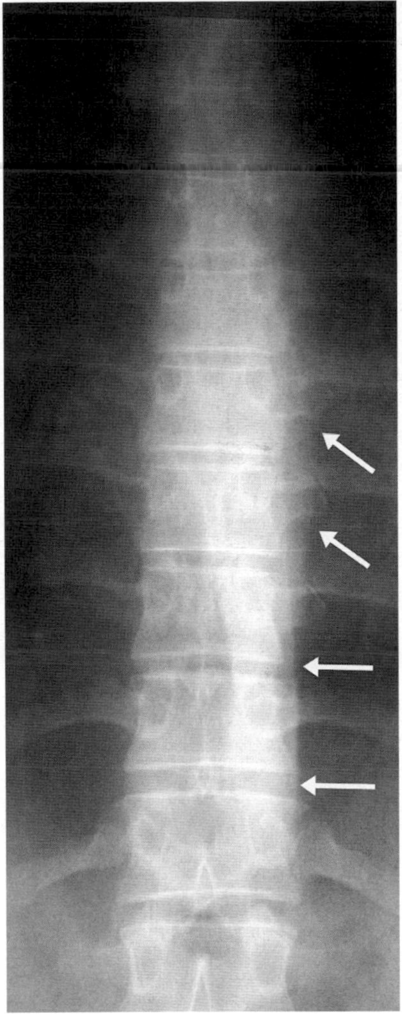

Fig. 4.3 *Normal paraspinal line (horizontal arrows) and lateral margin of the descending thoracic aorta (oblique arrows). The necessity for adequate penetration just to see these crucial structures on a chest X-ray is obvious.*

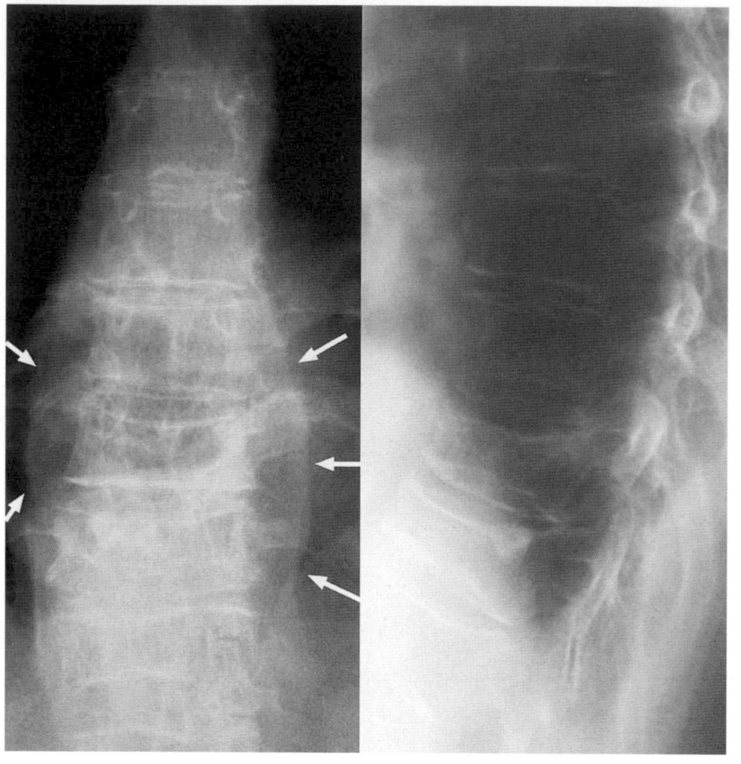

Fig. 4.4 **A** *AP and* **B** *lateral showing a spindle-shaped 'paraspinal mass' around collapsed vertebrae. This means it is likely to be acute (e.g. due to a haematoma.*

Fracture dislocations of the thoracic spine

The concept of columns

As elsewhere in the body, multiple classifications exist for injuries to the thoracic spine. One of the most useful is where the spine is divided up into columns in the lateral projection, thus:

1. Anterior two-thirds of a vertebral body and its ligaments.
2. Posterior one-third of a vertebral body and its associated ligaments.
3. Everything posterior to the posterior longitudinal ligament.

The guiding principle is that involvement of only one column is stable, involvement of three is unstable, and involvement of two, stable or unstable.

Thoracic fracture dislocations are therefore usually associated with a multiplicity of flexion/extension and shearing forces; they are essentially due to a disruption of all three columns of the spine and are by definition unstable and likely to involve paraplegia from the outset. Displacements may be forwards or backwards, often with fractures at multiple levels, or disruption through a disc in lieu of a fracture component. See Figure 9.15, (p. 220) for an image of complete disruption of the thoracic spine. The best initial appreciation comes from lateral X-rays followed by the mandatory CT/MRI scans for complete evaluation.

Typical aetiologies would include:

- Sky diving with late deployment of the parachute.
- A parachute that fails to open completely (a 'Roman candle').
- Falling from a height (e.g. off the Matterhorn – see below).
- Masonry falling on to a flexed spine (e.g. during an earthquake).
- Car crash.
- Plane crash.
- Motor cycle crash.
- Trying to hold back a ship, riding the tide with your feet, and with your back against the harbour wall, when you have fallen into the water.

Point of interest: During the descent from the Matterhorn, following its first conquest by Edward Whymper in 1865, the rope broke and four of the climbers plunged down the face of the mountain, bouncing off the outcrops as they fell. At the bottom their mangled remains were found, one with a crucifix sticking through his jaw. Some people pay a high price for conquering a mountain or indulging in a dangerous sport.

Fracture types

Compression fractures

- These are similar to those in the neck; when purely traumatic in normal bone, two-thirds of them occur around the thoracolumbar junction where the spinal curvature changes direction. The thoracic spine being curved concave anteriorly, any vertically directed vector will tend to force sudden forward flexion. Associated features may include retropulsion of bone and disc fragments.
- These injuries may occur after a fall, or jumping from a height, when the impact is transmitted up through the feet. Potential spinal injury should therefore be considered in a patient who presents with a fractured calcaneum. (The pelvis should also be assessed.)
- Elderly osteoporotic patients who fall may also sustain such injuries, exacerbated by the fragility of their bones, or the injuries may occur spontaneously. Pre-existing fractures may also be present, especially at and around the keystone vertebra at the apex of the thoracic curve (Fig. 4.5).
- Epilepsy with convulsions, electrocution and electroconvulsive therapy (ECT), used occasionally in psychiatry, may also induce fractures in the spine due to violent uncontrolled muscular contractions.
- *Burst fractures.* As in the neck, a burst fracture may occur in the thoracic spine due to a primarily axial force sending bony fragments out in all directions. These can be stable or unstable.
- *Sagittal slice fractures.* These occur when the vertebra above telescopes into the one below and forces fragments out laterally.

NB The thoracolumbar spine, where the relatively rigid thoracic spine meets the mobile lumbar spine, suffers similar problems to those occurring at the cervicothoracic junction, i.e. increased susceptibility to injury at this level.

Seat belt fractures (and Chance fractures)

The introduction in 1983 of the legal requirement to wear car seat belts in the UK was greeted with resistance in many quarters, but the idea was to restrain passengers on impact and stop them flying out through the windscreen.

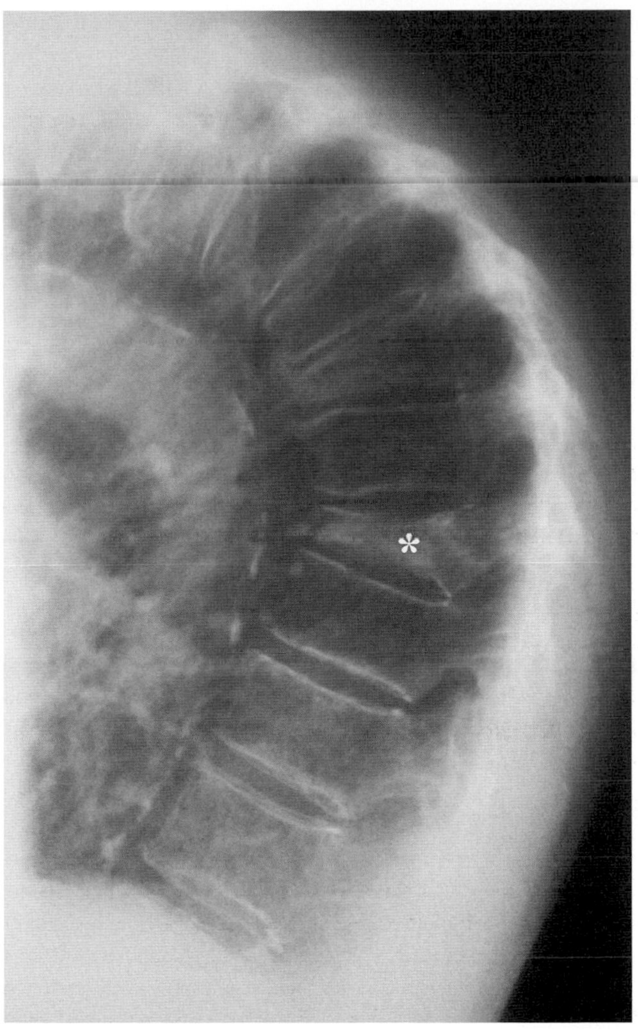

Fig. 4.5 *Typical osteoporotic fracture with severe kyphosis (asterisk). Note there are some more above.*

Seat belt fractures refer primarily to the effects of wearing only a lap strap, so that on impact the upper body and spine sustain sudden forward movement with instant flexion of the upper spine relative to the lower spine pivoting around the belt. Distraction of the spine causes a horizontal crack extending forwards from the posterior components of a vertebra, causing a horizontal split. This is the so-called classic *Chance fracture*.

Gold medal point: A similar injury may be seen as a result of extensive ligamentous injury with separation of the spinous processes and facet joints, and widening of the posterior disc spaces, but no fracture. This is known as the *chance equivalent*.

Inevitably, however, drivers who pile into one another head on at a closing speed of 150 m.p.h. (240 k.p.h.) will sustain even more serious disruption than this and will probably not survive.

Almost all cars nowadays incorporate a diagonal inertia reel belt to restrain the upper torso. Even so, light aircraft pilots would still distinguish between this arrangement and a full harness consisting of thick straps over each shoulder and a thick band at the waist secured centrally by a simple lock, or even a five-point harness with five straps, two of which go round the legs. These are essential for restraint during aerobatics (as some pilots have fallen out at the top of a loop) and increase survivability in accidents. A helmet also protects the pilot in survivable accidents, as it does in rallying motor cars. The seat-belt diagonal in cars is associated with certain specific injuries like rib fractures along the line of the belt, vascular injuries to the carotids, aorta and mesenteric vessels, and various visceral injuries.

A special kind of injury: the ejection seat

The ejection seat is a potent cause of injury to the thoracic spine. It is a fact, however, that the highly reliable Martin–Baker ejection seat has saved the lives of thousands of pilots of all nations, but each rocket-propelled ejection takes its toll on an airman's spine. Under typical acceleration normal bone begins to break at 30G (i.e. 30 times the force of gravity) and one or more vertebral fractures are the norm after each ejection, with a consequent loss of an individual's height. The Royal Air Force has protocols in place for the medical evaluation of any aircrew who eject, including a thorough neurological assessment and MRI of the spine at a dedicated centre, but initially they may be brought to the nearest A & E department. There is a limit to the number of ejections allowed, based on the degree of trauma sustained on each occasion; lumbar vertebrae may of course also fracture. Fortunately, bills are not issued for the cost of lost aircraft, but guilt and depression can follow such incidents, especially if a fellow crewman is lost. The latest version of this seat is the 'Mark XVI', and is a very sophisticated device being virtually 100% reliable.

Chapter 5

The lumbar spine

Background

The guidelines for the lumbar spine are similar to the thoracic spine. You may think you know the limitations of lumbar spine movements – until you see a ballerina, acrobat or contortionist at work.

The lumbar spine can execute forward, backward, left and right flexion and limited rotational movements. The thoracolumbar junction is particularly prone to injury because this is where the relatively immobile thoracic spine changes direction to meet the more mobile lumbar spine, so cord damage can therefore occur here. The spinal canal below L2 contains only the cauda equina, and not the cord, so only lower motor neurone and sensory fibres are affected at these levels. In addition, the prognosis in cauda equina lesions is better than in cord lesions. Powerful muscles are attached to the lumbar spine, including the long flexors of the hip (iliopsoas), which can break off the transverse processes. Recent work has also shown that lumbar spine injuries may be associated with occult injury to the abdominal aorta.

Traumatic lesions can vary from relatively minor compression injuries to severe 'burst' fractures and gross shearing fracture dislocations. As at higher levels, early progress to CT or MRI may be indicated for complete evaluation of fragments, displacements, cord and root damage.

Radiography

- The conventional X-ray views are the AP and lateral projections (Fig. 5.1). These should be 'coned', i.e. localized to the relevant areas, both to minimize radiation and optimize clarity by reducing radiation scatter (which reduces contrast).
- Ideally the AP film should include the lowermost thoracic spine superiorly and sacroiliac joints inferiorly.

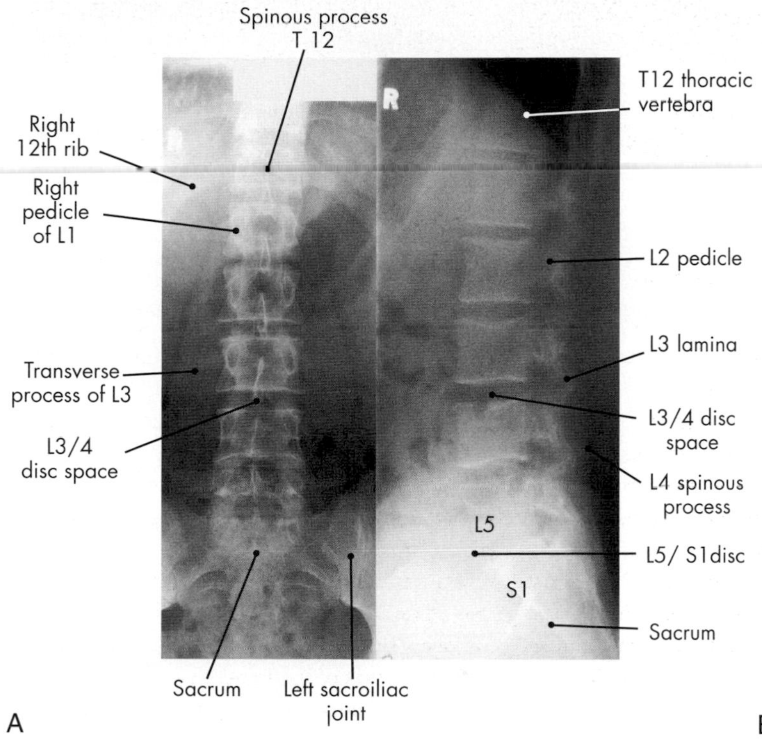

Fig. 5.1 ***A** AP and **B** lateral views of the lumbosacral spine.*

- The long lateral view is usually coned off just in front of the vertebral bodies. In older patients it is helpful to the observer if a little more of the prevertebral area can be included; this greatly assists in the assessment of a calcified and at times *aneurysmal* aorta, which may be a life-threatening cause of backache. In extremely hyperlordotic patients the front of the vertebrae may go off the film.
- In many patients the long lateral view may demonstrate the L5/S1 disc satisfactorily (Fig. 5.2) but sometimes it does not; for example, it is too pale to see or too distorted to interpret properly. If you accept such a film for

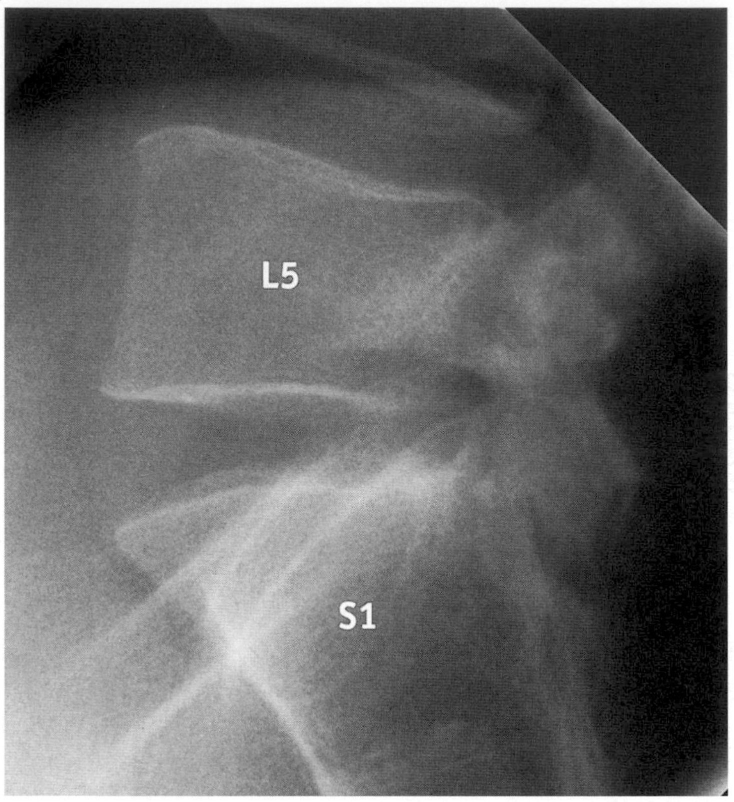

Fig. 5.2 *Localized lateral view of L5/S1. The posterior convergence of the disc space at this level is normal but L5 and S1 should not come into contact.*

diagnostic purposes the responsibility for its interpretation will be yours. Sometimes it is a matter of opinion as to whether or not the L5/S1 disc has been adequately demonstrated, and certainly a great deal of heated discussion has centred on this in the past. If necessary go and discuss it with the radiographer. 'Radiation' may be offered as a reason for not doing a coned view of L5/S1, but if the AP and long lateral have already been 'justified' and carried out, this is a difficult argument to sustain, even in a female. The patient's pregnancy status should already have been established **before** any X-rays were embarked upon.

Oblique views

In some patients with spontaneous pain 45° oblique views can be very helpful in elucidating certain conditions, e.g. a spondylolysis and spondylolisthesis (a defect in the pars interarticularis and slipping of a vertebra).

Anatomy

Configuration of L5/S1 disc: a special case

The anatomical configuration which enables this disc to be identified radiographically is important. Normal lumbar disc spaces have a basically parallel profile sandwiched between the end-plates of their adjacent vertebrae. The L5/S1 disc normally has a V-shaped configuration (Fig. 5.2), opening anteriorly like a trumpet, which should not be interpreted as an abnormality. A *parallel* disc space at this level is *abnormal*, however, and contact between the posterior bony margins of L5 and S1 is also indicative of disc space narrowing.

An important common normal variant

Spina bifida occulta Twenty-five per cent of patients will have incomplete fusion of the posterior elements at the L5/S1 junction to a greater or lesser degree. Rarely it may also be visible at the cervicothoracic junction and is usually without clinical significance. The margins are smooth and often sclerotic so this should not be mistaken for trauma.

Trauma to the lumbar spine

As higher levels in the spine, the lumbar vertebrae are subjected to flexion, extension, shearing and mixed forces, causing, for example, wedge-type injuries and Chance fractures.

Burst fractures

As has already been alluded to in discussion of the cervical and thoracic spine, when a large component of the force is axial, the involved vertebra effectively explodes and both disc material and bone splinters may be driven by retropulsion into the spinal canal, rendering the patient paraplegic. The consequences of these injuries are therefore often devastating and their full severity only visible on CT. The bone, of course, is bursting in all directions.

Look at Figure 5.3. This patient fell 20 feet (6 metres) off a ladder and then hit the top of a wall. Note:

- The acute curve of the spine concave to the right.
- The disruption of the cortical margins of the body of L3.
- The lateral expansion of the vertebral body.
- The decreased height of the vertebral body.
- The increased interpedicular distance at L3.
- The separation of the facet joint on the right side.

CT scanning will optimally demonstrate any splinter incursions into the thecal sac and is mandatory in such injuries. Vertical reformatting and 3D reconstruction can give even better spatial information to help decide on optimum treatment (Fig. 5.4).

A word to the wise

While A & E doctors may quite rightly regard themselves as being there primarily to deal with trauma, it is well known that patients can walk in off the street with absolutely anything the matter with them. 'Pain in the back' is a case in point. This may be due to anything from an exacerbation of long-standing degenerative disease ('I couldn't see my own doctor') to acute life-threatening disease (e.g. a leaking aortic aneurysm) or some distinctly unusual condition (like sickle cell anaemia) with bony involvement. **Once through the door, however, patients are your responsibility**. All doctors are conditioned by the environment in which they work – but you need to be able to do a lot of lateral thinking.

The important thing for the A & E doctor is to be able to unlock himself or herself from the mental straightjacket of the purely traumatic mode, and be able to consider both medical and surgical conditions when confronted with a new patient, and beware of diagnostic labels already attached to patients. That patient sent in as a 'myocardial infarction' may actually have a spontaneous rupture of

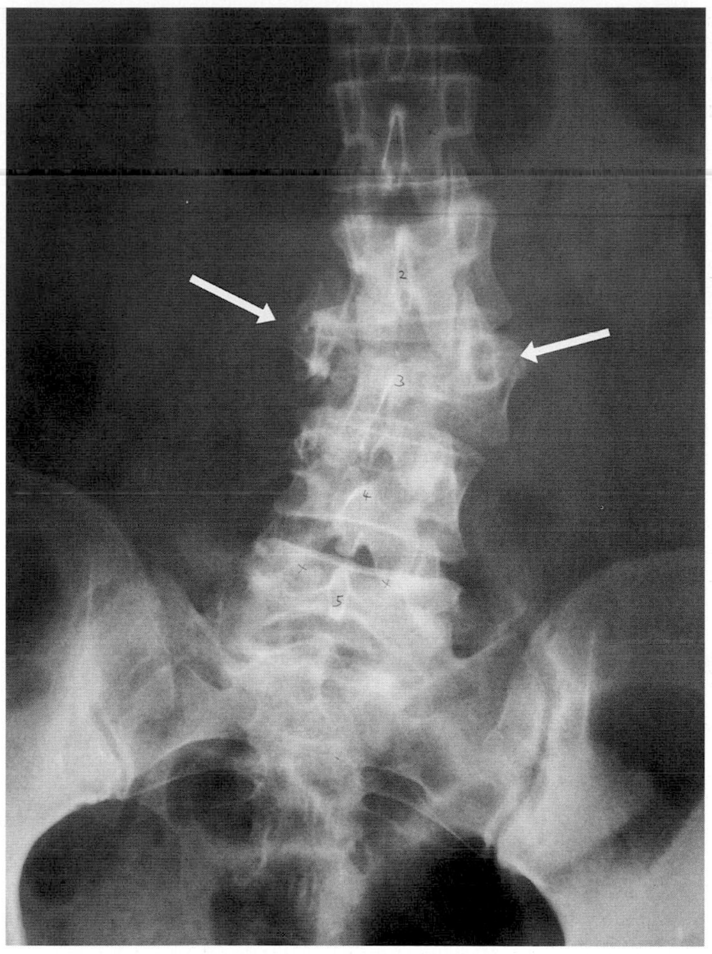

Fig. 5.3 *AP lumbar spine showing burst fracture of L3 (arrows).*

the oesophagus or pancreatitis, and the 'renal colic' may have an acute appendicitis causing irritation of the ureter. **Make up your own mind about what is wrong with the patient and do not be boxed in by other people's presumptive diagnoses.** There are plenty of other causes of backache apart from

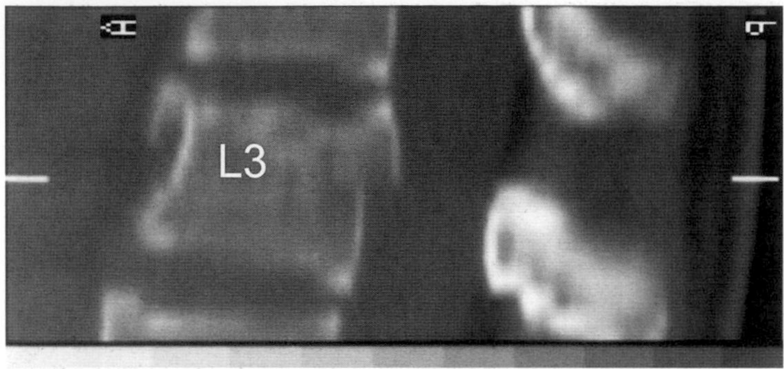

Fig. 5.4 Sagittal electronic reformatting of L3. Note the fragments extruding anteriorly, and particularly posteriorly into the spinal canal.

a 'slipped disc': spontaneous osteoporotic collapse, metastatic disease, juvenile osteochondritis, osteomyelitis, infective discitis and myeloma are some other examples (Figs 5.5, 5.6), so keep your eyes open – and your mind! Remember too that other conditions like a leaking aortic aneurysm or pancreatic carcinoma can present with backache.

Injuries to the sacrum

Background

The sacrum is a strong and deep-set bone which requires a lot of force to break it. It also forms part of the greater pelvic ring, so trauma to the sacrum or the sacroiliac joints should prompt a careful search for fractures elsewhere in the pelvis or at the symphysis pubis. Falls and direct impacts are frequent causative factors.

Radiography

AP and lateral views. The AP is, of course, visible on a full AP pelvis.

Anatomy (Fig. 5.7)

The sacrum is a triangular wedge of bone which sits like a keystone suspended by its 'wings' or alae between the left and right iliac bones, gripped by the

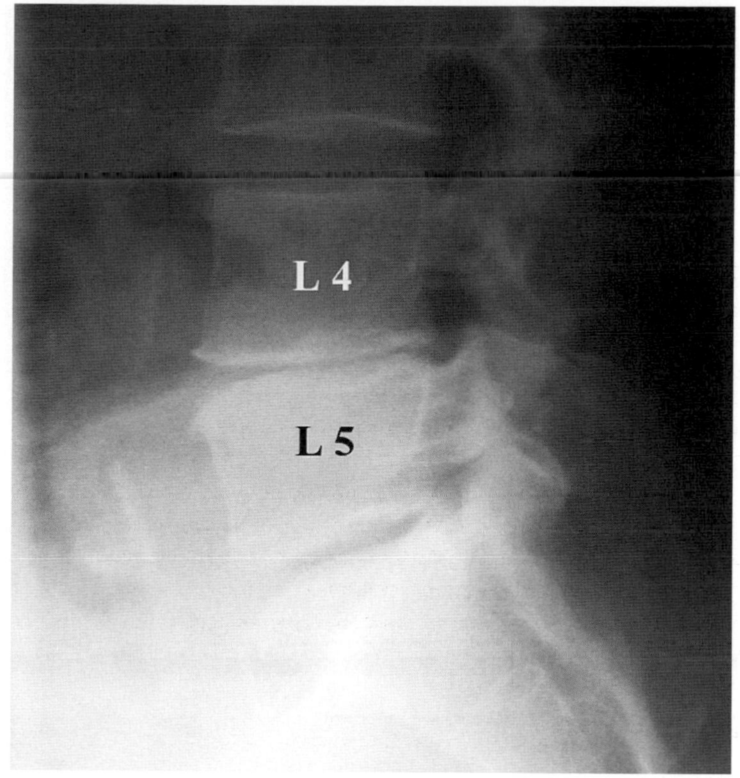

Fig. 5.5 *Patient presented with backache. Severe degenerative disc disease at L4/5. Note that the end-plates are intact.*

undulating surfaces of the sacroiliac joints and the powerful binding ligaments between these bones. Large foramina are present on its anterior aspect, the upper margins of these forming dense white edges (the arcuate lines). The oval-shaped upper surface, which articulates with L5, is known as the sacral promontory.

Normal variants Varying degrees of spina bifida occulta, lumbarization of S1 (giving six lumbar vertebrae) or sacralization of L5 (giving four lumbar vertebrae) can occur.

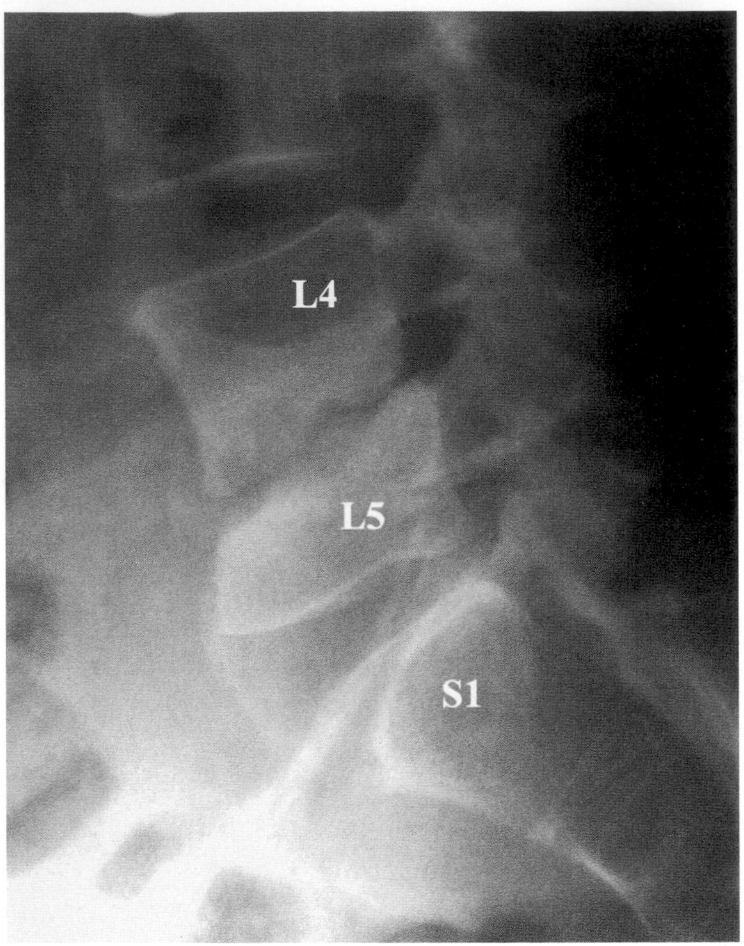

Fig. 5.6 *A mistake not to make! Patient presented with backache. Infective discitis at L4/5. Note the destruction of both end-plates. The potential exists for a posterior rupture into the spinal canal, causing meningitis. Commoner in drug addicts and immunosuppressed patients. Do not mistake it for osteoarthritis.*

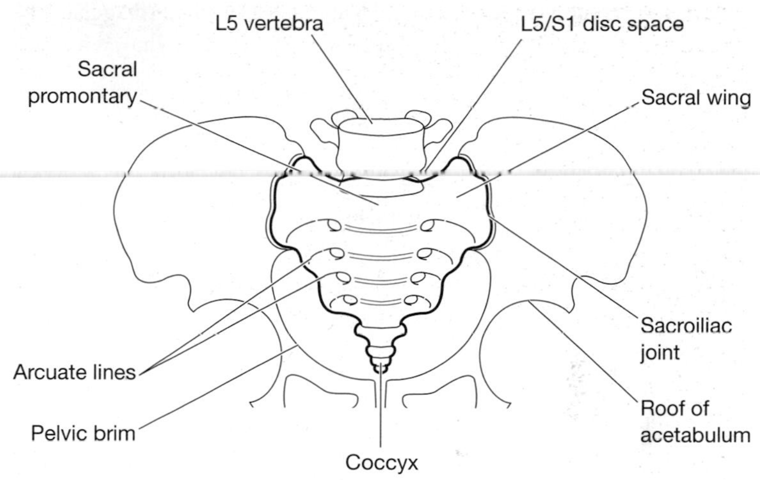

Fig. 5.7 *Anatomy of the sacrum.*

Anatomy

Look for:

- Continuous outlines of the sacral margins.
- Symmetrical positioning of upper and lower sacroiliac joint margins.
- Symmetrical width of the sacroiliac joints.
- Smooth continuity of the arcuate lines (disruption of these means there is a fracture present).

NB On a good day many or all of the above features may be visible. On a bad day, however:

- The sacrum as a distinct bony structure can often be almost completely invisible on an X-ray due to the large amounts of bowel gas which may be lying in front of it, so that you are more likely to miss a fracture than to find one!
- Gas tends to accumulate in the gut after trauma (secondary ileus) and the mucosal margins and dark pockets of gas can both mimic normal foramina, as

well as simulating disruption of the arcuate lines and sacral foramina, while simultaneously obscuring genuine trauma but a lateral may show a fracture.

- Slight obliquity and anatomical variation often makes parts of even the normal sacroiliac joints asymmetrical and invisible.

What to do? Look for mass effects in the pelvis. These may indicate bleeding. A fracture elsewhere in the pelvis or a disrupted symphysis pubis increases the likelihood of a sacral fracture. Maintain a high index of suspicion and consider CT/MRI, especially if there is clinical evidence of neuropathy following trauma.

NB A stress fracture of the sacrum in a sports person or army recruit may be a cause of severe pain, requiring a bone scan or MRI for demonstration or confirmation.

A memorable patient (who was brought to A & E)

Look at Figure 5.8. This 75-year-old female patient fell and developed excruciating pain in her back low down on the right side, which she told the doctor was 'due to arthritis'. Following inspection of the film a diagnosis of 'arthritis of the spine' was 'confirmed'; the patient was informed accordingly and discharged with analgesia.

Comments

- A subluxation of the right sacroiliac joint was completely missed in A & E.
- Not only that, the upper part of the sacrum is missing, having been destroyed by a metastasis from an undiagnosed carcinoma of the breast which the patient was concealing, although interpreting this as 'bowel gas' is very understandable.
- The patient attributed her increasing pain, even before the fall, to her underlying arthritis.
- The doctor was content to go along with this.
- An unexpected and previously unencountered injury (by this doctor) of a subluxed sacroiliac joint was completely overlooked, due to inexperience, i.e. he wasn't looking for it!
- In retrospect its presence is obvious – but it always is through the 'retrospectoscope'.

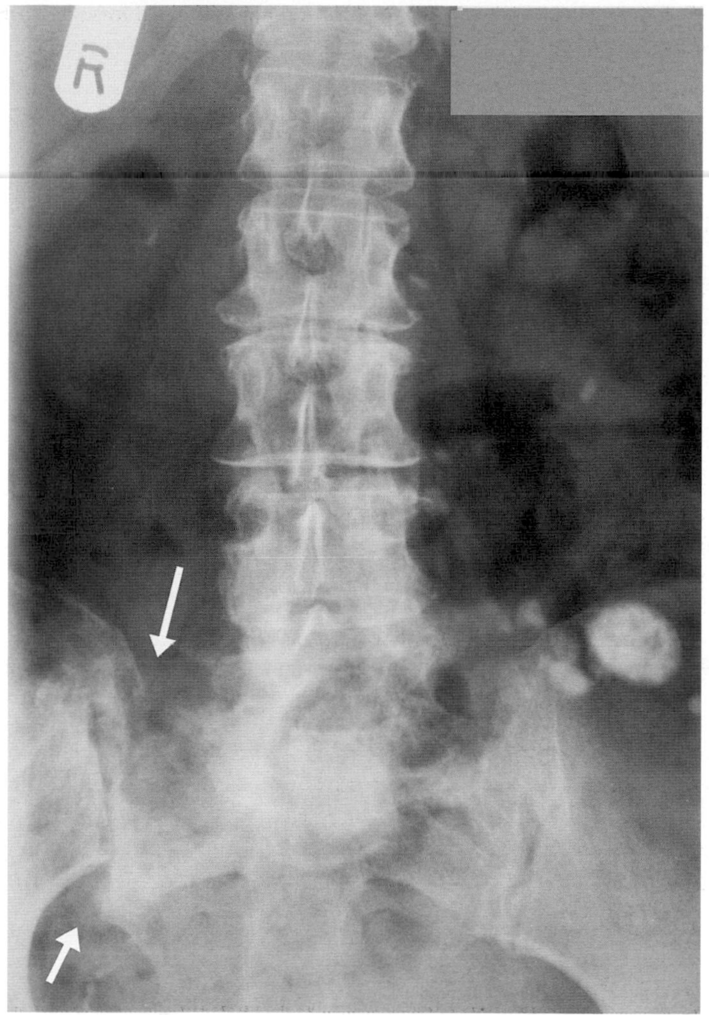

Fig. 5.8 *Inferior subluxation of right sacroiliac joint (arrows).*

- The observer had simply gazed at the film and waited for something to happen – **this is very dangerous**. Looking at X-rays is an **active** process.
- Obeying the simple rule of looking right round the edge of every bone and checking for the congruity of joints should have enabled this abnormality to have been detected.
- The subluxation was picked up the next day by more experienced A & E staff at their daily review.
- The destructive metastasis was picked up (after they missed it) by the radiologist.
- This sacroiliac joint had already been weakened by the destructive metastasis, which increased its susceptibility to trauma. (Would you have spotted it yourself without the arrows?). Bowel gas, however, could easily have mimicked this abnormality or concealed it. Eventually bone destruction was confirmed by CT scanning.

Morals

- If you are not looking for something, you are much less likely to see it.
- Do not always take the path of least resistance from information which seems to fit the bill. Always maintain a sceptical outlook on all information supplied.

And remember: We are all looking for the signs that stop us thinking!

The coccyx

The good news is that the coccyx has gone seriously out of fashion, so we need not dwell on it.

- Even in all its normal configurations the coccyx can look grossly abnormal and traumatized (see Keats & Anderson 2001).
- Even if you do break it, nobody is going to do anything about it (except very rarely).
- X-raying the coccyx irradiates the gonads of both males and females (not wise).
- The treatment for the pain is painkillers – not an X-ray poultice.

Chapter 6

The shoulder girdle

Sternoclavicular joints

Background

The heads of the clavicles are tightly bound to the manubrium sterni by their joint capsules and ligaments and movement is very restricted. Nevertheless, dislocations can occur, either forwards or backwards, usually caused by a fall on the outstretched hand, or a direct blow. (Fractures, often comminuted, may also occur in this position.)

Radiography

AP oblique views are usually attempted to get the sternoclavicular articulations projected off the spine.

Strange fact

Exquisite views of the sternoclavicular joints are frequently obtained inadvertently by radiographers and radiologists doing other things, e.g. barium swallows; they are often shown in greater clarity than in views recommended by standard texts. This is an example of Sod's law in radiology: getting a fantastic view of something when you are not particularly looking for it. A renal artery on ultrasound is another common example. The converse, of course, is also true.

Radiology and clinical aspects

It can be extremely difficult, if not impossible, to decide from plain films alone whether or not the head of the clavicle is dislocated – mainly because you cannot get 'beneath it' and into the requisite plane relative to the sternum to see if it has gone forwards or back.

Clinically, gross swelling usually accompanies a forward dislocation; with a posterior dislocation the patient is likely to be in some considerable distress due to compression of the trachea, leading to stridor, or injury to the larynx, causing dysphonia (a distorted voice) due to direct injury, or a 'helium voice' associated with surgical emphysema.

Important point: This is a job for CT, which can get into the requisite axial plane to confirm or exclude a dislocation, demonstrate any coexistent fractures and associated soft tissue injuries and do it *well*.

The clavicle

Gold medal point: The clavicle is the first bone in the body to ossify during development.

Background

Fractures of the clavicle can occur throughout life – indeed during the act of birth itself when the baby is compressed in the birth canal. In times past doctors would sometimes cut the clavicles with an instrument called a 'cleidotome' to allow the birth of a baby whose shoulders were too broad to allow delivery. Such fractures in an infant would, however, mend and remodel extremely quickly.

In adolescents, rough and tumble with falls on the outstretched hand or direct blows can lead to injuries to the clavicle; in adults, road traffic accidents, falls and sports inevitably take their toll. Injuries to the brachial plexus and subclavian artery and vein may also be associated with fractured clavicles, and should be sought or excluded clinically at presentation.

Good news for cats Because the feline clavicle is not directly attached to the shoulder girdle, Puss can usually absorb a hard landing on her front paws without breaking her clavicles.

Anatomy

See Figure 6.1.

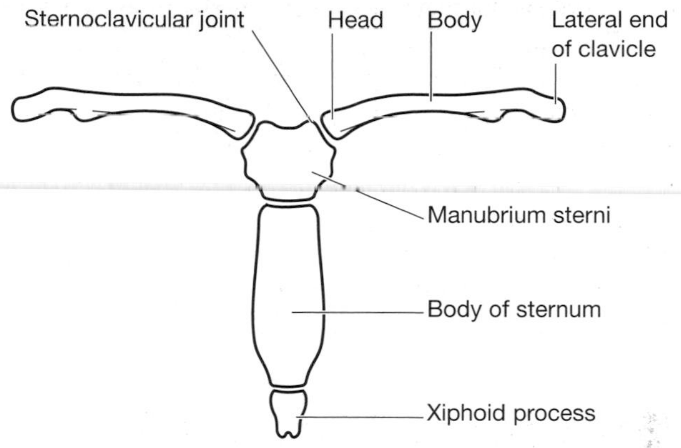

Fig. 6.1 *Anatomy of the clavicles.*

Radiography

An AP or AP oblique view will show most clavicular fractures. Unfortunately, the fracture line may not be visible on one view and without displacement of the fragments it will not be diagnosed. A second film with cranial angulation will usually solve this problem by exaggerating small degrees of separation.

Megahint: Do not fall into the common trap of asking the radiographer for an 'AP and lateral' of the clavicle! This will just show your ignorance as a 'lateral' clavicular view is virtually useless, and largely overlapped by the opposite side.

Moral: Always tell the radiographer what you want to see, i.e. 'right clavicle', rather than trying to specify fancy views which you may not fully understand. (X-ray departments regularly get such requests – a constant source of amusement – so don't let it be at your expense.) A conscientious radiographer will repeat any inadequate views or automatically take any further ones which she feels will help, but you must understand the strong pressure to minimize radiation under current IRMER regulations.

Radiology (see Fig. 1.1)

Diagnosis is usually easy, as long as the cortical margins are thoroughly checked. The clavicle is traditionally divided into thirds, and the middle third is the

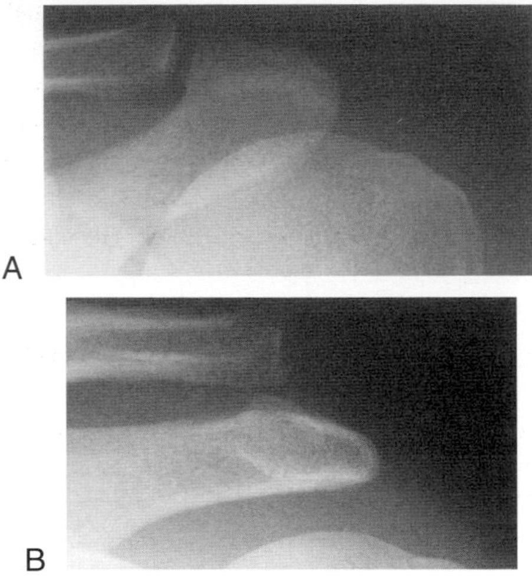

Fig. 6.2 ***A*** *Normal acromioclavicular joint.* ***B*** *Weight-bearing view of opposite side, electronically reversed for ease of comparison, showing upward dislocation of the lateral end of the clavicle.*

commonest site for a fracture. Next is the lateral end, and then the medial end. Fractures at the medial end may be overlooked because of underlying bones (e.g. the spine), so look very carefully round the edge of every bone.

Something to look for

Once the clavicle is broken right through, the weight of the arm usually drags the lateral component down so that there is a step effect at the fracture site. A third fracture fragment may also be present at right angles to the main axis of the bone.

Often fractures of the clavicle are left alone and treated just by a sling, but in some patients upward angulation of a fragment may occur, causing severe tenting of the skin with the risk of necrosis or perforation. Surgical reduction and internal fixation may then be required. In young ladies, conscious of perfection, avoiding an ugly lump of callus may bring cosmetic considerations to bear on the orthopaedic surgeon. Malunion or non-union are occasional sequelae to trauma, and surgery will be necessary.

Point of interest: The infraclavicular fossa, at the medial aspect of the shoulder girdle is, of course, 'the Hollywood safe spot'. This means, among other things, that it is a respectable place for a lady to take an arrow during a Commanche raid on a wagon train, mainly because it preserves her modesty and will not disturb her make-up. Similarly, the cowboy hero of the movie can safely be shot here too (apart from being 'winged' in the deltoid, or 'creased' in the scalp), as it enables him to keep moving, is not one of those nasty 'gut shots', and spares both his heart and angular jawline.

The idea that you could actually take a bullet clean through the axilla from a Winchester rifle without it completely carrying off your axillary artery, vein, and brachial plexus and smashing your ribs and scapula is all part of the entertainment, as is the notion that the injury can be readily cured by a simple sling which can be cast off after 3 days and the stricken limb remobilized just in time for the 'clinch' at the end of the movie!

Acromioclavicular joints

Background

The usual problem here occurs after a fall on to the point of the shoulder, or working overhead, disrupting the ligaments to varying degrees, leading to either subluxation or complete dislocation. Adjacent fractures may be in evidence and clinically there may already be a palpable step.

Radiography

Coned AP views are often taken before and after weight-bearing (see Fig. 6.2) in order to reveal a latent subluxation due to rupture of the ligaments at the affected joint. If necessary a comparative view of the opposite side is also taken.

NB The acromioclavicular joints should be visible on conventional shoulder films, both AP/obliques and axials; it may require a bright light to see them – but they will be there. Frequently they will be visible on chest films but are often fortuitously obscured by the name badge or L/R markers (Sod's law), which have to go somewhere.

Anatomy

The essential features are the smooth apposition of the lateral end of the clavicle to the acromion process of the scapula, which comes forwards and round from behind to meet the clavicle, with a variable gap between them, not usually greater than 1 cm.

Important points: Use only the lowermost margin of the clavicle, which should lie flush with the lower acromial edge, to assess displacement. The upper margin of the clavicle often sits higher than the acromion, creating a spurious impression of displacement when none exists.

A comparative view of the opposite side can be very useful but slightly different degrees of angulation between projections can impede interpretation. Take a long hard look again at the inferior acromioclavicular joint margins, which will normally stay constant, before 'confirming separation', as they say on the space launches. It can be a big help when the radiographer gets the two views alongside on one film, or by laterally inverting the normal one for direct comparison electronically (Fig. 6.2).

Some important medical facts

Pre-existing conditions can affect the appearance of the acromioclavicular joints, for example:

- *Osteoarthritis* – when osteophytes distort the apparent bony edges. Extrapolate from the main body of the bone to work out where it should be without them.
- *Rheumatoid arthritis* – causes tapering of the lateral end of the clavicle, called 'the pencil deformity' in the UK, with typical British reserve, and 'the sucked candy deformity' in the USA.
- *Post-traumatic osteolysis* – following a previous fracture or dislocation the lateral end of the clavicle may disappear. Try and obtain the relevant history from the patient.

Gold medal point: Patients with *cleidocranial dysostosis* have rudimentary or even no clavicles and can bring their shoulders to apposition in front of them. Do not mistake rudimentary clavicles for recent or old trauma.

The scapula

Background

The blade of the scapula is like a poppadom – easily cracked by direct trauma – and many muscles of the shoulder girdle are attached to it. Sudden abduction or forceful movement at the shoulder can easily cause fractures of the acromion, coracoid, glenoid or neck of the scapula. **Fractures of the scapula should be conscientiously sought with every shoulder injury**.

Radiography

The views taken are the AP, lateral, transthoracic (the worst) and, best of all, the axial or tangential view (Fig. 6.3).

Anatomy (Fig. 6.4)

The scapula is a thin bone. If you hold one up to the sky on a clear day the sun will shine through it.

Normal variants

Developing or unfused epiphyses at the tips of the acromion and coracoid may be present. Look for lack of displacement and marginal sclerosis (Fig. 6.7).

Trauma

The thinness of the scapula makes fractures hard to see; in addition, the overlapping ribs, vessles and soft tissues all get in the way. If spot on, the Y-view gets the blade off the chest. The axial view is good for checking the acromion but critical for providing unequivocal confirmation of the glenohumeral relationship.

Important point: Surgical emphysema of the chest wall can obscure real, or generate spurious, scapular blade fractures. CT, however, excels at assessing the shoulder girdle, with or without coexistent chest trauma.

Gold medal point: *Scapulothoracic dissociation* mentioned in an oral examination might cause eyebrows to rise. The scapula here is smashed and torn from many of its attachments – expect serious vascular and brachial plexus injuries, and to graduate *summa cum laude!*

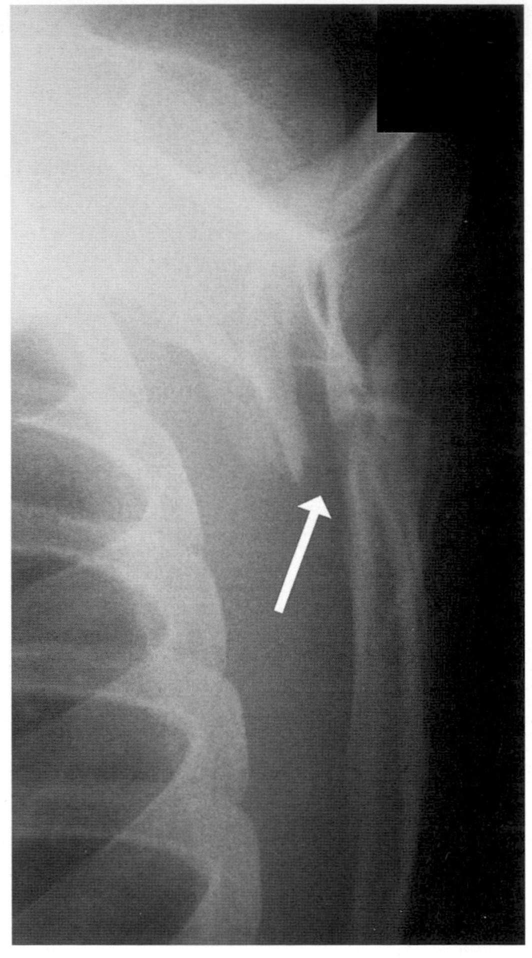

Fig. 6.3 *Tangential view showing comminuted fracture (arrow) of blade of the scapula.*

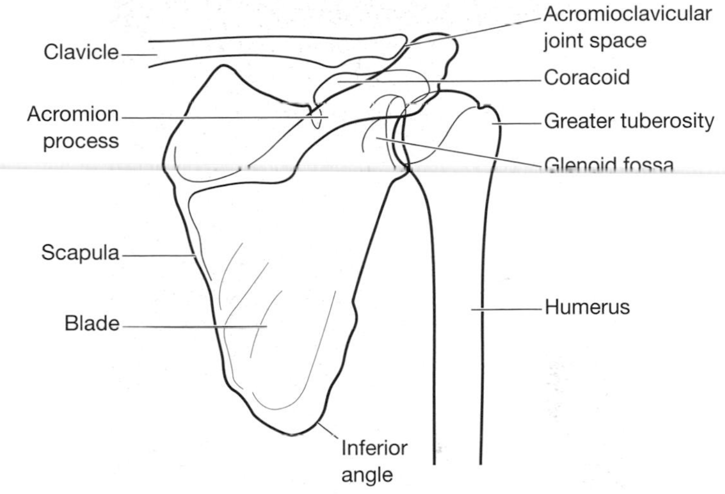

Fig. 6.4 *Anatomy of the scapula (posterior view).*

The shoulder

Background

The shoulder is the most mobile joint in the body (just watch someone waving a chequered flag), with its shallow ball and socket configuration, but the penalty of this mobility is that it is also the most common joint of all to suffer a dislocation; in fact around 50% of all dislocations occur at the shoulder joint. The falls causing dislocations may or may not be associated with fractures.

Radiography

Look at Figure 6.5:

- This view is usually referred to as an 'AP view' of the shoulder but in fact, in terms of the direction of the X-ray beam relative to the joint space, it is actually an AP oblique view. The glenoid fossa points anterolaterally like a satellite dish, as also does the coracoid process.

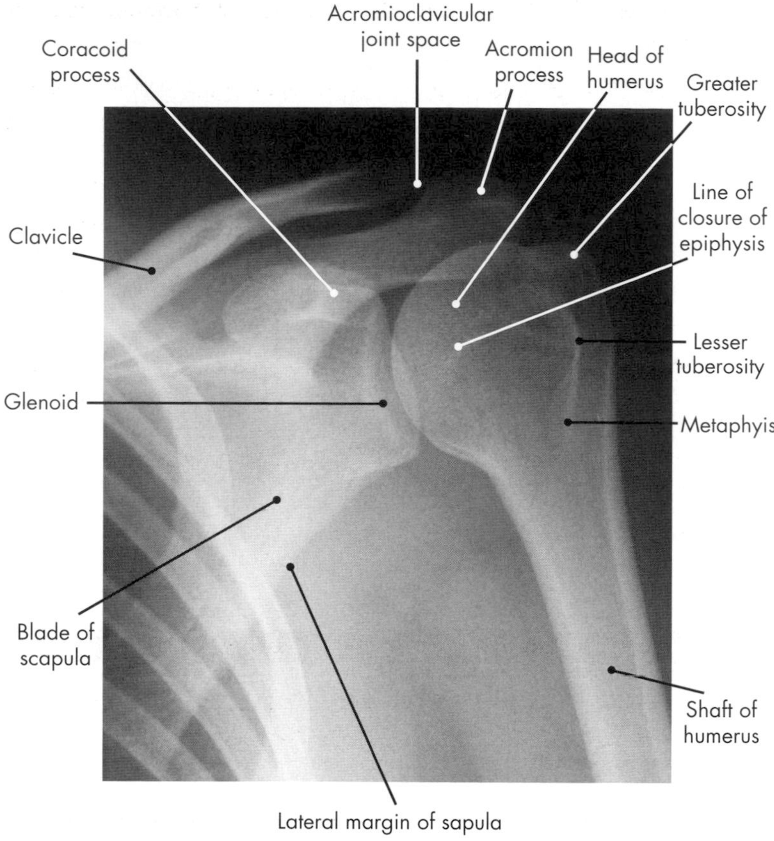

Fig. 6.5 *Normal shoulder joint.*

- To reduce radiation the AP oblique view alone is often now used for the initial survey of a spontaneously symptomatic or painful shoulder. This view has serious limitations and **does not suffice alone** in the context of trauma because a **posterior dislocation may look virtually normal to the untrained eye**, and is the one injury to the shoulder that is particularly likely to be missed. Additionally, the basic concept of two views at right angles, or at least a second view from some other direction, applies just as much to the shoulder as to anywhere else for the adequate demonstration of fractures, subtle or otherwise.

- Alternative views include the transthoracic but often the glenoid cannot be identified, and unless the radiographer can bracket the shoulder at optimum exposure between the spine and the sternum for you, you will find yourself totally confused. A good view is the tangential or Y-view of the scapula, which, if successful, will show the humeral head centred over the glenoid like a catapult or the hub of a propeller (Fig. 6.6), or displacement anteriorly or posteriorly depending on the nature of the dislocation. Ultimately an axial or Garth view may be required (see below).
- **NB** There is no 'lateral' of the shoulder joint to be had. All you would get is a meaningless jumble of underpenetrated upper thorax. (So do not make a fool of yourself by asking for one.)

Normal variants

- The developing juvenile shoulder (Fig. 7.3, p. 146).
- Os acromiale (Fig. 6.7).

Anterior dislocation of the shoulder

Look at Figure 6.8. Note that the head of the humerus is no longer parallel or congruous with the glenoid, having been displaced downwards and medially to sit under the coracoid process.

- This is an anterior (subcoracoid) dislocation of the shoulder and represents around 90% of all dislocations. This diagnosis is relatively easy and should not be missed. Further views may confirm the presence or otherwise of fractures of the shoulder, which should always be looked for.
- Clinically the patient will have lost the rounded contour of the shoulder and have fullness of the soft tissues anteriorly. The usual cause is forced external rotation in abduction during sports or other vigorous activities. With practice you should be able to identify one of these clinically, galloping past on a horse or coming through the doors of A & E.
- Damage to the axillary nerve can occur with this injury, leading to paralysis of the deltoid and numbness over the upper outer arm or 'regimental badge

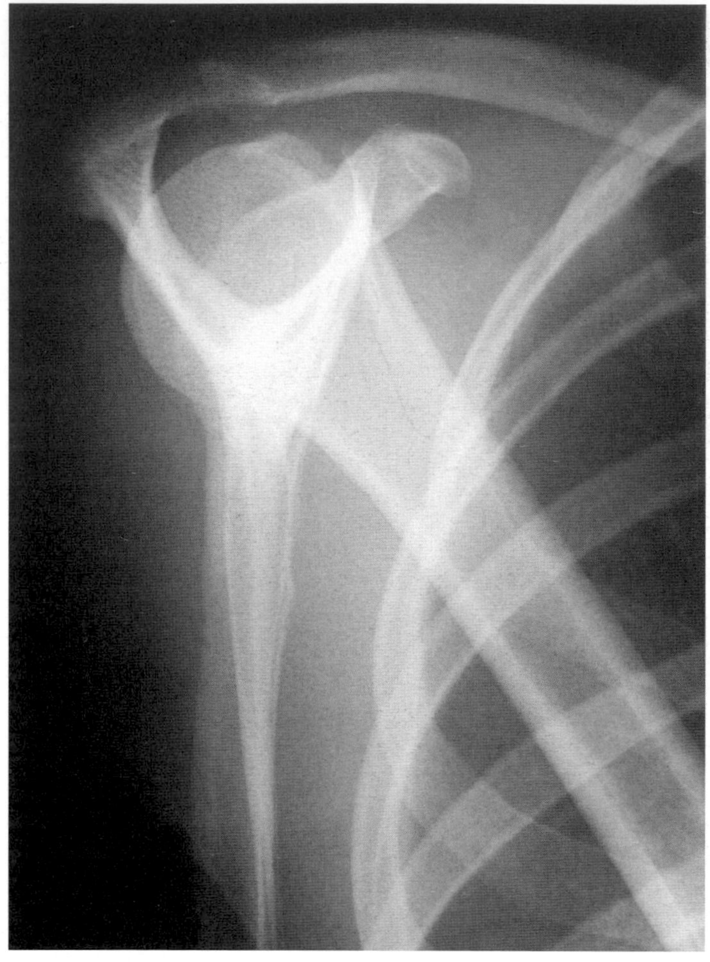

Fig. 6.6 *Normal Y-view of scapula showing central positioning of humeral head articulating with the glenoid.*

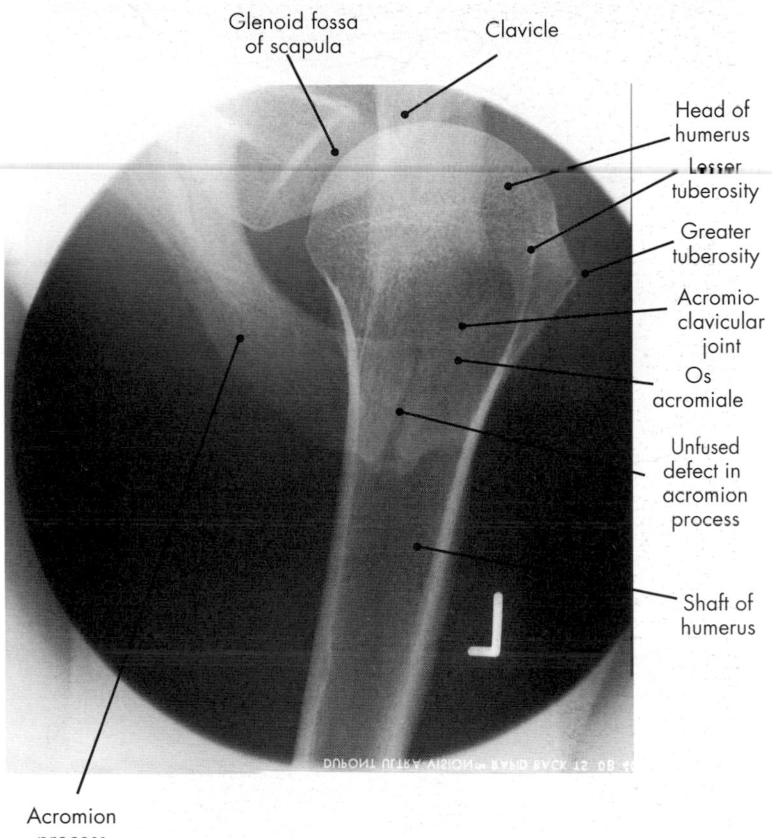

Fig. 6.7 *Axial view of Os acromiale. Note the sclerotically-marginated tip of the acromion process which has not fused – seen through the proximal humerus.*

area'. Bruising of the axillary artery and vein may also occur, leading to vascular complications (thrombosis or deep vein arm thrombosis).

- Prompt reduction is advised as delay can make reduction impossible, although in the longer term recurrent dislocation can occur. Occasionally the

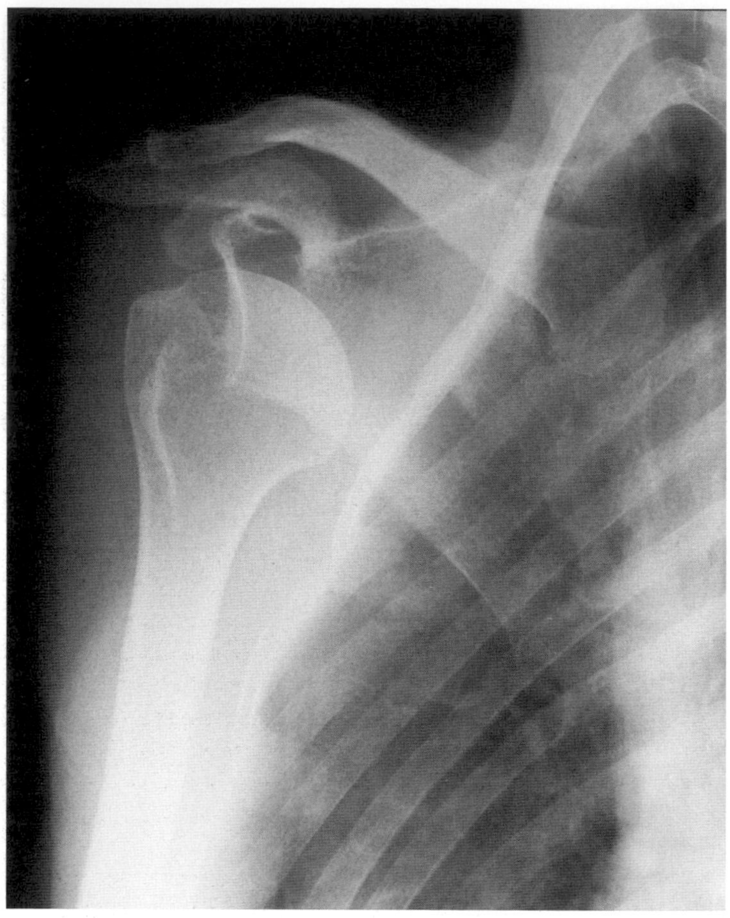

Fig. 6.8 *Anterior subcoracoid dislocation of the shoulder.*

humeral head will stick and 'buttonhole' in the subscapularis muscle, requiring operative reduction.

- Various degrees of impaction by the humeral head against the glenoid can occur causing the so-called Hill–Sachs and Bankart lesions, i.e. impacted fractures of the humeral head or glenoid rims, respectively. These are best seen on an axial view.

- **Point of interest:** The 'Former Naval Person' Sir Winston Churchill suffered a dislocation of his shoulder after a fall when he was a young man in India. The fear of recurrent dislocation caused him to bind his arm in a sling while playing polo; it was also a worry when, as First Sea Lord visiting various cruisers and battleships, he would be hauled from small launches on to a ship or ashore by naval ratings grasping his outstretched arm.
- **NB** One or more dislocations of the humerus may lead to chronic instability.
- **Point of interest:** It is said that Hippocrates would treat a chronically dislocated shoulder by thrusting a flaming torch into the armpit. No doubt the jolt put it back and the scar tissue kept it there!

Posterior dislocation of the shoulder

The posterior dislocation – this is the facer! This is the one which is ten times less likely to occur than the anterior dislocation and many times more likely to be missed. The problem is that a film of a posterior dislocation can look deceptively normal. Over 50% of these get overlooked and often take a year to be diagnosed, the patient being jollied along and told he has a 'frozen shoulder'.

Look at Figure 6.9. At first glance the humerus appears to sit normally alongside the glenoid. But look at the shape of the humeral head: it is like a light bulb or balloon, as the humerus is now internally rotated, and the normally prominent greater tuberosity is no longer on the horizon. This is the 'light-bulb sign'.

NB The light-bulb sign is not, however, totally reliable, as internal rotation when the humeral head is in the normal position can look very similar.

How to avoid missing it

The radiographer will do his or her best to get you another view such as the transthoracic or axial scapular Y-view, which require the patient to sit up and, if successful, may be of considerable help but these require skilled interpretation. For the novice dealing with A & E films, the most convincing way to obtain unequivocal confirmation of the glenohumeral relationship is the axial view (Fig. 6.10). Patient pain and discomfort may militate against attempting this but only

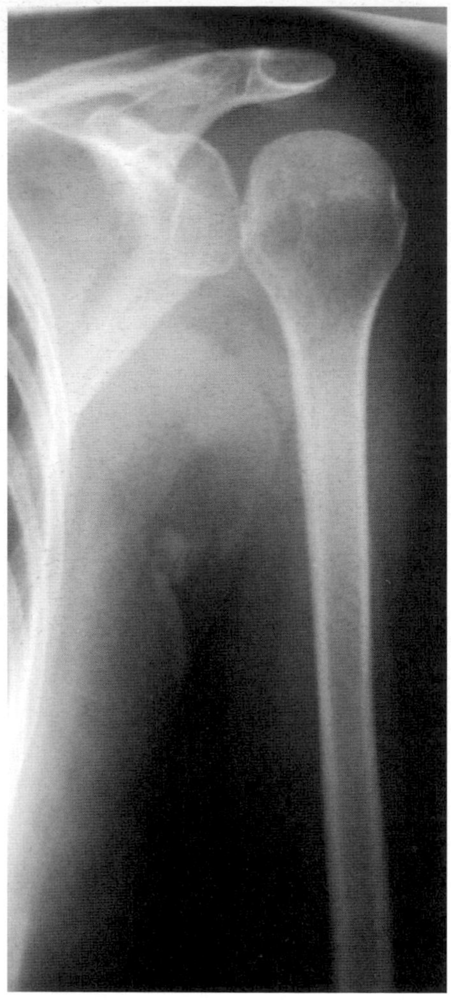

Fig. 6.9 *The 'light bulb sign' – a posterior dislocation of the shoulder.*

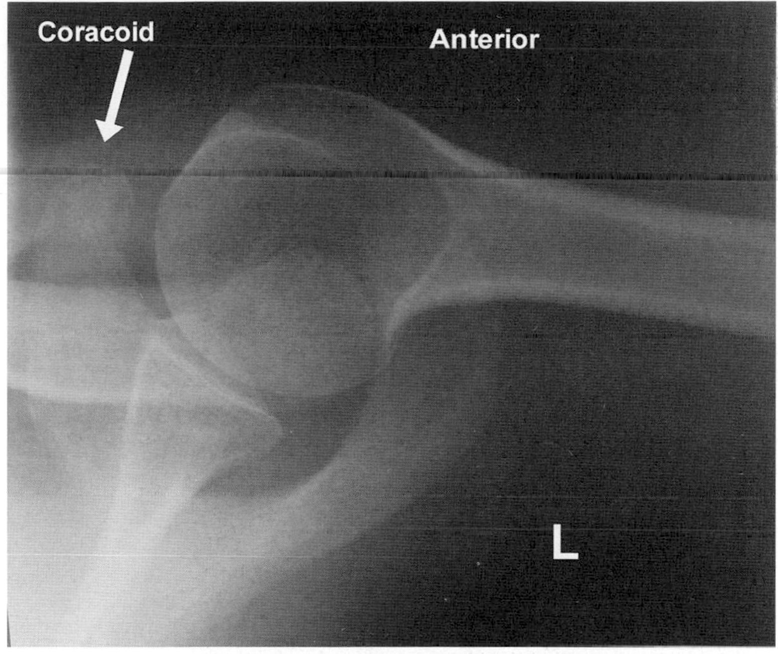

Fig. 6.10 *Normal axial view of the shoulder. The coracoid points anteriorly (as does the acromion).*

10–15° abduction of the arm from the side is needed to get the tube pointing upwards between them, with the cassette placed across the top of the shoulder and the beam fired up from below – or vice versa with (ideally) a curved cassette to fit into the armpit.

Often these films will be dark, so make optimum use of the bright light. With digital equipment the relevant anatomy can be displayed electronically.

Hint: Make sure you know the anatomy on the axial view. Use the coracoid process as a landmark and remember it basically **points forwards.** Then you should be able to work out what is going on.

The Garth view This is a steep 45° oblique superoinferior, rotated, angulated projection which demonstrates the glenohumeral relationship without requiring the patient to abduct what may be a very painful arm; however, it is more difficult to assess than the axial view.

Rarer forms of dislocation

- *Luxatio erecta*. This extremely rare but occasional presentation is of an *inferior* dislocation of the shoulder usually caused by a fall – classically down an open manhole. The arm is caught on the rim of the aperture and suddenly thrown upwards from the elbow, resulting in the head of the humerus locking under the glenoid. This then results in the unfortunate situation of someone with an arm stuck up in the air – the so-called 'erect subluxation'; if really unlucky, both arms will be up in the air.
- *Traumatic pseudodislocation*. Following a fracture of the head of the humerus, the bleeding into the joint can be so intense within the capsule that the humeral head can literally be pushed outwards and downwards from the joint by a *tension haemarthrosis*, effectively dislocating it from within. If performed with the patient upright, careful inspection on occasion may also reveal a *lipohaemarthrosis*, if you think about it and look for it, and of course a fracture.
- *Recurrent dislocation*. Some patients who suffer chronic instability can pop their shoulders 'out' at will as a party piece, thus making the evening go with a bang.

Other spurious dislocations

- *Chest X-rays*. Shoulder joints can often look bizarre on chest X-rays for projectional reasons. With the hands on the hips and the elbows brought forward to get the scapulae off the lung fields, the humerus goes into full internal rotation and produces a false-positive light-bulb sign. The shoulder joint cavity can also look falsely narrowed on chest X-rays – don't rely on them! **NB** A genuine shoulder dislocation, usually of the anterior subcoracoid variety, can, however, still be present on a chest X-ray but the gross separation of humerus and glenoid is usually obvious and unequivocal.
- *Stroke patients*. Patients who have suffered cerebrovascular accidents can lose power and muscle tone, the affected humeral head lying low and limp in the shoulder joint, simulating a traumatic displacement. In those of long standing, look for concomitant muscle wasting (increased soft tissue lucency) and cortical thinning (reflecting disuse osteoporosis).

- *Impingement syndrome*. In this situation, with rupture of the supraspinatus tendon the humerus may sit high up in the joint, grinding against the undersurface of the acromion (look for reactive sclerosis and osteophyte formation).

A legal anecdote

The famous advocate F.E. Smith (Lord Birkenhead) once challenged a young man who was suing his employers for an injury allegedly sustained in an accident, following which he claimed he could no longer raise his arm above the level of his shoulder.

'Show the court how high you can lift your arm now' came the instruction. With a lot of wincing and grunting the boy slowly struggled to abduct his arm just up to shoulder level.

'Now show the court how high you could lift it before the accident' said F.E. Smith. In a flash the arm shot upwards to the vertical!

'Case dismissed!' said the Judge.

Moral: Beware of smart lawyers!

The power within

Look at Figure 6.11. This is the X-ray of an epileptic patient who complained of severe pain in the shoulder following a grand mal attack.

Note: The AP film shows:

- A positive light-bulb sign.

The axial view shows:

- Loss of congruity of the glenoid and humeral head, i.e. the patient has also suffered a partial posterior displacement, together with a compression fracture with impaction and partial collapse of the humeral head.

NB Such injuries may also occur with electrocution or electroconvulsive therapy and may be bilateral. These fractures are due to the strength of the patient's own muscular contractions.

Moral: Axial views to assess the glenohumeral relationship can be critical in the assessment of trauma to the shoulder especially posterior dislocations.

And finally: spontaneous pain in the shoulder

Patients who walk into A & E off the street because they 'couldn't see their own doctor' may have:

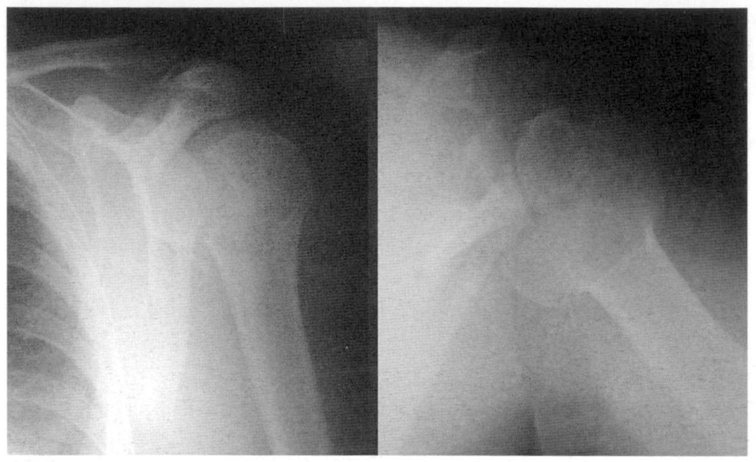

Fig. 6.11 ***A*** *AP and* ***B*** *axial view showing an impacted posterior fracture subluxation of the shoulder.*

- Supraspinatus tendinitis (Fig. 6.12).
- Exacerbations of osteoarthritis or rheumatoid arthritis.
- Pathological fractures.
- Acromioclavicular osteoarthritis.

Some words about fracture types

Before considering fractures of the humerus (a classic long bone), it is appropriate to review the different kinds of fracture that may occur.

Firstly, fractures are either *open* or *closed*, i.e. the fragments either stick out through the skin or they remain within the tissues and do not connect with the atmosphere (or by implication, infection).

Fractures are also subdivided by their appearance (Fig. 6.13):

1. *Transverse* – due to direct trauma, across the shaft of a bone.
2. *Oblique* – due to oblique impact.
3. *Spiral* – due to twisting injury.

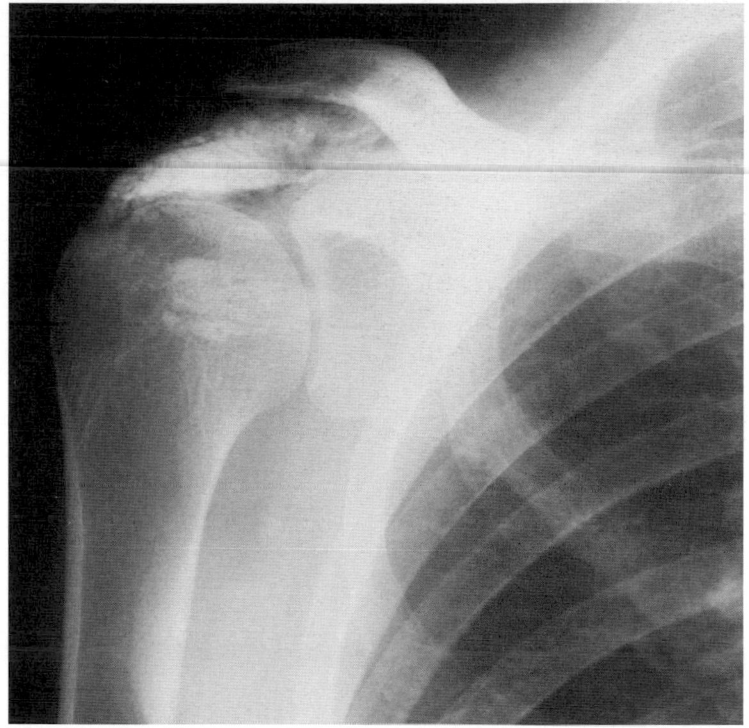

Fig. 6.12 *Massive supraspinatus and capsular shoulder calcification. Often just a small focus presents above the greater tuberosity.*

4. *Comminuted* – smashed into more than two and often many pieces.
5. *Segmental* – broken in two places.
6. *Torus* – buckling of cortices. (Latin *Torus* = swelling).
7. *Greenstick* – breaking of one cortex and bending of the other.
8. *Plastic bowing* – bending of whole bone.
9. *Pathological* – clue to underlying bone lesion.

6, 7, and 8 occur only in children.

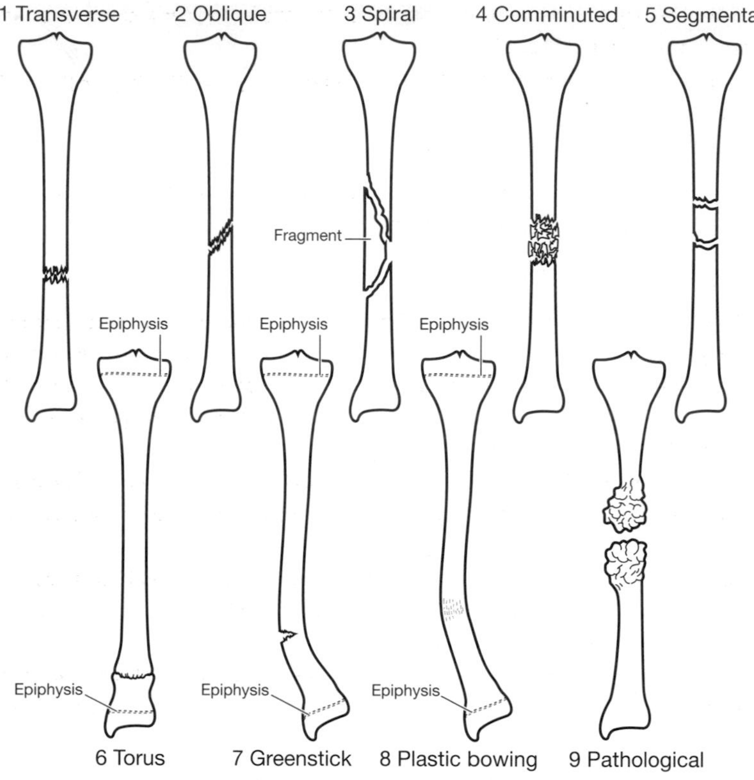

Fig. 6.13 *Types of fracture. 1, transverse; 2, oblique; 3, spiral; 4, comminuted; 5, segmental; 6, torus; 7, greenstick; 8, plastic bowing; 9, pathological.*

Pathological fractures may occur through sites of weakness where metastases have grown, e.g. the humerus, or the bone is weakened by osteoporosis, e.g. the femoral neck. Take a chest X-ray to look for a primary tumour or more secondaries – something useful you can do while the patient is in the hospital, if you think there is a malignancy.

Stress fractures are due to repeated submaximal trauma in normal bone, e.g. the neck of the second metatarsal after running a marathon. They may not show up immediately but only become visible 10–14 days later after a cloud of callus appears (see Fig. 13.27, p. 301).

Insufficiency fractures are due to normal stresses on weakened bone, e.g. in the pelvis.

Some other terms in common use include:

- *Impacted fractures* – e.g. the hip when the cancellous bone is driven into itself and causes a dense line of impaction.
- *Crush fracture* – e.g. in the spine.

NB Check every fracture for **alignment, separation** and **angulation**. Angulation is described by reference to the distal component relative to the proximal one. Make sure the joints at both ends of a long bone are on each film so that rotational deformities are not overlooked. 'Valgus' means angled *out* the way. 'Varus' means angled *in* the way.

Non-accidental injury: This is a huge issue, which includes fractures, touching on child abuse and its important differential of osteogenesis imperfecta (p. 315).

Crucial fact about fractures: The associated damage to soft tissues, i.e. arteries, veins, nerves, ligaments, muscles and the articular cartilage in joints must always be uppermost in your mind.

Ultimately various forms of *malunion* and *non-union* may complicate fractures. The late complication of a Sudeck's atrophy is also important (intense osteoporosis).

Developing epiphyses and the Salter–Harris classification

Special attention is required in regard to epiphyseal injuries occurring at the growing ends of bones in children, as, if there is disturbed growth, arrest or severe deformity may occur.

The classification devised by Salter and Harris is a pillar of orthopaedics and you could be asked about it. It comprises five types of injury (Fig. 6.14):

1. A fracture horizontally through the line of the growth plate itself, sometimes with a slip or angulation.
2. A fracture through the growth plate with a small triangular piece of bone separated from the proximal main shaft.

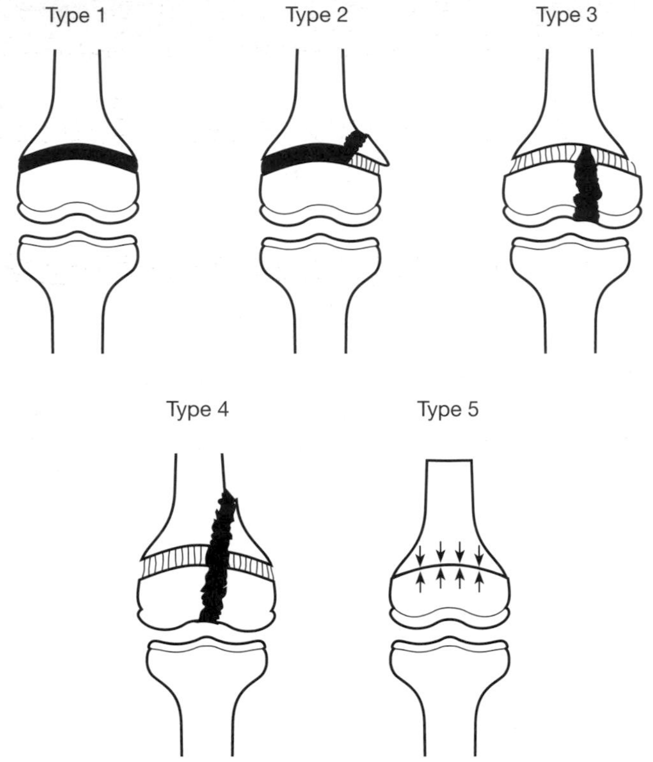

Fig. 6.14 *Injuries to growth plate: Salter–Harris classification (see text).*

3. Fracture separation of part of the epiphysis with part of it remaining attached to the shaft.

4. A fracture through the distal shaft and the epiphysis.

5. Compression injury to all or part of the epiphysis – which may be hard to diagnose at the time. Growth problems will start later.

Rule of thumb: The lower the Salter–Harris number the better the prognosis. See page 289 for Salter–Harris type 2 fracture of the ankle.

Chapter 7

The upper limb

The humerus

Background

Proximally, fractures at this level in the humerus are usually caused by falls, either on the outstretched hand or against a solid object. Fractures should be sought (i.e. X-rayed) with every dislocation of the shoulder, and vice versa. Most injuries here reunite well, but some may be so comminuted and displaced that they never reunite.

Radiography

As for dislocation:

- AP obliques
- Y laterals
- axial – far and away the best
- Garth view
- transthoracic.

Anatomy

The humeral head is a hemisphere directed upwards and medially like a blob of ice-cream slightly offset on its cone (Fig. 7.1). Where the blob meets the cone is the anatomical neck. A couple of cherries are stuck on to the lateral aspects of this delicious strawberry ice, one beneath the other, i.e. the greater and lesser tuberosities.

Beneath the anatomical neck is the surgical neck, which is usually where the humerus actually breaks (Fig. 7.2), just as your crispy ice-cream cone does if someone suddenly slams into the back of you.

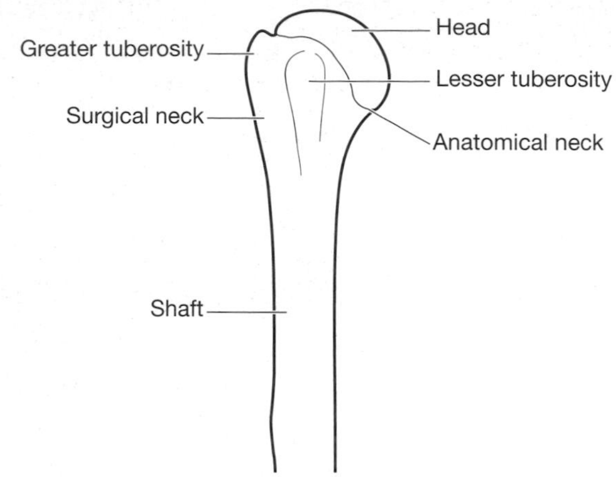

Fig. 7.1 *Anatomy of the humerus.*

Normal variants The main differential problem is the unfused proximal humeral epiphysis, which fuses in the late teens. When still present this forms an inverted V with a sclerotic margin (Fig. 7.3).

Fractures

- The commonest fracture is an impacted surgical neck of the humerus, which causes a dense band in the bone and usually slight cortical discontinuity.
- Separation injuries may also occur, causing lucent lines, cortical disruption and variable numbers of fragments; the greater the number of fragments, the greater the instability.

NB This is an important concept which applies to all fractures, i.e. **separation = lucency and impaction = increased density.**

- Occasionally the humerus will break at the *anatomical neck*; as in the hip, this can lead to avascular necrosis of the humeral head (the 'snow cap sign'), but is very rare.
- The greater tuberosity may be avulsed if the supraspinatus gets a jolt.

NB Displacement of the proximal humeral epiphysis may be an indication of non-accidental injury in children.

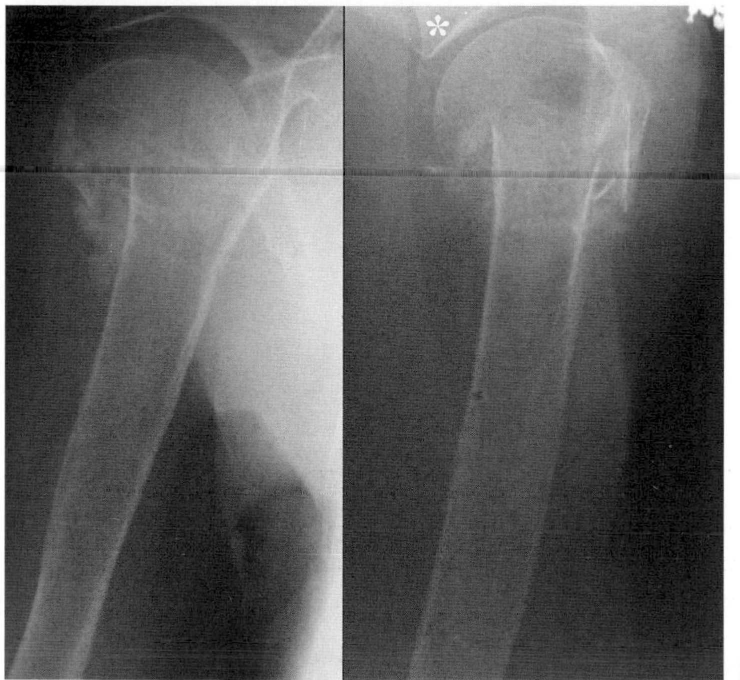

Fig. 7.2 ***A*** *AP and* ***B*** *axial views. Comminuted fracture separation of humeral head at the surgical neck. The glenoid (asterisk) is just visible on the axial view, confirming the head remains in the joint.*

Humeral shaft

Radiography

The ideal views are full AP and full laterals with 'the joint above and the joint below' (i.e. the shoulder and elbow) clearly visible on each film. This enables optimum assessment of any fracture with regard to angulation, alignment, rotational effects, etc. In multiply-injured patients, or patients in great pain, ideal views may be hard to achieve, but every effort will be made to obtain such films. Occasionally, however, you will just have to do your best with 'running obliques' and incomplete views (Fig. 7.4).

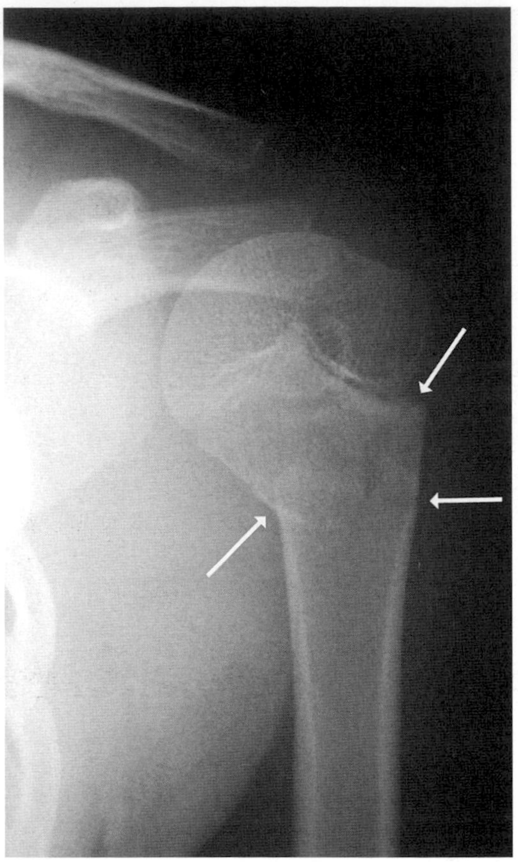

Fig. 7.3 *Injury to juvenile shoulder. Upper arrow shows normal epiphysis – note inverted V configuration and sclerotic margins. Do not mistake this for a fracture. Lower arrows show a genuine fracture through the proximal shaft.*

Crucial fact: When both humeri have been X-rayed, make sure you check left and right when assessing each film. **Do not use the right AP with the left lateral to assess a broken right side (or vice versa).**

Clinical aspects: These are crucial here. Long slivers of bone can result from comminutions and rotational injuries. So in any humeral shaft fracture check radial nerve function – that is, the brachialis muscle. Ultimately it may have to be explored. Check also the arterial and venous status of the arm.

Normal variants

- The deltoid tuberosity on the upper lateral aspect of the humerus is a raised rough area. Do not mistake it for a tumour.
- The nutrient canal enters the cortex from above and outside the bone and passes through it downwards towards the elbow **('To the elbow I run, from the knee I flee!').** Do not mistake it for a fracture.

NB Pathological fractures due to metastatic disease, for example from the breast or bronchus, have a predilection for the proximal humerus, although there should be a history of pain before the final 'crack'. The femur is also a target for metastases, like the so-called 'banana fracture'.

The elbow

Background

This joint is subject to fractures and dislocations due to falls, impacts and traction injuries, but most fractures are relatively easily detected in adults by X-ray, either directly or indirectly.

Paediatric elbow injuries are, however, a completely different matter. They are a frequent source of considerable anxiety among junior doctors, as indeed they are to everyone involved with them, not least of all the tiny tots who sustain these excruciating injuries and their overwrought parents.

NB The biggest worry is the list of nasty complications which may ensue from fractured elbows in children, particularly damage to the brachial artery and ischaemia of the forearm.

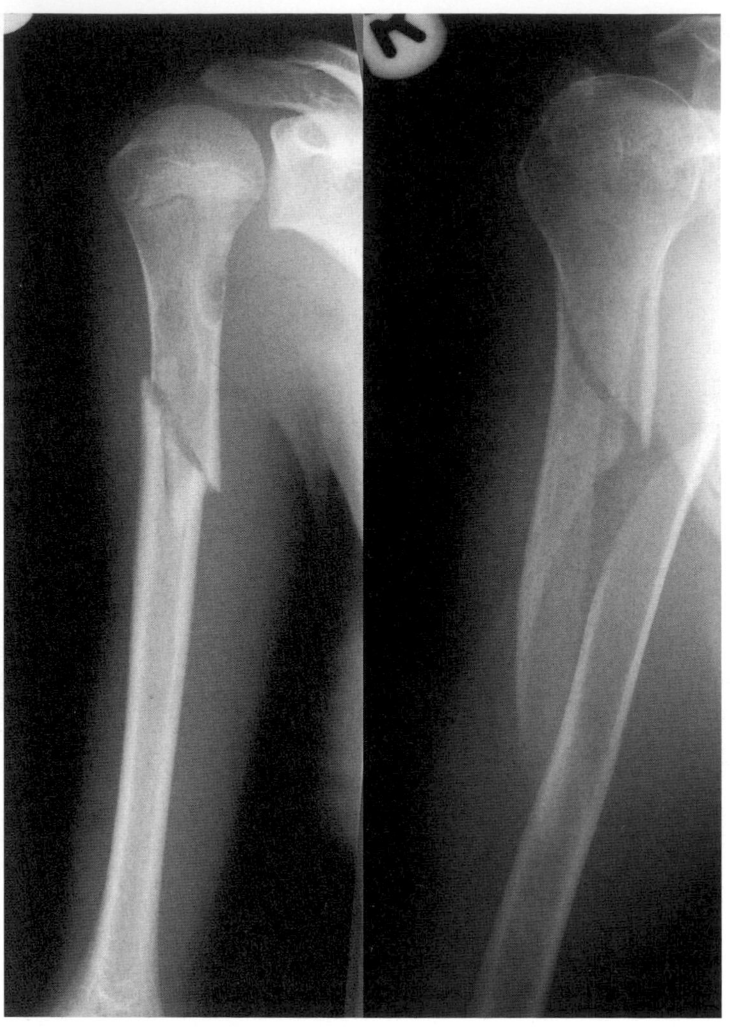

Fig. 7.4 ***A*** *AP and* ***B*** *lateral views of a spiral fracture of the humerus. Note how much more information the lateral view adds in terms of fragmentation, separation and angulation. Note also that the elbow is not on these films.*

Radiography

In theory this is straightforward:

1. A good AP in full extension.

2. A nice lateral in 90° of flexion.

In reality patients with fractured or dislocated elbows are often locked in various degrees of angulation and the AP, or both films, may have to wait in a young patient until the child is under sedation, and the screaming has subsided.

NB Ultrasound, CT and MRI, as elsewhere, may be useful in complex injuries, moving on from conventional radiography.

Anatomy

The anatomy of the fully developed adult elbow is shown in Figure 7.5.

Important points to remember

- **NB The head of the radius is at the elbow.** The radial styloid at the wrist is frequently incorrectly referred to as the 'head' on X-ray request forms by junior doctors and others who should know better.
- The humerus has 'epicondyles', not 'condyles' like the femur.
- The word 'trochlea' means 'pulley'. Just picture the forearm being hauled up by the biceps. This lies on the medial side.
- The radial head and coronoid process overlap on the lateral view but can be separated by a steep 45° oblique view.

Fat pads

- A small dark triangular fat pad sits in front of the lower humerus and is often visible, with a slightly concave or straight anterior margin (Fig. 7.6).
- There is another fat pad at the back of the joint but this is not visible in normal circumstances.
- These fat pads billow out like sails when an effusion fills the joint in trauma.

Facts about fat pads

- Fat pads are not seen in everybody.

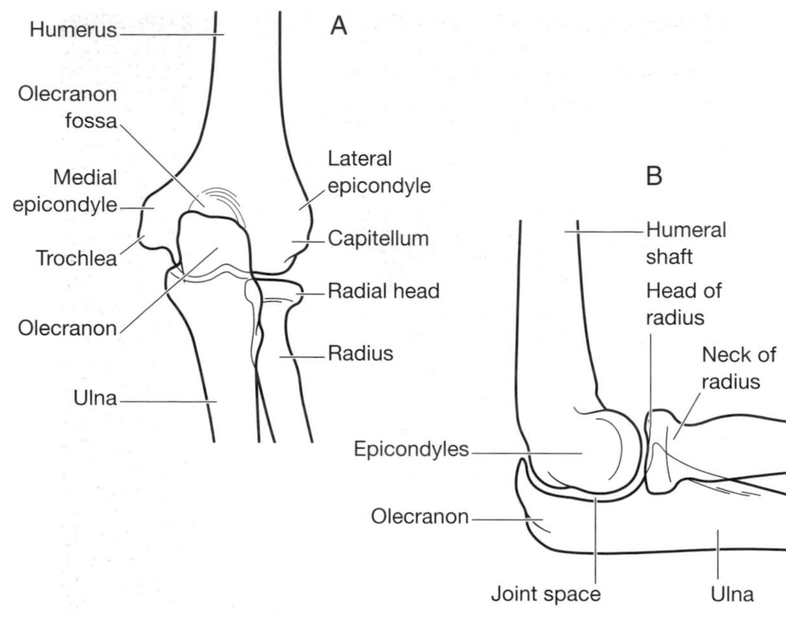

Fig. 7.5 *Anatomy of adult elbow.* ***A*** *AP;* ***B****, lateral.*

- Thin people can have good fat pads (i.e. easy to see).
- Fat people can have poor fat pads (i.e hard to see). (Increased X-ray scatter and decreased contrast.)
- An undisplaced anterior fat pad is normal.
- Any visible posterior fat pad is abnormal, as it is by definition displaced.
- A displaced anterior fat pad is abnormal.
- Displaced fat pads (Fig. 7.7) are caused by effusions or haemarthroses into the joint and in trauma should be regarded as due to a fracture until proved otherwise, but synovial thickening in rheumatoid disease, or infected pyarthrosis can also have this effect, so obtain a proper history.

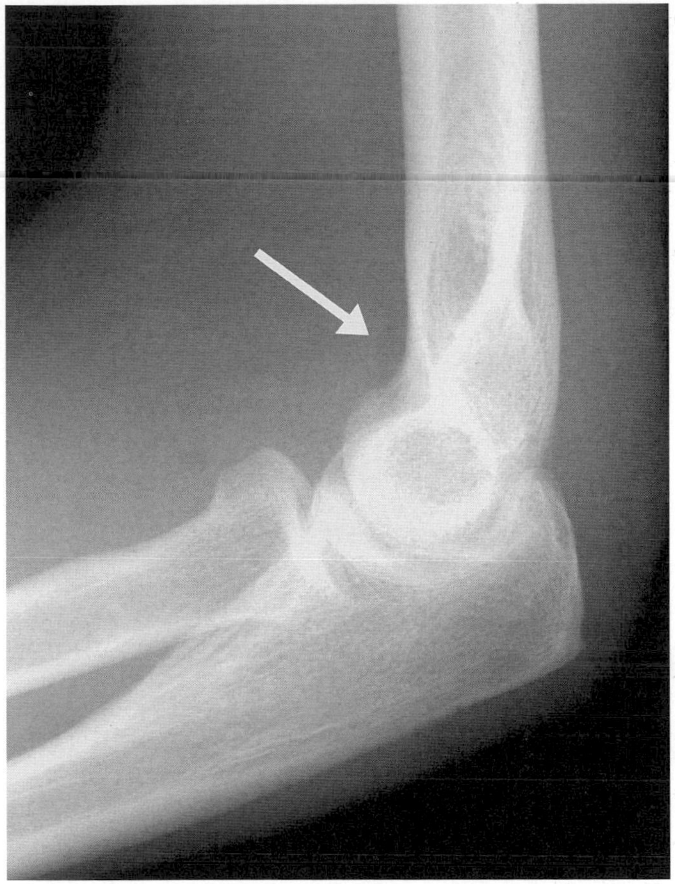

Fig. 7.6 *Elbow – the normal anterior fat pad.*

- Rupture of the joint capsule (a severe injury) may prevent displacement of the fat pads, as the effusion or blood will have leaked out of the joint. Any fracture should, however, be visible.
- **NB** The absence of fat pad displacement does not exclude a fracture.

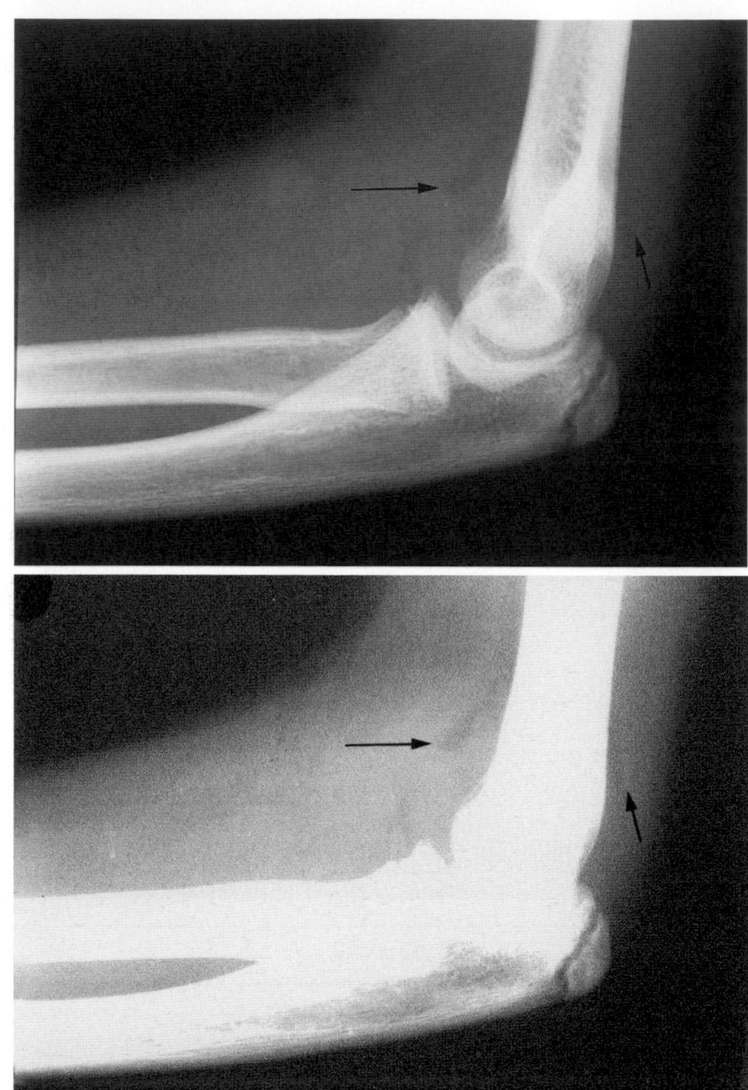

Fig. 7.7 *Elbow – displaced fat pads. Lateral views:* **A** *for bone density;* **B** *set to highlight soft tissue structures. Dark films may require bright lights to see them.*

- If you cannot see a fracture but do see an effusion it is probably due to a crack fracture of the radial head in an adult and a supracondylar fracture in a child.
- **NB** Oblique views of an elbow might obscure the fat pads but may show a fracture.

Hint. Radiologists' eyes hunt straight away for displaced fat pads when confronted with elbow films, before they even look at the bones. Just seeing a normal anterior fat pad usually means that you are probably not dealing with a fracture.

Dislocation of the elbow (Fig. 7.8)

NB Fifty per cent of elbow dislocations have associated fractures. The X-ray diagnosis of dislocation is relatively easy, although gross swelling may impede the clinical examination. The purpose of an X-ray is to document the injury and to confirm or exclude any coexistent fractures.

Complications Check for vascular and neurological injuries. Considerable stiffness of the joint may be a long-term sequel following reduction.

Fractures of the adult elbow

- As usual, fractures may only be visible on one view, hence the need for a minimum of two (ideally two views at right angles, or as close to this as possible). Remember the aphorism 'one view is no view', or may effectively turn out to be pretty close to it (Fig. 13.15, p. 285).
- Dramatic fractures visible at first sight obviate the need for assessing the fat pads.
- Remember with elbow fractures that the proximal radius and ulna are part of a ring (see below) so be sure you have considered, and if necessary X-rayed, **the forearm right down to the wrist** in case of an associated fracture or dislocation at the distal ends or on the way down there.

Exotic views exist to isolate the head and neck of the radius, and 'round the clock' views were taken at one time to hunt for fractures, **but you will not find a fracture in every case. Besides you must know when to stop pouring radiation**

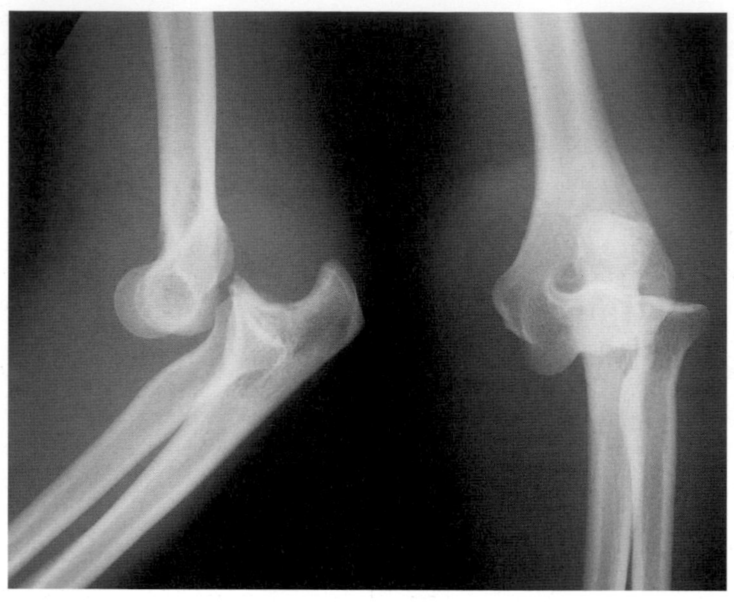

Fig. 7.8 ***A*** *Lateral and* ***B*** *AP showing posterior dislocation of the elbow.*

into patients. If you are stuck go and ask someone with a bigger brain than yourself what the films show. He or she may see the fracture you missed.

A word about ossification centres

In babies, there is only a large radiolucent gap (due to cartilage) where later the familiar adult bony elbow will be. The elbow develops as bony ossification centres appear **in predetermined sequence,** usually conforming to the well-known acronym and mnemonic 'CRITOL', which stands for:

Capitellum
Radial head
Internal (medial) epicondyle
Trochlea
Olecranon
Lateral (external) epicondyle

The times of appearance can vary by as much as 2 years and there are typically differences between girls and boys, but all should be visible by the age of 12 years and later coalesce. The crucial fact, however, is that the trochlea usually only appears after the medial epicondyle. **So if the trochlear epiphysis is visible, there should already be a medial epicondyle present as well.**

The normal medial epicondyle

Look carefully at Figure 7.9, the normal paediatric elbow, and study carefully the appearance and position of the medial epicondyle. This can be avulsed and separated from the main body of the humerus – 'little leaguer's elbow' – and is fairly easy to spot if you know what you are looking for. In extreme cases, however, it drops right down into the elbow joint and the novice observer mistakes it for a 'normal epiphysis' of the capitellum (Fig. 7.10).

Avoid this mistake!

The developing paediatric elbow in A & E

It is probably true to say that more than one A & E doctor over the years has prayed that those paediatric elbow films requested at 4.45 p.m. would not come back until after 5 p.m. when he or she was off duty. Such is the fear of the paediatric elbow. This fear, while understandable, is not really necessary, as long as a few simple facts are understood and major questions about the medial epicondyle are answered at the outset. So, in summary:

Question 1: Does this child have a trochlear epiphysis?
Answer: If yes, he will also already have a visible epiphysis for the medial epicondyle.

Question 2: Where is the epiphysis of the medial epicondyle?
Possible answers:

1. Normal position

2. Avulsed and partially displaced

3. Avulsed, totally displaced and dropped into the medial joint compartment.

If (2) or (3) obtain, the child requires active treatment and reduction with referral to orthopaedics.

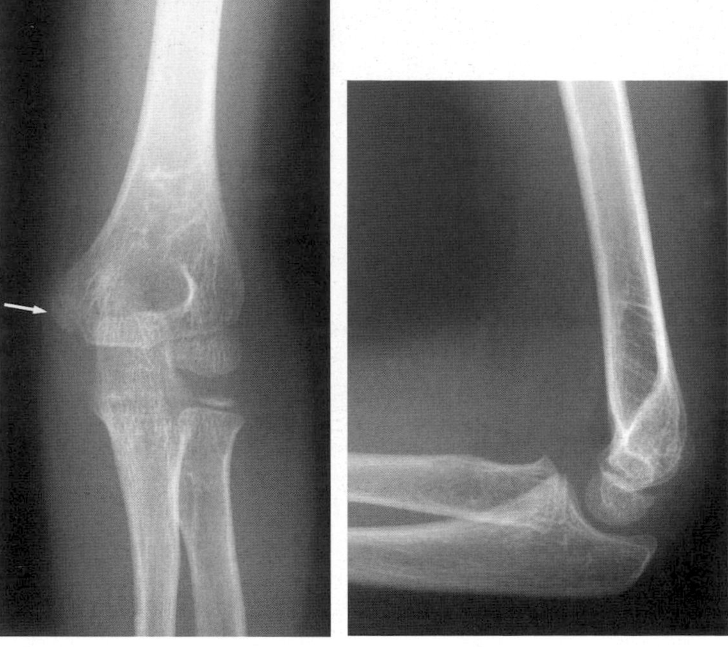

Fig. 7.9 ***A*** *AP and* ***B*** *lateral of a normal developing paediatric elbow. Note the position of the medial epicondyle (arrow) and that the trochlear epiphysis has already appeared.*

The elbow: normal variants

Obviously the paediatric elbow in all its phases of development is demonstrating normal variation. This creates the option of taking a comparative view of the opposite side in difficult cases of suspected fracture but do not expect perfect symmetry on the contralateral side, and get senior advice before re-irradiating a child.

In the elbow a multiplicity of variants exists to make your life difficult. A common one is the incompletely fused olecranon epiphysis (Fig. 7.11). Others include:

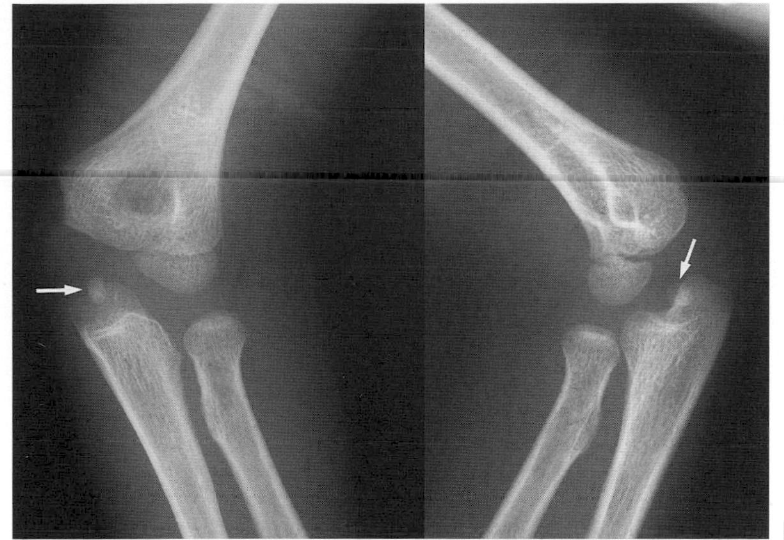

Fig. 7.10 ***A*** *AP and* ***B*** *lateral of a 'little leaguer's elbow'. Avulsed medial epicondyle in joint (note its absence from the normal position).*

- *Skin creases* at the elbow on films in extension, causing false 'fractures' due to lucent lines; these can usually be followed beyond the bones (you also see them at the hip).
- *Faulty positioning* on conventional views, which may cause apparent yawning gaps to appear in epiphyseal lines. A repeat may be necessary.
- *Irregular ossification centres,* which can look traumatized.
- *Thin flanges of bone* above the lateral epicondyle looking like a cortical fracture.

More of this? There is plenty in Keats & Anderson (2001).

Some important geometry

The distal humerus is angulated forwards with a 45° kilter on the lateral view. Absence of this finding is abnormal.

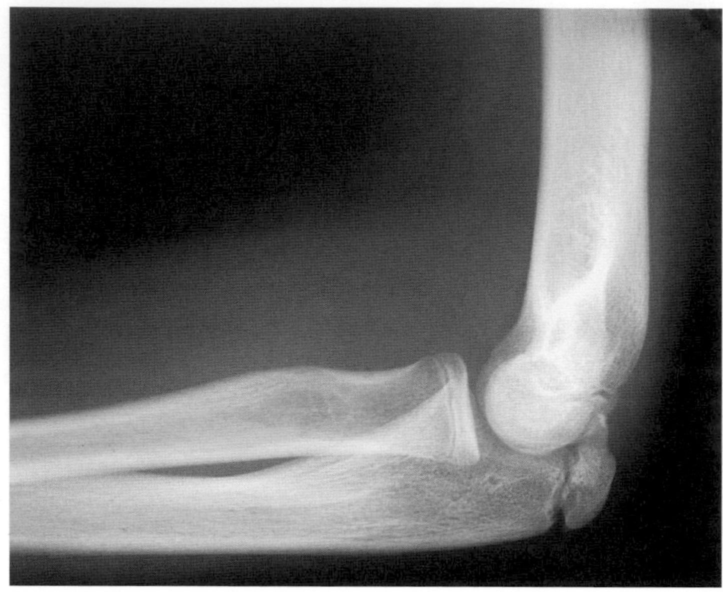

Fig. 7.11 *Normal olecranon epiphysis simulating a fracture.*

- Astute observers in the past have noticed that a line drawn down the anterior edge of the humerus normally traverses the capitellum at a position that still leaves one-third of this structure ahead of it (Fig. 7.12). This applies to adults and childrens' epiphyses. Less than one-third ahead of the line will represent backward displacement and a supracondylar fracture in children.
- A line drawn up the axis of the radius will bisect the capitellum. If it does not, then the radial head is out of position.
- **Crucial fact: Non-displacement of the distal humerus does not exclude a supracondylar fracture;** 45% will have a normal anterior humeral line relationship. This is one of nature's dirty tricks!

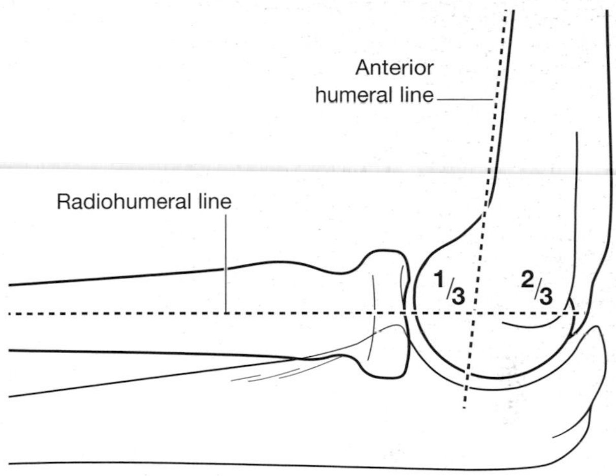

Fig. 7.12 *The anterior humeral and radiohumeral lines (lateral projection).*

Complications of a supracondylar fracture

The worst case scenario is irretrievable occlusion of the brachial artery leading to a 'compartment syndrome', with necrosis of the flexor muscle bellies of the forearm giving rise to the dreaded *Volkmann's ischaemic contracture*. This causes a deformed and useless claw hand and the remains of the muscles may calcify (Fig. 7.14).

Hint: Keep this picture in the front of your mind every time you are dealing with a supracondylar fracture.

NB With an evolving anterior muscle compartment syndrome, **even in the presence of good radial and ulnar pulses,** check for nerve function (motor and sensory) and ask about pain here if the patient has not already volunteered it, as it probably indicates ischaemia.

Pulled elbow

It is natural at times for parents to give their 2–4-year-olds a tug on the arm when they hang back at the sight of a big dog, trip up or want a spin round in the

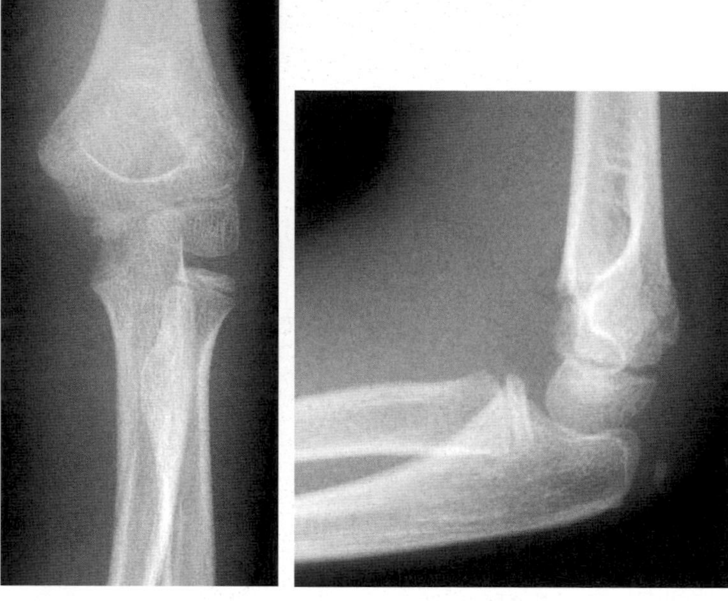

Fig. 7.13 ***A*** *AP and* ***B*** *lateral showing a supracondylar fracture. Note the loss of forward angulation of the distal humerus behind the anterior humeral line. You need a true lateral to make this assessment.*

garden. This can result in the radial head being pulled out of its annular ligament. With a clear history the radial head can potentially just be manipulated back into place, but in these litigious times it is a good idea to X-ray the joint first to prove there is no fracture there. The X-ray should look normal.

Another problem

'He's not using his arm, Doctor.' This can be due to many things, from a fractured clavicle to osteomyelitis of a bone, from a pulled elbow to a non-accidental injury, and includes every cause you can think of from the shoulder

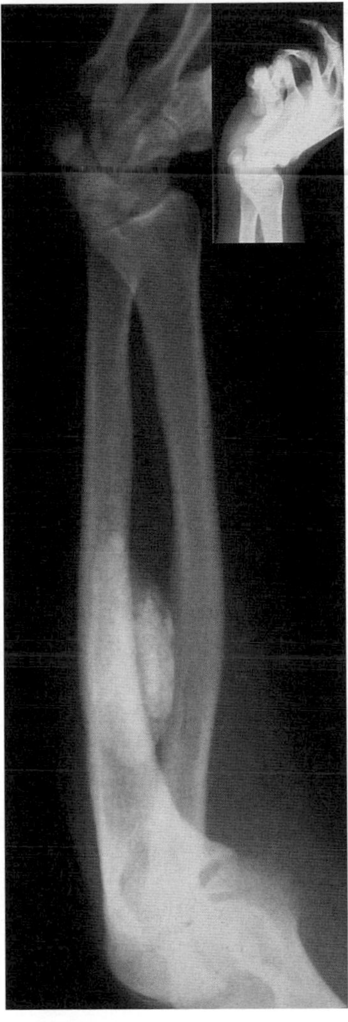

Fig. 7.14 *The dreaded Volkmann's ischaemic contracture. Note the calcified flexor muscle bellies and permanent claw hand (insert).*

girdle down. Time to get your thinking cap on and your brain into top gear. X-rays often get taken as 'an excludogram'.

The forearm

Background

This area comprises the radius and the ulna plus the joints which they form and articulate with at both ends, i.e. the elbow, wrist, the proximal and distal radioulnar joints.

These are classic long bones which largely stand alone on X-rays, but are part of a ring because of their anatomical and functional ligamentous attachments. This means that **after a fall a fracture in one bone or at one end is likely to be associated with a fracture or dislocation at the other**. Think of them therefore as a unit, and if a recognized pattern of trauma appears proximally, make sure you also have X-rays of the lower end taken.

Strangely, this pearl of wisdom is usually universally ignored with Colles' fractures at the wrist!

Radiography

AP and lateral views are the starting points. The position needed to uncross the radius and ulna is with the forearm and hand face up on the cassette. The beam enters from the front (remember the anatomical position?), which makes it an AP. So do not ask for a 'PA and lateral', here. Just request 'forearm please', or 'radius and ulna'. Similarly the frontal view of the knee is an AP. Why?

Crucial point: Long length radius and ulnar films are centred in the middle so the elbow and wrist get projectionally distorted, leading to worries about their unusual appearance at the joints. Optimum assessment may require localized views centred on the joints in question.

Normal variations

Nutrient arterial canals cause thin oblique parallel lucent lines to run through the cortices of the radius and the ulna. A nutrient canal's inner opening will always be more proximal than its distal one in the arm. **Mnemonic:** 'To the elbow I run, from the knee I flee.' Try not to misdiagnose these as fractures, but you will not see them in every patient. When entering the bone, only one cortex will show a lucent line, but never two, with a nutrient canal (see Keats & Anderson 2001). A fracture line will usually go through both.

Tho Italian fractures

There are two forms of injury specific to the forearm worthy of mention; they are named after the Italian surgeons who first described them.

The Galeazzi fracture (Fig. 7.15)

This is usually caused by a fall on the outstretched hand. The essential features are a fracture of the distal radius associated with a dorsally dislocated distal ulna, due to disruption of the distal radioulnar ligament.

NB The configuration of the distal ulna may be difficult to interpret on a lateral wrist film (Fig. 7.16) if the final 5° of supination from the apparent lateral to the true lateral position has not been achieved (p. 165), in which case the normal ulna may look dislocated. Do not fall for this!

Gold Medal point: Some patients have an excessively long ulna ('positive variance') which may normally sit out of place, but a comparative view of the opposite side may show an identical appearance. **NB** Shortening of the radius due to overlap at the fracture site may also simulate or accentuate this.

The Monteggia fracture (Fig. 7.17)

This is trauma to the proximal end of the forearm resulting in a fracture of the proximal ulnar shaft, with associated subluxation or dislocation of the radial head. It is usually caused by a fall on the outstretched hand or direct blow.

Radiology The displacement of the radial head may be subtle, but if necessary AP and lateral views centred on the elbow should be obtained, and, if you specifically look for it, it should be detectable. As usual in this area check the integrity of the radiocapitellar and radiohumeral lines (p. 159). Remember that if you miss this displacement, the patient may later sustain an avascular necrosis of the head of the radius. A positive anterior fat pad sign is also likely to be in evidence.

NB Because of its association with self-defence, this fracture is sometimes known as a 'parry' or 'night-stick injury' when the victim reflexly holds up the arm as a shield against a blow. It is also known as a 'side-swipe injury' due to the

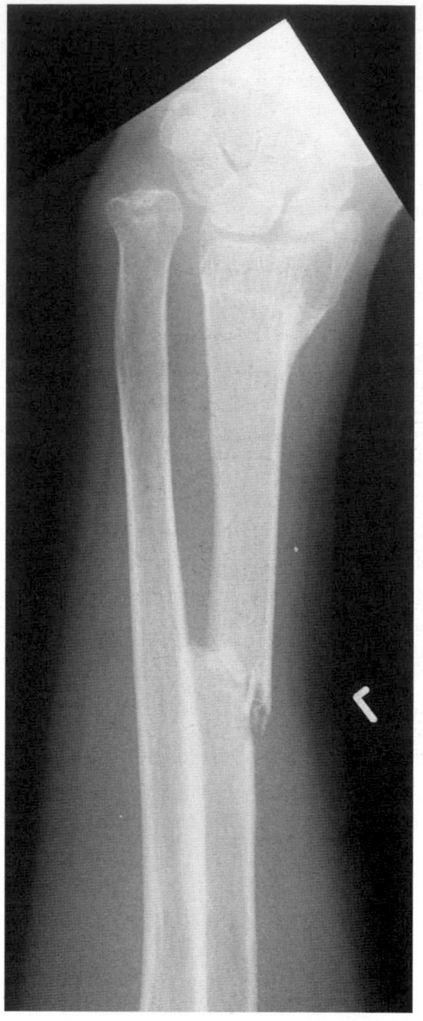

Fig. 7.15 *Galeazzi fracture. Note the dislocated distal radius.*

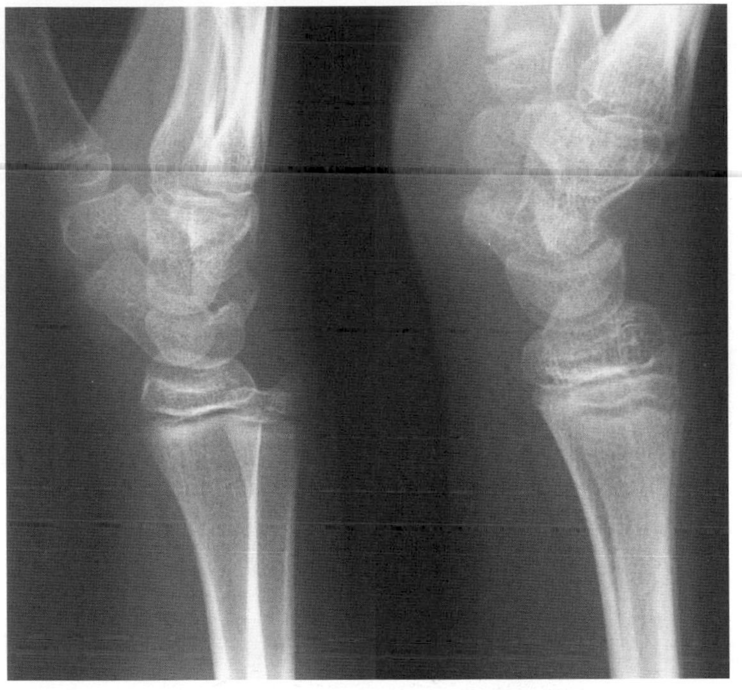

Fig. 7.16 *Spurious displacement of the distal ulna.* ***A*** *Attempted lateral and* ***B*** *true lateral of wrist. The effect of faulty radiographic positioning. Don't fall for this old chestnut!*

habit of some drivers in letting their arms lean out of their cars on a hot day. Collision with an oncoming vehicle's extended mirror or a dog's head may then have serious consequences, especially for the dog!

Moral: 'Don't stick your elbow out too far, it may go home in another car!'

And finally:

Question: How will I remember which is the Monteggia fracture and which is the Galleazzi fracture?

Answer: You won't.

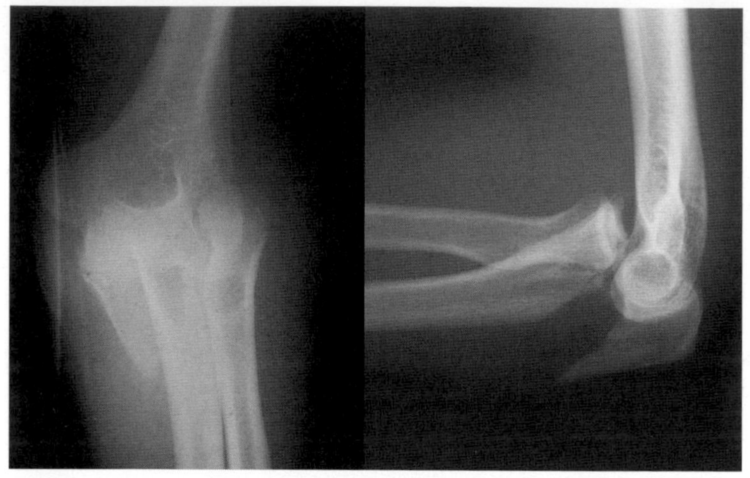

Fig. 7.17 **A** *AP and* **B** *lateral showing a Monteggia fracture.*

The wrist

Background

Wrist injuries constitute a significant proportion of the workload of an A & E department, especially elderly ladies on icy pavements in winter. Sports injuries and martial arts inevitably do their worst – tried breaking a brick in two with the edge of your hand recently?

Crucial point: If a middle-aged woman has broken her wrist she could already be *osteoporotic*, so consider her for further investigation, e.g. bone densitometry. You might later save her from a broken hip. This is called 'looking at the patient as a whole'.

Radiography

The simple PA and lateral views suffice for the initial evaluation of most wrist injuries. Problems arise when these ideal views are not achieved (e.g. due to multiple injuries), although as a basic principle radiographic assessment of peripheral fractures may on occasion be justifiably delayed while more pressing problems are sorted out. See also facial injuries (p. 44).

Attention is again drawn to the classic trap of the undersupinated 'lateral' causing an apparent but spurious 'dislocation' of the lower ulna (Fig. 7.16).

What about the scaphoid? Traditionally a scaphoid series incorporating a PA, lateral and two intermediate obliques have been taken for this (Fig. 7.21). More recently, just a PA, with the hand *in full ulnar deviation*, and a lateral have been advocated as giving reliable results. This opens up the scaphoid, which is foreshortened on the straight PA view. This can usefully be used in all hand and wrist views to give an optimum look at the scaphoid, but there is no doubt even so that if four views are taken the fracture may only show up on one of the projections.

Occult carpal injuries

Anyone who has felt the sting of a cricket bat when the ball strikes, or hit the ground with the bat instead of the ball, may have sustained an occult carpal injury. Carpal tunnel views, or better still CT scanning, may elucidate causes of initially 'X-ray negative' carpal and wrist pain (e.g. a fractured hook of hamate).

Anatomy

'The wrist' is actually a rather loose anatomical term. Strictly speaking it is the joint between the radius, ulna and proximal row of carpal bones. However, if you ask for a 'wrist X-ray', the films you get back will incorporate the wrist joint proper and much of the rest of the hand (Fig. 7.18).

Important points

- **NB** X-ray departments frequently receive requests for the wrist to be X-rayed to assess the 'radial head', by which the requester means the radial styloid.
- **The radial styloid process is not the 'head of radius' – that is at the elbow.** If you thought that it was, revise your anatomy. If you already knew where it was, however, put yourself down for a silver star!
- The carpal bones have names. Don't worry about them – just learn them. (See the mnemonic on page 173).

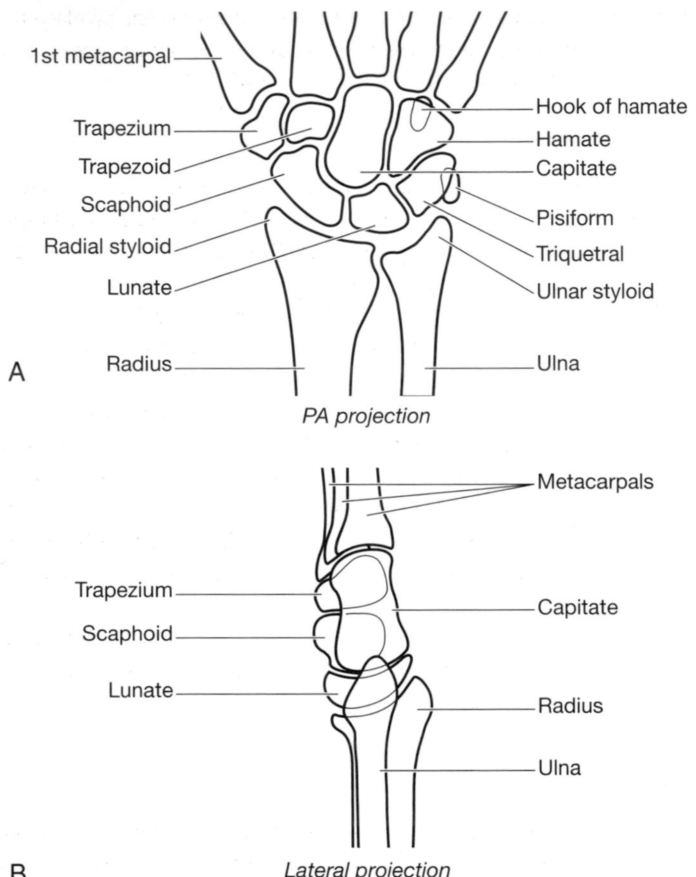

Fig. 7.18 *Anatomy of the wrist.* ***A*** *PA;* ***B*** *lateral.*

- As in the knee joint and ankle joint, for instance, the wrist has cartilage in it. Do not forget that it may have been injured although you cannot see it on an X-ray. Your patient may need an MRI scan to elucidate it.

Normal variants

Like the elbow, the wrist of a baby is just a dark cartilaginous space. Slowly the little round carpal bones pop out as they ossify. A chart showing their times of arrival is useful in A & E. If necessary, a comparative view of the opposite side is helpful in difficult cases (with senior permission).

The adolescent wrist can cause diagnostic problems: a small spicule of bone at the radial side of the line of closure of the distal radial epiphysis can be mistaken for a fracture, as can spicules within the line itself.

In the adult a multitude of accessory ossicles can infest the wrist right round the edge of every bone – each resplendent with its own Latin name from the 'os epilunatum' to the 'os styloideum'. These place you on the horns of an intellectual dilemma, usually just at the moment when the patient pipes up with 'Everything's alright, isn't it doctor?': are they the result of trauma or is it normal variation? Look for cortication, indicating oldness, then make a bee-line for Keats & Anderson (2001).

Be aware also that the position of closure of the distal radial epiphysis can leave a dense line or scar which **should not be mistaken for an impacted fracture**.

The Irish fractures

The names of two Dublin surgeons are perpetuated in a couple of important injuries which may occur at the wrist, namely the Colles' fracture and the Smith's fracture.

Colles' fracture (Fig. 7.19)

(Note: His name was Colles, hence the position of the apostrophe.) In simple terms this is a fracture of the distal radius due to a fall on the outstretched hand, classically with dorsal displacement of the distal fragment producing a 'dinner-fork deformity' on the lateral view. It may be associated with a fracture of the ulnar styloid process, impaction and/or various degrees of comminution.

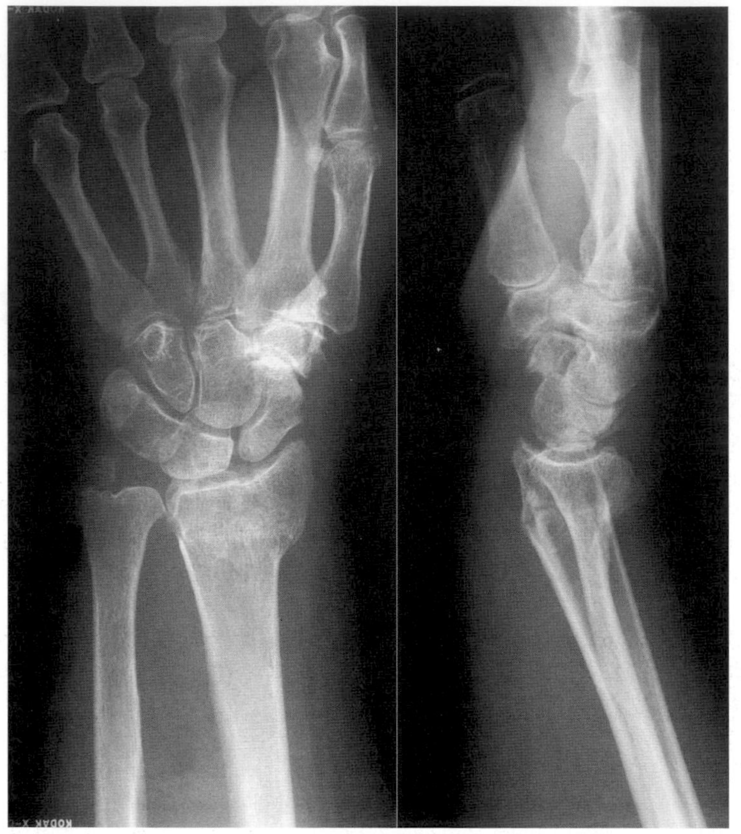

Fig. 7.19 ***A*** *PA and* ***B*** *lateral showing a Colles' fracture with typical 'dinner fork' deformity.*

Important point: An assessment needs to be made as to whether this injury needs to be reduced or can be left, usually with some residual dysfunction of flexion and supination. The distal articular surface of the radius normally points downwards 5°. More than 15° of dorsal angulation of the distal fragment relative to the main shaft will usually be regarded as an indication for reduction.

Point of interest: The Colles' fracture is known as a 'Pouteau fracture' in Europe.

Smith's fracture

Commonly known as a 'reverse Colles' fracture', this occurs when the distal fragment is forced forwards due to a fall impacting on the back of the hand.

So much for our trip to The Emerald Isle.

Other important wrist and carpal injuries

Barton's fracture This is a crack fracture on the dorsal aspect of the distal radius that extends into the wrist joint. A 'reverse Barton's fracture' occurs on the anterior aspect and also extends into the joint.

Crucial fact: Remember, fractures that extend to articular surfaces carry a less favourable prognosis than those that do not, due to the liklihood of associated articular cartilage injury and the early onset of osteoarthritis. Damage to the triangular fibrocartilage of the wrist may therefore occur, for example, and MRI is now the modality of choice in the further assessment of such injuries.

'The chauffeur's fracture' For those sufficiently well off to have done things in style and owned a Rolls Royce in the 'Good Old Days', the occasional sudden backfire of the starting handle at the front of the engine could easily fracture the chauffeur's radial styloid. Modern cars no longer offer this facility, and one has to make do with a rather vulgar ignition key.

NB Not all wrist fractures are obvious, particularly at the outset. If strongly symptomatic, repeat the films in 10–14 days, do a bone scan or MRI examination. **Once again: Treat the patient, not the X-ray.**

What about kids? (wrinkles and crinkles)

The wrist is a common place to see a 'torus' fracture in children (Fig. 7.20), i.e. a wrinkle across the distal radius, or a greenstick injury with crinkling of the cortex on one side and plastic bowing on the other. (Fracture types, p. 140).

Greater trauma in children may cause more serious fractures and displacements of the distal radial epiphysis, at which point you need to revisit the Salter–Harris classification (p. 142).

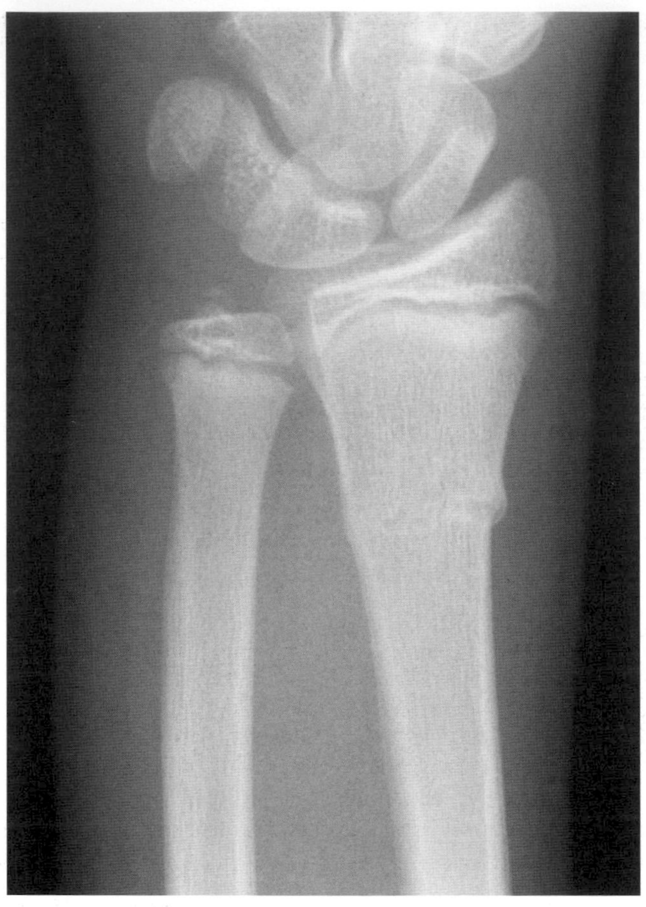

Fig. 7.20 *Torus fracture.*

Revelations about the carpus

Consider this. With the de-emphasis of anatomy now so endemic in many UK medical schools, many students can qualify as junior doctors and still be unable to confidently point out the names of the bones of the carpus, and are quite open about it. In a way this is understandable because, apart from the early instruction in bone anatomy at the beginning of the course, there is little application for this knowledge unless one is later going to be an anatomist, an orthopaedic surgeon, a radiologist – or an A & E doctor.

Mnemonics abound to help scholars try to remember the names of the bones in the hand; here is one:

Some	Scaphoid
Lawyers	Lunate
Take	Triquetral
Physicians	Pisiform
To	Trapezium
The	Trapezoid
Court	Capitate
House	Hamate

The medicolegal overtones will not be lost upon you during your trip to the Royal Courts of Justice!

Carpus injuries

- Like the paediatric elbow (and the tarsal bones in the foot), X-rays of the carpal bones of the hand can induce a phobic reaction in the new A & E doctor.
- **Megahint: If you haven't learnt them before you start in A & E, each time you are confronted with a wrist X-ray force yourself to point out and name each bone in the carpus to yourself until it becomes second nature.** Then do the same with the tarsal bones in the foot. When you have learnt them all, put yourself down for a silver star!
- It is also a good idea to **count** them. There should be eight. Finding 'nine' may suddenly reveal that you are dealing with an old ununited fracture of the scaphoid, accessory ossicle or foreign body (p. 310).

- There are two neat smooth rows of carpal bones like pieces of a plastic puzzle sweeping out in graceful arcs and articulating together. About 2 mm normally separates each bone from the other in each direction.
- The most important common fracture to look for is in the scaphoid and the most common dislocations are of (1) the lunate, and (2) the rest of the carpal bones around the lunate (perilunar dislocation).

The scaphoid

The overwhelming majority of carpal fractures (around 90%) occur in the scaphoid, a dinky little bone shaped like a cashew nut; however, around 20% of scaphoid fractures are invisible at the first X-ray examination and many patients initially suspected of having a scaphoid fracture turn out not to do so, despite yelping when the anatomical snuff box is pressed.

Radiography

PA, lateral and two obliques – the scaphoid series (Fig. 7.21).

Traditionally the approach to the dilemma outlined above was to treat every clinically suspect fracture of the scaphoid as a definite fracture, i.e. put it in a plaster and re-X-ray it in 10–14 days. If a fracture was then visualized by way of a lucent or dense line which was not there before, its presence was regarded as established and the plaster (removed for the second X-ray examination) reapplied. If no fracture was found, the patient was discharged. However, it is now known that it can actually take 6 weeks for an initially radio-occult fractured scaphoid to appear on X-ray.

More recent attempts to evaluate the traumatized scaphoid have shown that MRI can be exquisitely sensitive in picking up fresh fractures at the first examination, i.e. after just a few days, with a dedicated extremity unit. If a patient is still symptomatic at 14 days but radiologically negative at that time, an MRI will then be justified and the beauty of it is you do not even have to remove the plaster.

A bone scan can also be helpful if X-rays remain negative and MRI is not available, and others have used ultrasound and CT to look at this problem.

Inevitably MRI will, on occasion, show up injuries in the adjacent carpal bones that have also gone undetected on X-ray. By the time you are a consultant or a professor, of course, everything in A & E may well be done by MRI. Junior doctors will then really have their work cut out, being first to try to read the films.

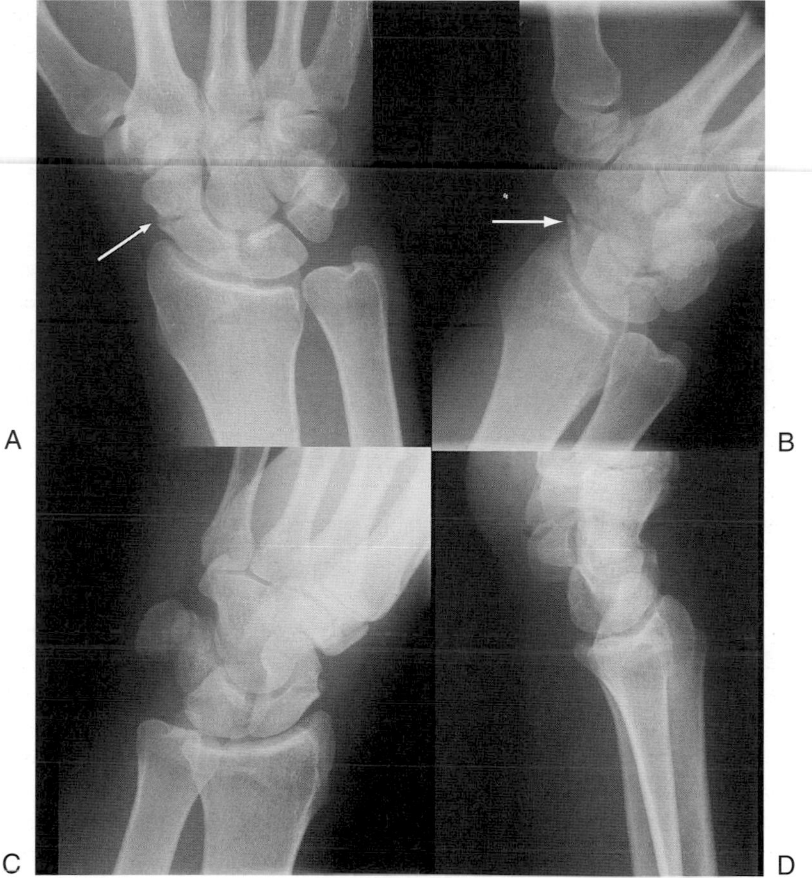

Fig. 7.21 *Scaphoid series with a fracture through the waist of the scaphoid (arrow).* ***A*** *PA,* ***B*** *PA oblique,* ***C*** *AP oblique,* ***D*** *lateral.*

Just be glad that we are still using the old 'steam X-rays' in the meantime.

X-ray appearances

Trying to decide whether or not there is a fracture in the scaphoid can be very difficult. If you gaze at it long enough, as with any other bone the 'fortuitous alignment of trabeculae' will often erroneously cause the brain to join up the dark bits between the trabeculae and lead to the false perception of a fracture – one of the hazards of staring at a film for too long.

Other normal variants include notches in and bumps on the scaphoid, and accessory carpal bones alongside the scaphoid itself. An old ununited scaphoid fracture will occasionally be present in some patients but this should have sclerotic margins – do not mistake it for another normal carpal joint. Counting the bones should prevent this. An old avascular necrosis will involve the proximal half of the bone as the scaphoid frequently has a dodgy blood supply entering from the distal pole, so it is the proximal part that disintegrates. (Great multiple choice question!)

Hint: Look hard at the scaphoid on routine wrist films (PA and lateral) and encourage your radiographers to put the hand into 'ulnar deviation' for these, so that you get an optimum view of the scaphoid.

If in doubt, treat a suspicious scaphoid as a fracture and proceed accordingly.

The triquetral

Golden rule: Look carefully at the dorsum of the carpus on wrist films. Flake fractures from the back of the carpus come off the triquetral.

Other carpal bones

Any of the other carpal bones may fracture, but less commonly than the scaphoid. 'Carpal tunnel views' are dated but may occasionally reveal an initially radio-occult fracture; a CT scan of the carpus would nowadays be preferable, easier for the patient to bear and for a high-tech trained radiographer to do.

Dislocations of the carpus

Warning! These are likely to be missed without an eagle eye and a keen knowledge of the relevant anatomy, but are relatively easy to pick up if you know what you're looking for. (This of course is true of *every* abnormality on *every* X-ray.)

Dislocated lunate

Look at Figure 7.22. On the PA film note:

- The overall positioning is good.
- No joint space is visible between the scaphoid and lunate bones and the dark space between the proximal and distal row is interrupted.
- Instead of having a rounded quadrilateral appearance, the lunate has become triangular and shaped like an onion.

On the lateral view note:

- The distal radius has no close bony surface running parallel to it.

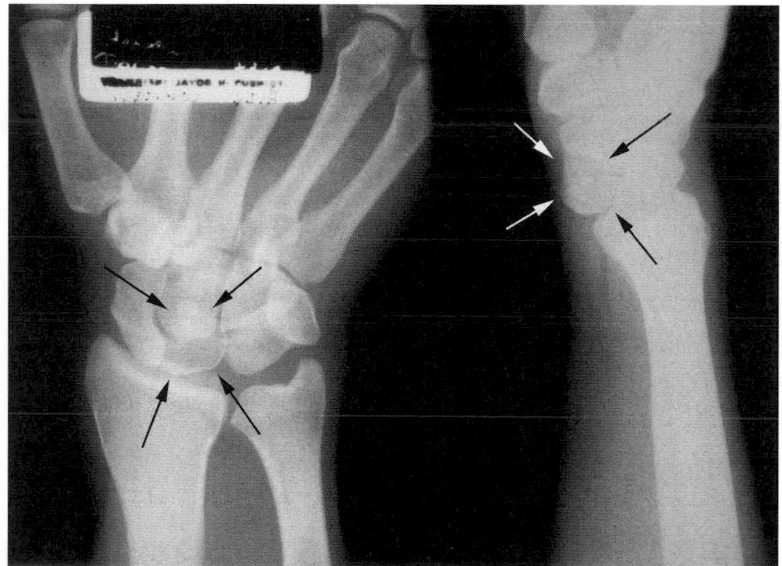

Fig. 7.22 ***A*** *PA and* ***B*** *lateral showing anterior dislocation of the lunate.*

- The lunate has up-ended itself, like a banana or slice of orange standing on its end, and has popped out forwards from the carpus, filling the space anteriorly, which is usually empty.

Conclusion: This is an *anterior dislocation of the lunate* (the rest of the carpal bones are where they should be). Learn to recognize it.

Perilunar dislocation

In this injury the lunate stays put but the rest of the carpus moves back en bloc, leaving the concavity of the lunate empty again and nothing to articulate with distally (Fig. 7.23), although it is still parked normally with the radius behind it.

The diagnosis comes from the lateral view where the large capitate bone dominates and overhangs the lunate posteriorly, being offset like a bayonet.

NB The concavity of the lunate should always be articulating distally with another bone. If it is not, there is a dislocation.

Crucial point: With any dislocation, look for a fracture. Often the scaphoid fractures in this clinical situation, giving rise to a so-called *trans-scaphoid perilunar dislocation*.

Further carpal subluxations

As we have seen, there is a fairly uniform smooth separation of the joints of the wrist and carpus of about 2 mm, although different projections may apparently diminish this. Occasionally gaps wider than this will be seen, particularly between the scaphoid and the lunate, and following trauma this should be regarded as a scapholunate subluxation or *rotary dislocation of the scaphoid*, and further advice sought. Clinically a 'clunk' may occur on moving the hand from the radial to the ulnar side. This gap is known as the 'Terry Thomas sign' after the suave and sophisticated (but now deceased) English actor, renowned for his cravat, cigarette holder and the famous gap between his front teeth.

Point of interest: Such an appearance can sometimes be seen in certain individuals without trauma as a sign of degeneration.

Carpometacarpal and metacarpal injuries

When a hand X-ray is requested, the standard PA and PA oblique views between

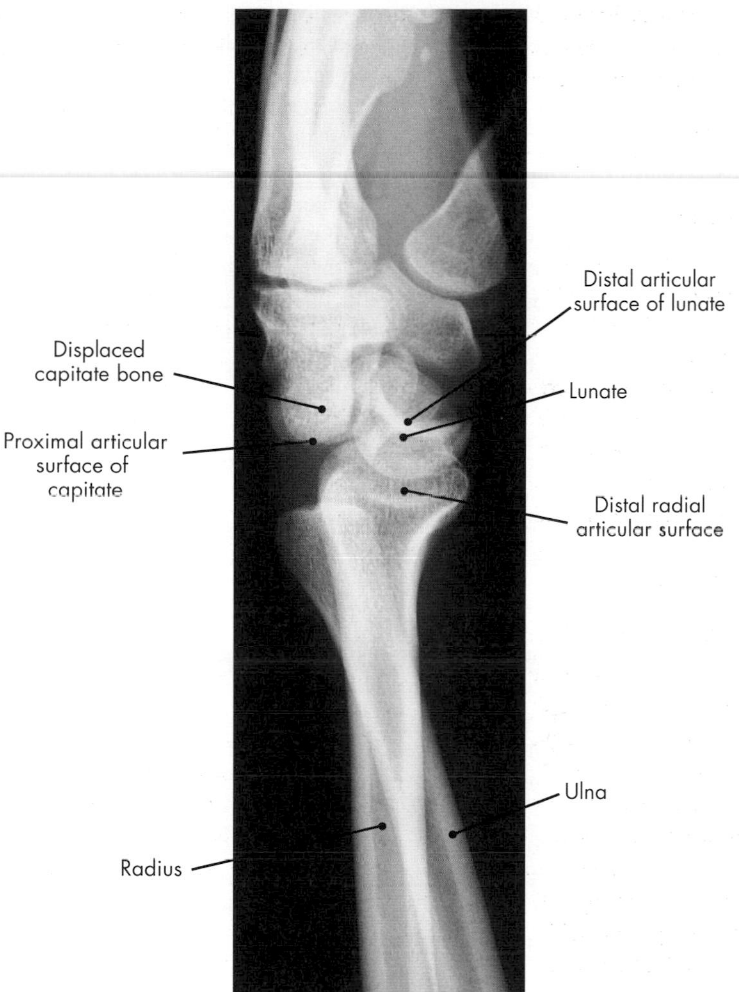

Fig. 7.23 *Perilunar dislocation.*

them will normally permit visualization of all the carpometacarpal joints. If one or more of these joints cannot be discerned between the two views due to bony overlap, a dislocation is likely and further advice should be sought. Remember, as you will see in the foot, the first three metacarpals each rest on their own carpal bone, trapezium, trapezoid and capitate, and the last two (4th and 5th) share the hamate at their base (p. 168).

Important point: This is a difficult location to inspect, with the temptation just to let the eye slide over it and the naughty voice inside you say 'It's probably OK' so that you can write 'No gross abnormality' in the notes. Don't do it! You know your job is to find the joint lines, so do it! Fractures may also complicate the issue but if you obey the golden rule and **look right round the edge of every bone** you should find them, so always check for congruity at the joint margins.

Normal variants

Important diagnostic traps here include accessory secondary ossification centres in young children. Knowing these can occur is half the battle, and residual cortical clefts may persist into later life. Look for the old friends of rounded edges and corticated margins which will help you to arrive at the right conclusions.

Thumbs and things

NB Injuries to the thumb warrant individual X-ray examinations, i.e. a PA or AP, whichever the patient and radiographer can achieve, and a lateral view even though trauma to this structure may be visible on full hand films. Remember the thumb has only one interphalangeal joint, so do not call it the 'PIP' or 'DIP', proximal interphalangeal or distal interphalangeal joint.

Bennett's fracture This is a fracture of the base of the first metacarpal with extension into the carpometacarpal joint, usually disconnecting and displacing the main body of the first metacarpal from a smaller fragment. Because it is unstable it may necessitate internal fixation.

'Gamekeeper's thumb' (or 'skier's thumb') (Fig. 7.24) Due to sudden wrenching, the ulnar collateral ligament of the metacarpophalangeal joint of the thumb may rupture, with or without a bony avulsion. If no fracture has occurred, the initial X-ray may look normal. A stress view (if necessary with sedation) will, however, demonstrate instability of the joint and the need for surgical repair.

Point of interest: One can quite easily imagine a ski-stick wrenching a 'hot

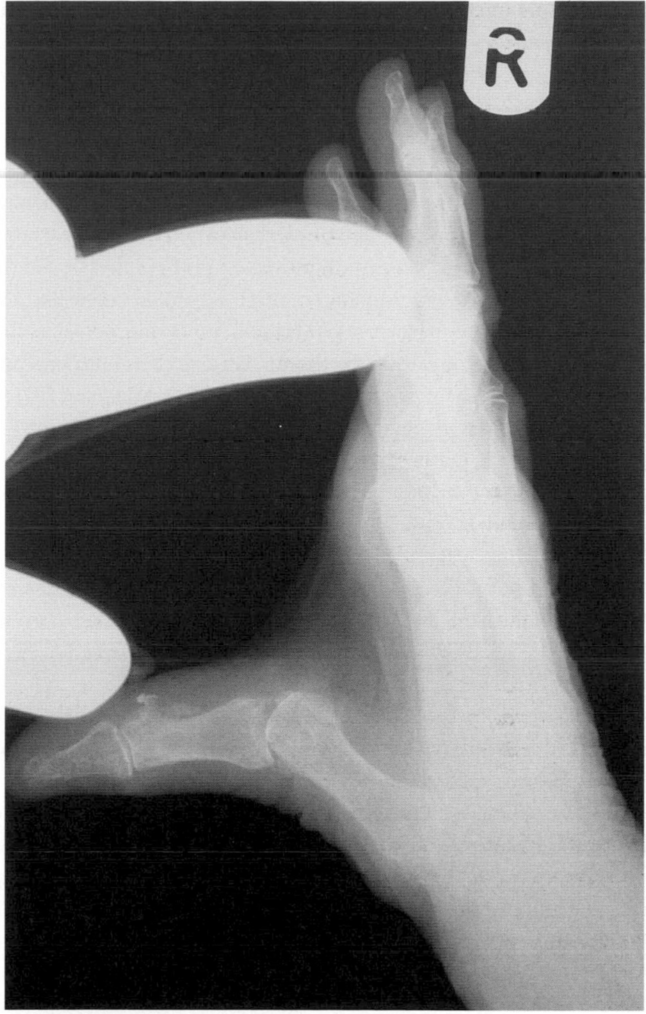

Fig. 7.24 *Gamekeeper's or skier's thumb. The joint is being stressed by the hand of the radiologist wearing a lead glove.*

dogging' skier's thumb as he tries to emulate James Bond being pursued by the bad guys in the snow.

Metacarpals and phalanges

NB A completely mangled hand is a job for a hand surgeon from the outset and, although X-rays will be needed, a careful neurovascular assessment must be made. Most A & E cases comprise fractures, dislocations and avulsions of lesser degree. The juvenile hand contains multiple developing epiphyses, and the adult thumb and digits will frequently contain multiple sesamoid ('seed-like') bones in the flexor tendons, at the metacarpophalangeal joints and occasionally at the interphalangeal joints, especially in the thumb. Various clefts, nutrient canals and tiny particles of bone also infest this region (see Keats & Anderson 2001).

NB The bones of the fingers are frequently found to have receded into the moonlight of a hand X-ray because the wrist and hand are much thicker and denser than the fingers but are subjected to the same exposures. So if you are not 'on digital', use the bright light.

Inspection of the bones of the hand is laborious; if you do not find it so, you are not doing it properly. There is a great deal of coastline to cover, but remember: do not just look at the hand as a whole, **look right round the edge of every bone.**

Metacarpal fractures (Fig. 7.25)

One of the commonest injuries is the *Boxer's fracture,* a fracture of the neck of the 5th metacarpal due to striking the opponent's jaw. This is usually associated with forward angulation. A steeper oblique will show angulation better, but ultimately a true lateral may be required to assess the actual degree of forward angulation and see whether it is such that reduction is required. Picking out the one you want from the 'row of soldiers' on the lateral film is not always easy, especially if there are two injuries, but usually the fracture can be seen. Tracing out the different lengths of each bone may help you to identify the one you want.

Spiral fractures These are common in the metacarpals but require careful clinical assessment to decide on the rotational component, as internal fixation may be required.

Phalangeal injuries

NB These are often *small* injuries that may cause *big* clinical problems of

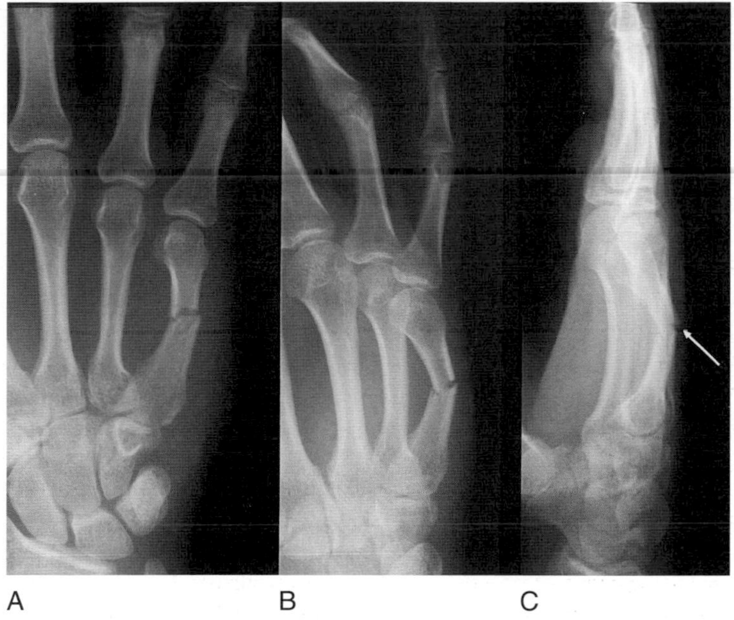

Fig. 7.25 ***A*** *PA,* ***B*** *oblique and* ***C*** *lateral views showing a fracture of the shaft of the 5th metacarpal. Note how the degree of forward angulation is optimally demonstrated on the lateral, and completely unappreciable on the PA.*

impaired hand function if missed. Some crucial soft tissue anatomy here relates to:

- *The collateral ligaments,* which bind the heads of each proximal or middle phalanx to the base of the next distal one.
- *The volar plate,* which is the thickened joint capsule on the palmar aspects of the joints between the phalanges.
- *The extensor tendons,* which insert into the bases of the phalanges on their dorsal aspects.

Crucial fact: Each of their attachments may be avulsed and the implications of tiny chip fractures at these positions should be appreciated and clinical integrity of the ligaments sought.

The mallet injury (Fig. 7.26) In this condition the extensor tendon is avulsed from the terminal phalanx, with or without a bony fragment, so that the end of the finger droops and loses its power of extension, or cannot be extended against resistance.

NB Only one-quarter of patients will take a bony fragment off the terminal phalanx as well, so a careful clinical examination is vital to assess whether an avulsion has occurred. An untreated or flail terminal phalanx can be surprisingly disabling for anyone, particularly, for example, for a dextrous manual worker or a professional pianist. A corresponding injury may occur on the flexor surface.

Moral: Do a thorough clinical examination of the hands and a meticulous assessment of the X-rays of the bones.

Interphalangeal dislocations These joints can be dislocated by trauma as well as arthropathies (Fig. 7.27). Note the malalignment on the PA view. Lateral views are needed for a full evaluation. Some unfortunates suffer double dislocations (as here).

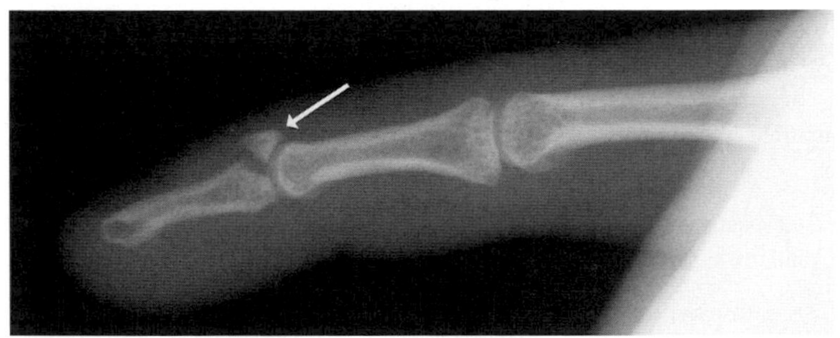

Fig. 7.26 *Mallet injury of terminal phalanx.*

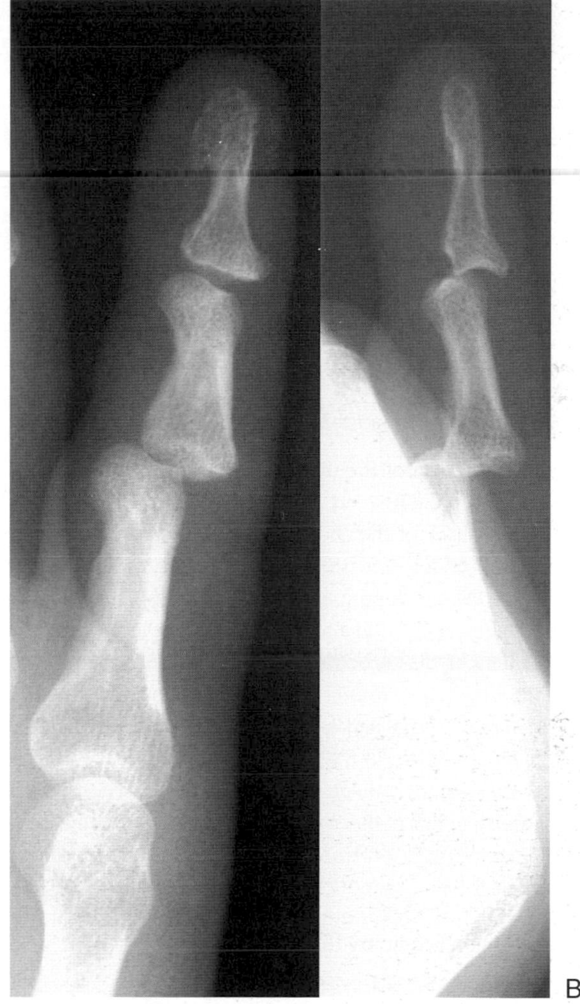

Fig. 7.27 ***A*** *PA film and* ***B*** *lateral film of a double interphalangeal dislocation of the 5th finger. Dislocations require laterals for optimum assessment.*

Chapter 8

Upper airway obstruction

Background: danger of sudden death

Foreign body obstruction of the upper airway is an **acute medical emergency** which may require urgent first aid, if you cannot extract the object by hand, such as a thump on the back of the chest in the head down position or a Heimlich manoeuvre, with sudden upward compression by your fist from below the xiphisternum via the enveloping arms from behind. Classically these incidents will not occur in hospital, but in a restaurant with a piece of meat, or in the home when a child inhales a plastic bottle top.

Usually the first-aiders among the other diners will have pounced on the 'obstructee' before you have had a chance to wipe the vegetable soup away and respond to 'Is there a doctor in the house?'

Hint: If the restaurant patient is a huge fat man whom you are unable to envelope for the Heimlich manoeuvre, sit him in a chair and compress him from the front against the wall. Stridor is a dangerous sign, so call the emergency services if you hear it and cannot clear the obstruction.

'There's something stuck in my throat, doctor!'

Much more common in A & E is the non-occluding but desperately unpleasant sensation of a fish bone or a chicken bone stuck in the throat.

Question: What if I inhale and choke on something when I am alone?
Answer: This requires great presence of mind. If you can 'keep the heid' (stay calm), as the Scots say, and breathe in very slowly past the obstruction you may get enough air behind to eject it with a big cough.

X-Rays of the upper airway

Usually only one film is required here, namely a good lateral view of the neck, but set for a *soft tissue exposure*. This gives a good view of the oropharynx, nasopharnyx and laryngeal regions, but the cervical spine will tend to look rather white. Occasionally you will have to go on to chest X-rays, plus or minus a lateral and abdominal X-rays for elusive foreign bodies (p. 305).

Anatomy and physiology

NB A lot of crucial anatomy *and physiology* can catch you out in this region.

Some normal structures

- *The larynx.* Look at Figure 8.1. This may look very dramatically and irregularly calcified; or there may just be calcification at the superior cornu of the thyroid lamina or an isolated sliver of calcification at the posterior cricoid lamina, both of which may be mistaken for chicken bones. On AP films of the neck, two obliquely lying and slightly diverging thyroid laminae may be visible over the lower cervical spine – laid back like a couple of opposing London Millennium Dome masts. Somebody sometime is sure to try and sell you these as 'calcified vertebral arteries'. The vertebral arteries *never* calcify.

- *The hyoid bone.* This sits horizontally at the level of the C3/4 disc and may be partially or completely ossified. Calcification in all or in parts of the stylohyoid ligaments (Fig. 8.1) may be present, extending from the styloid processes at the base of the skull to the hyoid bone, and simulate big chicken bones to novices.

- **Hint:** If the film is slightly oblique or angulated you should usually see *two!* This is a guiding principle. *Obliquity should duplicate normal structures.* There should only ever be one extraneous bone visible (unless it is a complete wishbone!).

- *The epiglottis.* Learn to recognize this like a bent pinkie pointing concave forwards in the upper airway – of soft tissue density. Remember in *epiglottitis,* this swells up in children like a red cherry, often due to *Haemophilus influenzae.* If you suspect this, get the child X-rayed erect – if held supine for too long the epiglottis may fall back and choke the child to death, courtesy of your good self.

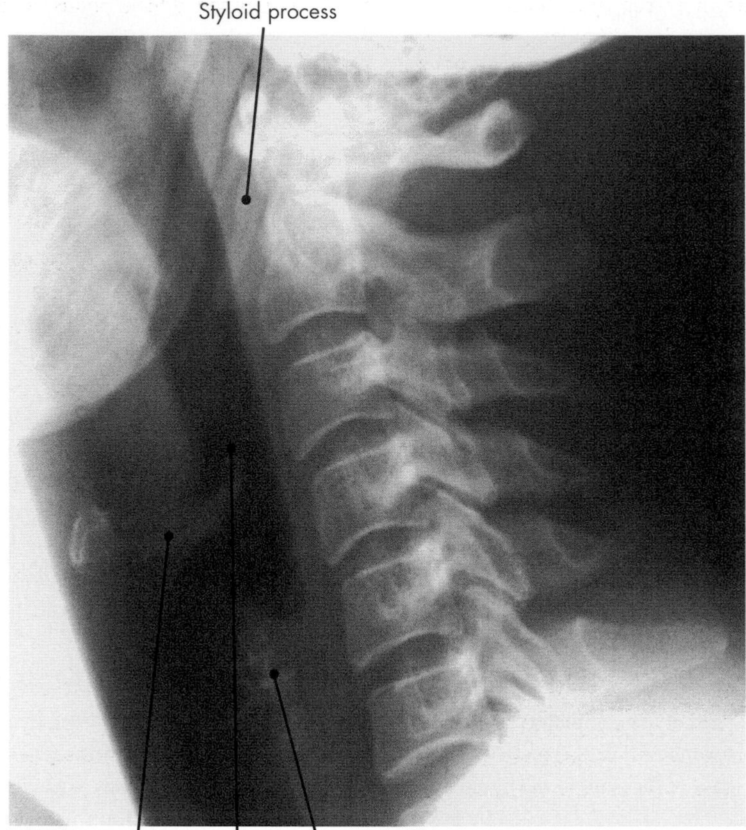

Fig. 8.1 *This is the normal anatomy of the upper airway.*

Important anatomy: the prevertebral tissues

The *retropharyngeal soft tissues* have been mentioned in the section on the neck; as a guide, they should not be more than 7 mm in an adult. Similarly the *retrotracheal soft tissues* should not be more than 22 mm in an adult or 14 mm in a child. These are, however, guidelines and it is often focal bulging which points to an abnormality, although generalized swelling can also occur.

NB Big osteophytes can displace these tissues and sometimes they are so big they can cause dysphagia, or look like foreign bodies themselves, especially if 'developmentally detached' from the vertebrae. But other signs of osteoarthritis should be present as well.

Important pathology and physiology

NB Some children have such enormous tonsils and adenoids that they can compromise the airway (causing mouth breathing due to nasal obstruction), and in babies and young children the pharyngeal tissues may be so lax and redundant that they cause apparent anatomical nasopharyngeal occlusion on expiration but immediately revert to normal and open up again on inspiration (Fig. 8.2).

Moral: Do not always rely on just one film. Sometimes it may actually be necessary to take a second one and a skilled paediatric radiographer may be able to capture the moment of inspiration for you. Ultimately, however, X-ray screening may be required.

So what about these foreign bodies?

- Is this an acute severe medical emergency, e.g. with stridor requiring emergency removal immediately?
- Obviously any object small enough can stick in the throat (Fig. 8.3). If you know what it is, you will know what you are looking for, e.g. a marble or a coin.
- Is there a good history?
- Has it actually been swallowed and do I need chest and abdominal films?
- Have I excluded anatomical structures? (easier said than done – consult Keats & Anderson 2001).
- Still in doubt? Call ENT to discuss a ? laryngoscopy. If clinically OK and if later than 3 a.m. – 'Come back tomorrow!'

Indirect signs of an impacted foreign body

Some foreign bodies are notoriously hard to see; for example a ring-pull, unless it is end-on, being made of relatively radiolucent aluminium. Other are

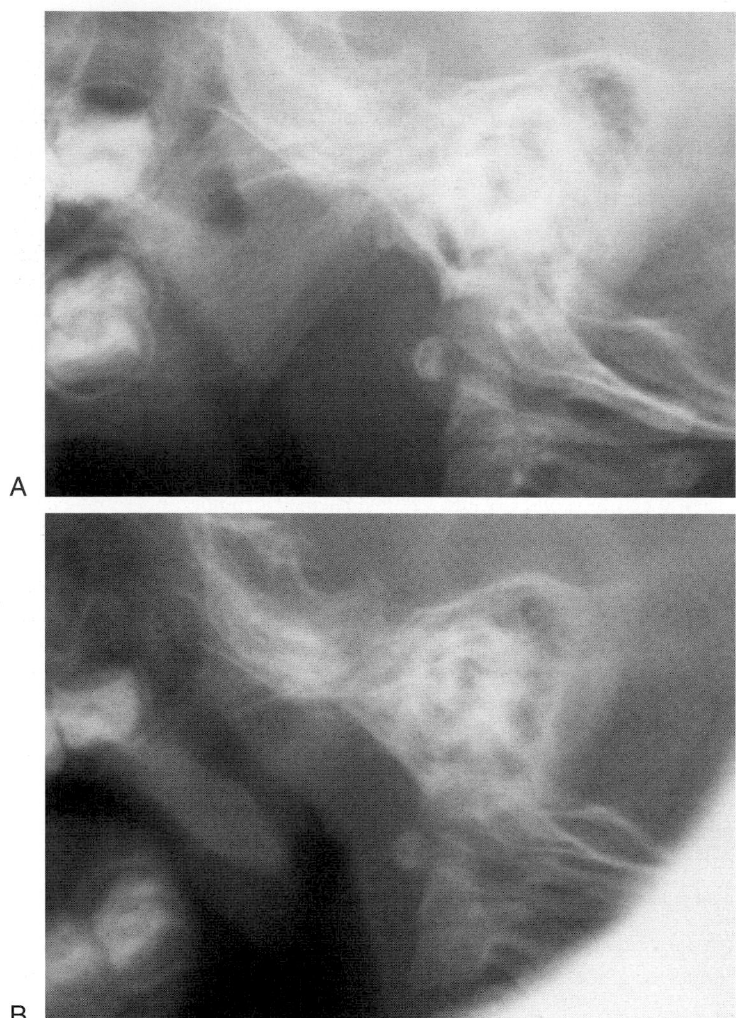

Fig. 8.2 ***A*** *Paediatric nasopharynx on expiration;* ***B*** *inspiration (note how the nasopharangeal airway is now open).*

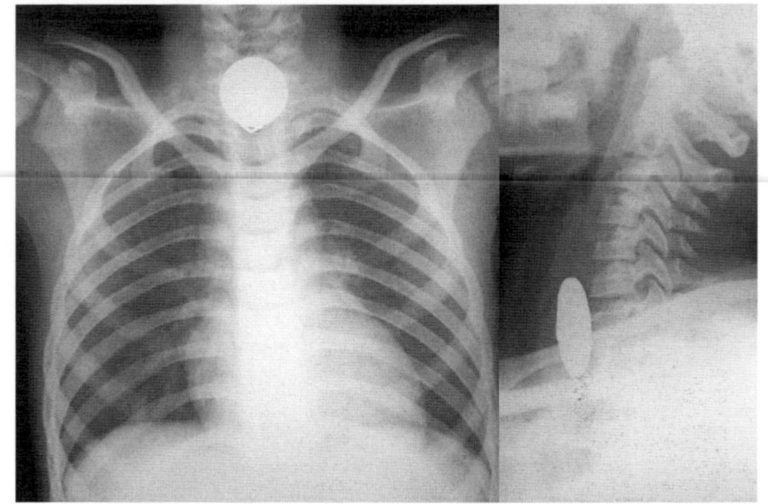

Fig. 8.3 *Medallion stuck in the throat. Note how on the AP film (**A**) it is lying transversely so, because it is too big to be in the trachea, it must be in the oesophagus (which begins at C6). Note: with swallowed coins a lateral (**B**) is a good idea because there may be a smaller coin hidden behind the big one!*

completely non-opaque (certain fish bones) but can provide indirect evidence of their presence, for example:

- Prevertebral swelling (abscess formation).
- Gas formation (also in an abscess).
- Surgical emphysema – if there is a perforation.
- Straightening of the neck or reversal of the normal cervical lordosis (e.g. due to the discomfort of an evolving abscess).

These, of course, occur later as complications arise.

Are chicken bones opaque? Yes, but that doesn't necessarily mean they are always easy to see (Fig. 8.4).

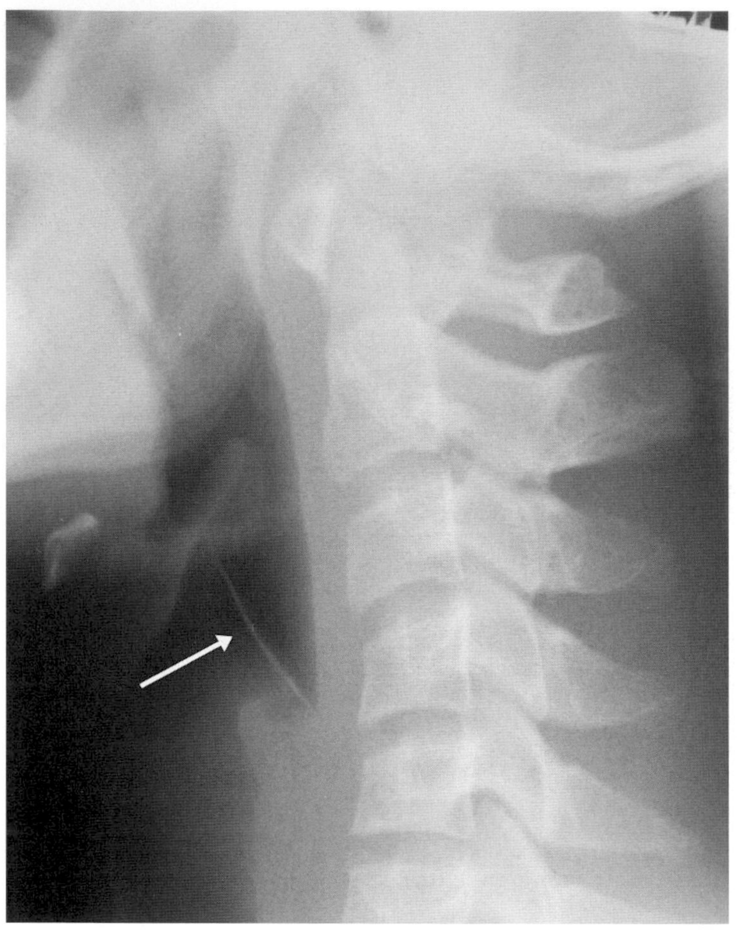

Fig. 8.4 *Chicken bone in throat. Note the reversal of the normal cervical lordosis, reflecting that the patient is in discomfort.*

Are fish bones opaque? Some are, e.g. cod, sole and haddock, but not kippers or salmon; it depends on the calcium content.

Some pathological causes of upper airway obstruction (giving stridor, etc.)

You must know about these – they may come in as acute medical emergencies:

- Croup (children); sublaryngeal oedema.
- Epiglottitis (as above).
- Prevertebral abscess.
- Bilateral fractured mandible (p. 57).
- Thyroid – goitre, carcinoma (may need emergency radiotherapy).
- Laryngeal oedema – following attempted homicide or suicide – strangulation.
- Angioneurotic oedema due to, for example, a penicillin reaction, peanut or latex allergy, bee sting, etc.

Important point Before you go to A & E make sure you know how to intubate, and find out as soon as you can how to do **an emergency tracheostomy.**

Chapter 9

The chest

NB Total command of the chest X-ray should be the goal of every hospital doctor who sees patients.

Background

The chest X-ray is at the centre of medicine and surgery, and most junior doctors who first come to work in A & E will be at senior house officer level and already have come face to face with them. In trauma, of course, their correct interpretation is critical. Nevertheless, experience shows that many such doctors still lack the total command and mental discipline necessary for the analysis of the chest X-ray, have limited understanding of the profound effects which technical factors play in their interpretation, and are easily led astray by such simple radiographic variables as rotation and underpenetration, which can lead in turn to the misdiagnosis of a 'thoracic aortic aneurysm' (which is not there) to the missing of a left lower lobe collapse (which *is* there!).

Since, by definition, anyone with any illness or injury can walk (crawl or be carried) in the door, every A & E doctor ought to have a thorough grasp of the basics of chest radiology, be totally conversant with the features of normality, be able to recognize and avoid the common pitfalls, and know precisely what he or she is looking for in terms of the common acute medical and surgical emergencies which present themselves and, of course, the manifestations of trauma.

Accordingly, a system of chest X-ray analysis is presented which should cover all the major eventualities that may arise, and all major departures from normality. **NB** This system should be committed to memory like an aircraft take-off checklist. **Aim to be red-hot on chest X-rays!**

Chest: a word of warning

One of the biggest mistakes you can make

Look at Figure 9.1A. Analysis of this film shows an increased cardiothoracic ratio CTR >50% by direct measurement, i.e. an enlarged heart, and clouding of both lung bases. The differential diagnosis includes:

- heart failure
- bilateral basal pneumonia
- pre-existing lung disease with pulmonary fibrosis, etc.

Now look at Figure 9.1B. This shows a heart size that is well within normal limits, and lungs that are totally clear to the bases.

Comment: These films were taken *just 2 minutes apart on the same patient, and both are normal*: (A) being taken on *full expiration*, and (B) being taken on *full inspiration*.

Guideline: On a well-inspired chest X-ray the left hemidiaphragm will clear $10\frac{1}{2}$ ribs posteriorly on the left side in a patient of average build.

Important points:

- Not realizing you are dealing with a poorly inspired film is one of the commonest and most dangerous errors you can make when trying to interpret a chest X-ray, almost on a par with failing to read the name of the patient. It is not, therefore, an intrinsic ignorance of the pathophysiology of heart failure or pneumonia, etc. that usually leads to this mistake, but a lack of knowledge of simple radiographic technique. **NB** You therefore have to make an allowance for the effects of poor inspiration on every such film.
- A well-inspired film requires a patient who is able to understand the instruction to 'take a deep breath in', and then do it. Not suprisingly, many critically ill and traumatized patients cannot achieve this. The ideal film is taken erect, but many A & E films will have to be taken supine, which in itself virtually precludes full inspiration.

Hitchhikers' guide to the chest X-ray

Check at the outset for quality and acceptability of the film, and demographic and technical information. This has been particularly emphasized in the chapters

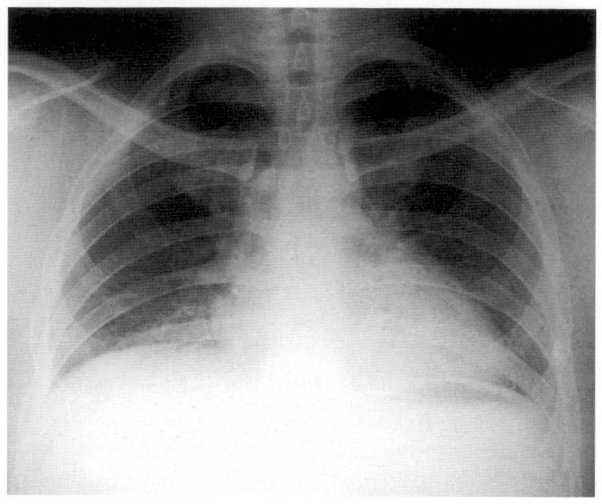

Fig. 9.1A *The 'killer film'. A normal chest X-ray in expiration. Note the false cardiomegaly and clouding of the bases.*

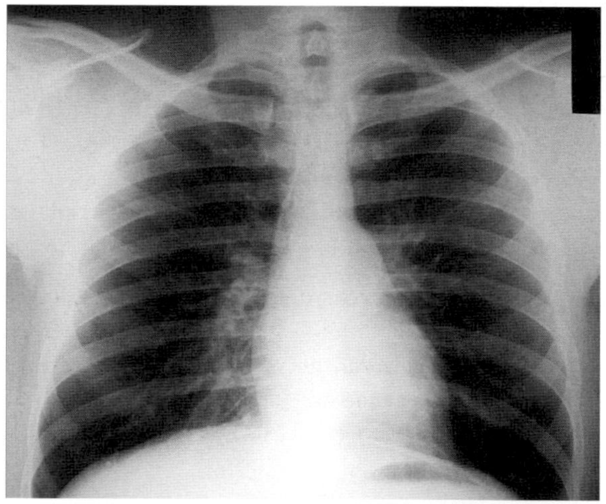

Fig. 9.1B *The same patient's film 2 minutes later on full inspiration. Crystal clear!*

on skull and neck X-rays but applies to all films – so it is being revisited and emphasized again here.

Check:

- *The name of the patient.* **This is the most important piece of information on the film, and you must check you have the correct patient's film up in front of you.** If you get this wrong, disaster may follow.
- **Warning:** Just occasionally, the wrong name gets on a patient's film. This is rare but it happens. Therefore **check for gross error** – your patient may have no history of surgery, but the film you are looking at has sternal metal sutures clearly visible.
- *Visible anatomy.* Is all the relevant anatomy on the film? If not and a part has been missed off, that is the part that will contain an abnormality, e.g. a fractured rib. A repeat to include the missing part may therefore be required if time and the patient's condition permit.
- *Date of the film.* You must check you are dealing with the current film. Usually in A & E you will only have the current ones to deal with, but sometimes old films will be available. You must still check the date anyway as a matter of course. Sometimes patients will arrive with films from abroad. Remember the American system of dating is to give the month before the day, i.e. 4/3/2005 in the USA corresponds to 3 April 2005 in the UK. Some UK marking systems will also give the date in reverse, e.g. 05/03/04 for the 4 March 2005, so be on your guard.
- *Check date of birth/hospital number.* This gives further confirmation of the age and identity of the patient.
- *Sex.* Make sure you know the sex of every patient. Many names can belong to either males or females, e.g. Frances/Francis, Jessie/Jesse, Jackie, etc. Some names may be foreign and their gender implications unknown to you. Someone else may ask your opinion on a film when you have not seen the patient and you may not realize you are dealing with a female who has had a bilateral mastectomy.
- *Breasts.* Consciously look for and confirm or exclude evidence of visible breasts, which help to confirm the sex. The best time to do this is immediately after you read the name of the patient, especially if the patient is female.

- Large or asymmetric breasts and breast prostheses can mimic pneumonia (get the history). Patients often do not volunteer that they have breast implants.

- *PA or AP projection?* (Posteroanterior or anteroposterior refers to the direction of the beam through the patient). PA films are done on relatively fit patients who can sit or stand up. AP films are done on sick patients who may be sitting up or lying down. **All supine films are AP.** An AP film excessively magnifies the heart size, giving false cardiomegaly. In many hospitals the radiographer will mark the film for you by hand 'AP erect' or 'AP supine', or the positioning may be incorporated in the name badge. If you are unsure, the radiographer will usually be able to work out from the various parameters how a given film was done, even if he or she did not take it personally. **Hint:** If in an exam and not sure whether a film is AP or PA, just call it a 'frontal chest X-ray' and avoid an unnecessary argument!

- *Position.* Look for clues, e.g. a gas–liquid level in the gastric fundus will indicate an erect chest film. A multiply-injured patient with several tubes inserted is unlikely to be erect. A haemothorax will just cause a veil of increased density in the supine position having tracked out posteriorly behind the lung.

- *Rotation.* It is essential that you know how to work out if a chest X-ray is rotated, and if so, which way. This is done by assessing the distances from the medial aspects of the clavicular heads to the midline, as determined by the spinous processes, i.e. **the side with the greater distance between the medial aspect of the head of the clavicle and the spinous process is the side to which the patient is rotated.**

Effects of rotation

- *Distortion of heart size and shape.* Spurious chamber enlargement.

- *Altered relative prominence of hila.* One may disappear while the other sticks out more and everybody starts suggesting '?neoplasm'.

- *Spurious 'displacement' of trachea.* The lower trachea normally curves to the right in older patients, where it has to negotiate the aorta; this is accentuated by rotation to the right. Rotation to the left will also cause spurious displacement.

- *Altered apparent size and arc of aorta* (greater rotation to the right unfolds the arch more, simulating aneurysm).

- *Altered relative density of hemithoraces.* Rotation to the right causes increased opacification of the opposite side, and vice versa, as the beam has to traverse more tissue.

Crucial point. If the trachea is 'central' on a rotated film it must actually be displaced, as it will move away when the patient is straightened.

- *Ward/Unit/Hospital.* This is included because it is so vital always to go through the mental discipline of identifying the source, and therefore potential nature, of the illness of a patient, e.g. renal, cardiac, orthopaedic, etc., when assessing films. Obviously if films are requested in A & E and being viewed there, that is how they will be marked.
- *Left/right marker.* This is the classic major potential disaster in medicolegal litigation and recent high profile cases have confirmed this in the media. Not checking this can probably lead to more grief than just about anything else when dealing with A & E films, especially extremities, but chest X-rays are no exception. To the radiologist, left/right discrepancies occur with alarming frequency in piles of A & E films which come for reporting. Frequently a 'left foot' is requested; this is challenged by the radiographer when confronted by a patient who says 'No, it's the *right* one!' and a film marked 'right' has been taken, but this goes unnoticed by the doctor and nothing appears about this contradiction in the clinical notes. So – find the L/R marker on the chest X-ray and check that it is compatible with the visible anatomy. The commonest cause of an apparent 'dextrocardia' is radiographic error, so re-examine your patient for an apex beat, etc. and go and check with the radiographer. If confirmed correctly to have a dextrocardia, however, your patient may be presenting with a *left-sided appendicitis, due to situs inversus,* or it may explain that crazy-looking ECG.

Quick L/R anatomical checklist

- Heart predominates to the left.
- Right *hemidiaphragm* is higher than the left.
- Left *hilum* normally higher than right.
- *Gastric fundal air shadow* on the left.
- *Aortic knuckle* should be on the left (some patients have a right-sided arch, but this is how you find it – by checking).

- *Horizontal fissure* on the right.
- Left *main bronchus* – steeper angle of take-off from trachea than the right (peanuts therefore tend to go down the right main bronchus).

Moral: You cannot afford to be careless about left and right.

- *Scapulae.* You must locate the positions of the scapulae and it is the *medial margins* you are interested in. On an ideal film, in fit patients, they are off the lung fields. In sick patients and on supine films, the medial scapular margins will inevitably intrude into the lung fields. Once identified, **they must not be misinterpreted as the edge of a pneumothorax or pleural thickening,** and an unnecessary drain put in which then gives the patient a pneumothorax that he did not have in the first place.
- *Inspiration.* Check for full inspiration or take account of its absence.
- *Penetration.* 'Penetration' refers to your ability to 'see through' the patient to the retrocardiac anatomy (i.e. spine, ribs and parts of the right and left lower lobes) on a chest X-ray. The inexperienced observer may be given a film where the heart just looks like a snowman and nothing is visible within its borders but a 'white-out'. **NB Underpenetrated films are very dangerous and may lead to the missing of serious pathology, like an aneurysm, metastasis or left lower lobe collapse.** A film that is overpenetrated (i.e. too dark) can be resurrected with a bright light, but little can be done to retrieve the anatomy from an excessively pale conventional film – apart from tilting it and looking at it obliquely, which slightly increases the contrast. With a digital image, however, you can set the picture to show you anything you want and most A & E departments are rapidly transferring to the digital format, converting conventional X-rays to relics of the past but the necessity to view behind the heart remains critical.

Structures you should be able to see on well-penetrated chest films of diagnostic quality

- The lower thoracic intervertebral disc spaces (without undue effort) and the adjacent vertebral bodies. This encompasses the definition of a well-penetrated film.
- The paraspinal line on the left side (see Fig. 4.3).

- The lateral margin of the descending thoracic aorta.
- The posterior ends of the ribs.
- The upper medial surface of the left hemidiaphragm.
- The vessels in the medial parts of both lower lobes

Sobering thought: Only now, having assimilated and understood the above technical aspects relating to chest X-ray analysis, are you safe to start looking for pathology. If you do not do these routine assessments on every film you will make some totally avoidable but catastrophic mistakes, some of which may have very serious consequences for both the patient and yourself.

Indications for chest X-rays in A & E

- Acute medical problems, e.g. chest pain and shortness of breath, the common causes of which should be known to you.
- Assessment of acute abdomen (for free air and anaesthetic assessment).
- Moderate chest trauma, i.e. for complications of rib fractures and following stab wounds.

NB Severe chest trauma should go to CT.

A word about pathology

The heart and lungs have a limited response to disease. The heart may become larger or smaller and the lungs become more or less opaque (i.e. dense); it is the pattern of the changes in the lungs that enables diagnostic deductions to be made.

Radiographic densities: important points

It is well worth knowing that only about five basic densities are visible on an X-ray:

- *Air* – black (e.g. the lungs and atmosphere outside the chest).
- *Fat* – thin dark grey lines between muscle layers (e.g. chest walls and supraclavicular fossae under trapezius).
- *Soft tissues* – grey, e.g. pulmonary vessels and chest wall (summation effect may make the heart look denser).

- *Bone* – white (e.g. ribs). This is not, however, as intense as metal.
- *Metal* – intense white (e.g. the L/R marker, or a bullet).

This means that when you have identified its density you know what something is made of.

The CTR measurement

A valid CTR measurement is defined as A + B divided by C on a well-inspired erect PA chest X-ray (Fig. 9.2). Up to 50% is normal in adults and 55% in young children. A measurement of, for example, 60% in an adult is a non-specific finding but implies there is something wrong with the heart. A pericardial effusion may enlarge the cardiac silhouette, while the underlying heart is actually normal. Elucidation of these problems requires echocardiography.

Do not be misled by cardiophrenic fat pads on one or both sides. The actual heart border usually remains visible medial to them, but is less clear. The position of the edge can be better assessed by viewing the film obliquely.

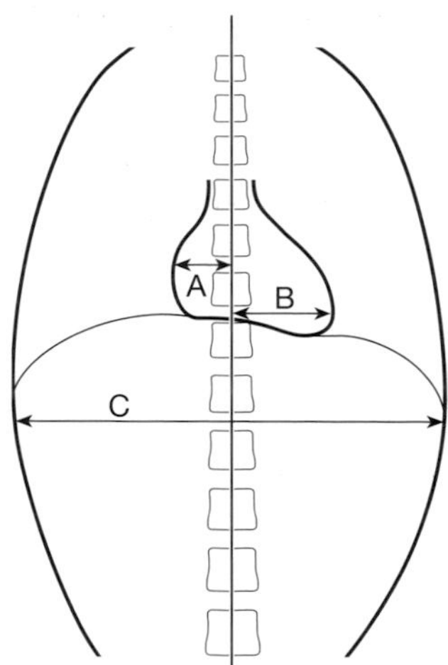

Fig. 9.2 *The CTR measurement. CTR = (A + B)/C, where A = distance of maximum convexity to midline on right; B = distance of maximum convexity to midline on left; C = maximum internal thoracic diameter. Note how these lines are usually not at the same level – it is a common misconception that they always are, although on occasion they can be.*

Diagnosis

The differential diagnosis of a patient's problem at presentation of course remains open, but usually by the time you have seen and examined him you will have a good idea of what is going on. With regard to the chest X-ray, **your duty is to know what radiological signs you are looking for, while remaining alert to any other findings that might modify or alter your diagnosis.** More than one doctor has had a nasty surprise when the films came out of the processor, to such a degree that he could not believe they had come from the patient he had just seen.

Acute myocardial infarction

This is the **number one differential diagnosis** for exclusion in any patient with sudden severe central chest, neck or arm pain. It is also the number two and number three differential diagnoses because it is such an important condition not to miss! More than one patient has been told he had just pulled a muscle' only to drop dead at the hospital gate. Nevertheless, two-thirds of chest pains in patients presenting to A & E are non-cardiac in origin.

On the chest X-ray look for heart size and signs of heart failure.

Heart size This will usually be normal at the first myocardial infarction but is often enlarged with subsequent episodes. Look for evidence of left ventricular enlargement due to aneurysm formation (may contain a thin rim of calcification).

Signs of heart failure

1. Normal or enlarged heart.
2. Bilateral or unilateral pleural effusions (usually on the right if unilateral).
3. Distended upper lobe veins (larger than lower lobe vessels on an erect film in full inspiration). **NB** A supine film will cause spurious physiological upper lobe diversion.
4. Interstitial opacification, i.e. pulmonary oedema due to alveolar flooding.
5. Kerley-B lines (small 1 mm thick horizontal lines at right angles to the pleura at and above the costophrenic angles. **NB** These can fibrose in chronic cases and become a permanent feature of the patient's film. They may also be seen in malignancy, i.e. lymphangitis carcinomata and mitral stenosis.
6. Fluid in the fissures. Instead of thin lines they take on a lenticular shape (Fig. 9.3).

Pulmonary embolism

Consider this in patients with pleuritic-type chest pain and breathlessness. Women on the contraceptive pill and travellers from long-haul flights are at particular risk. Many occur out of the blue or complicate deep vein thrombosis in patients with malignancy.

Crucial point: The chest X-ray may be normal, so a normal chest X-ray does not exclude a pulmonary embolism.

There are, however, several radiological signs that may occur. These include:

- A pleural effusion.
- Elevation of the ipsilateral hemidiaphragm.
- Enlargement of the ipsilateral pulmonary artery.

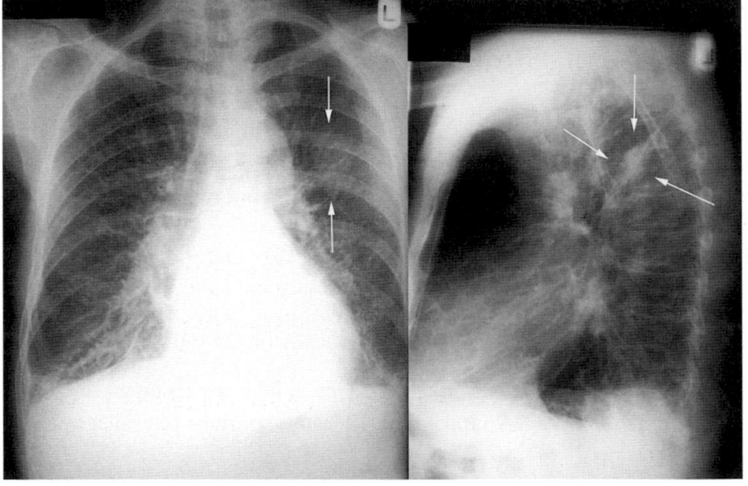

Fig. 9.3 ***A*** *Overt cardiac failure with enlarged heart and pulmonary congestion. Note the opacity (arrows) in the left upper lung field. Do not tell the patient he has a carcinoma.* ***B*** *Encysted great fissure effusion. Note the lenticular or galaxy-shaped object (arrows) in the upper end of the great fissure. This is encysted fluid due to cardiac failure and will disappear on treatment, hence the term 'vanishing lung tumour'.*

- Truncation of vessels beyond the occluded artery.
- Opacification of the costophrenic angle with convexity pointing back to hilum – 'Hampton's hump'.

These signs may take some time to evolve, and later cavitation may occur in an infarct.

Further investigations:

- Doppler ultrasound of legs for ?DVT.
- Ventilation/perfusion isotope scan for evidence of mismatch.
- CT pulmonary angiogram for definitive demonstration of a pulmonary embolus.

Acute asthma

Usually there is a history of this. The chest may be normal but look for:

- Hyperinflation, with flattening of hemidiaphragms, and separation of ribs.
- Increased radiolucency of the lungs.
- Peribronchial thickening or 'cuffing' around the hila.
- Signs of associated infection (which may have precipitated it).
- Check for a pneumothorax and mediastinal emphysema, which may complicate the clinical picture; the latter may extend up into the neck. Non-response to drugs should lead you to consider the presence of a pneumothorax and ensure a chest X-ray is done.
- **Gold Medal point:** Check for *Aspergillus* plugs in the upper lobe bronchi.

Bronchiolitis (babies)

Look for:

- Hyperinflation with bulging of lungs between ribs.
- Peribronchial cuffing.

Do not mistake a large thymus for a pathological mass on the chest X-rays of young children (see Keats & Anderson 2001).

Lobar pneumonia

Important points:

- Genuine lobar pneumonia is a dangerous condition, even for young adults, so never think of it as 'just pneumonia' in this context. For the elderly and babies it is particularly lethal. It may occur de novo due to underlying conditions, e.g. HIV or bronchial carcinoma, and (more recently) complicate the deadly SARS (severe acute respiratory syndrome) virus.
- Each lobar pneumonia has a characteristic appearance and each lobe of the lung collapses in its own way (Figs 9.4–9.8).
- 'Consolidation' of the lung means opacification (whiteness) due to fluid, cells or blood, etc. The terms 'collapse' and 'consolidation' are sometimes used as if they were synonymous but they are not. Consolidation is a component of collapse, but **collapse is only present when there is loss of volume and displacement of anatomical landmarks,** although it may of course be only partial.
- Although a patient may clinically have pneumonia, consolidation may not actually appear if the patient is severely dehydrated, but may show up the next day following the administration of intravenous fluids.

The 'silhouette sign' You must appreciate this phenomenon in order to understand chest X-rays.

The heart and hemidiaphragms are visible because they are in contact with air-filled lungs, which are of a different radiographic density, the contrast rendering them visible. The interior of the heart is not visible on chest X-rays because blood and myocardium have the same radiographic density (i.e. fluid = soft tissue), so no contrast is generated.

Important point: When an area of consolidated lung in contact with the heart becomes opaque, that part of the heart 'disappears' because the two structures have acquired the same density. This is called the 'silhouette sign', and enables, for instance, right middle lobe collapse and lingular consolidation to be localized.

Learn the lobar anatomy of the lungs so that you can correctly apply this principle.

Exacerbation of COPD (Fig. 9.9)

Look at:

- The small heart.

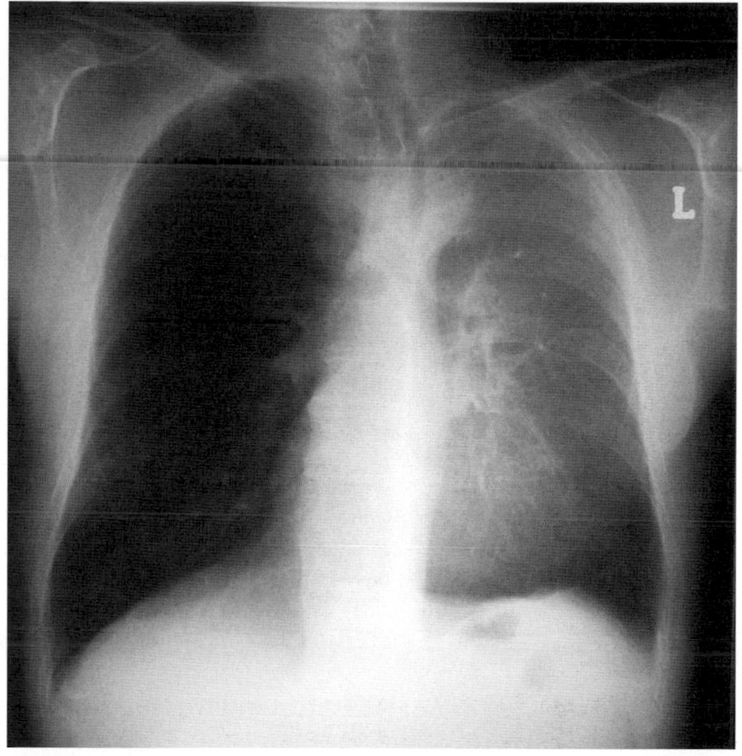

Fig. 9.4 *A PA chest film showing increased density on the left side, mediastinal diplacement to the left, tracheal deviation to the left and loss of clarity of the whole left heart border. Most junior doctors confronted with this for the first time have no idea what is going on.*

- Hyperinflation of the lung fields – low-set hemidiaphragms (> $10\frac{1}{2}$ posterior ribs on the left).
- Large central pulmonary arteries.
- **NB** Often no change from the chronic appearances is apparent at presentation, even if the patient harbours infection, but some focal consolidation may be visible.

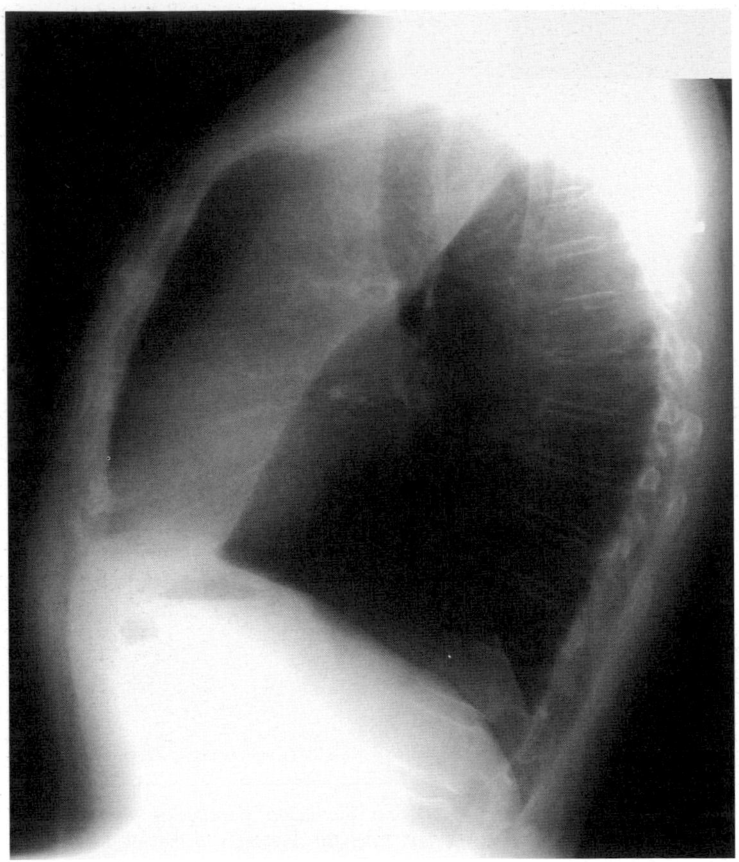

Fig. 9.5 *Lateral view of the same patient (Fig. 9.4), showing spectacular clarity of interface of the great fissure on the left and consolidation in the left upper lobe.*

Bronchopneumonia

Look for scattered irregular areas of opacification, often bilateral. If the organism is atypical, e.g. *Pneumocystis*, consider HIV, immunosuppression etc.

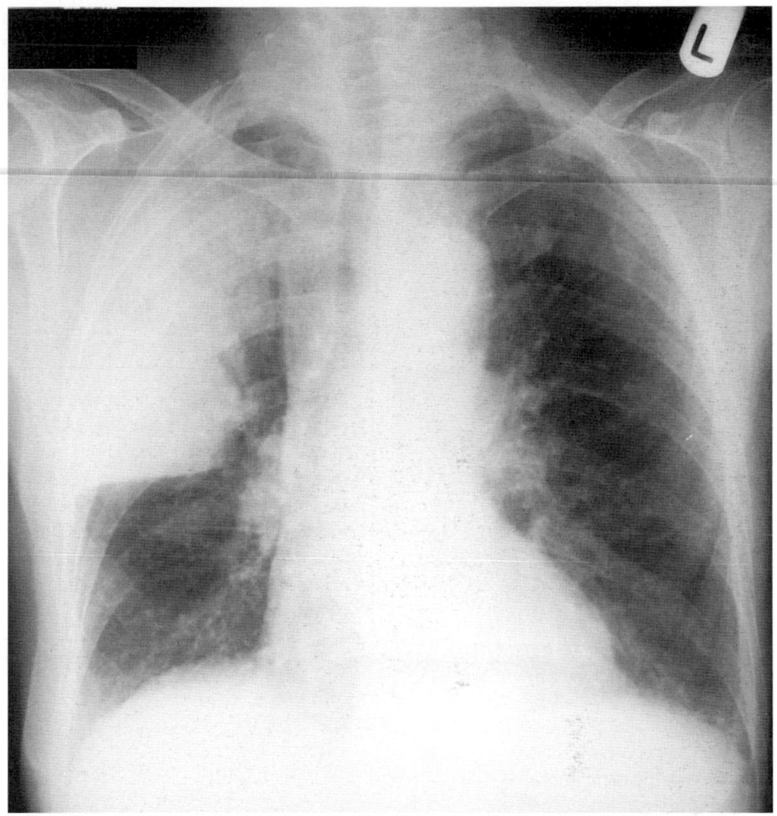

Fig. 9.6 *Right upper lobe pneumonia. Note the sharp inferior border due to the horizontal fissure (know your anatomy).*

Pulmonary abscess

Pulmonary abscesses present just as opaque nodules in the early stages; only after cavitation has occurred do you get the classic air–fluid levels within them. Malignancy may need to be excluded. Pulmonary abscesses can occur in drug addicts, who of course can frequent A & E departments.

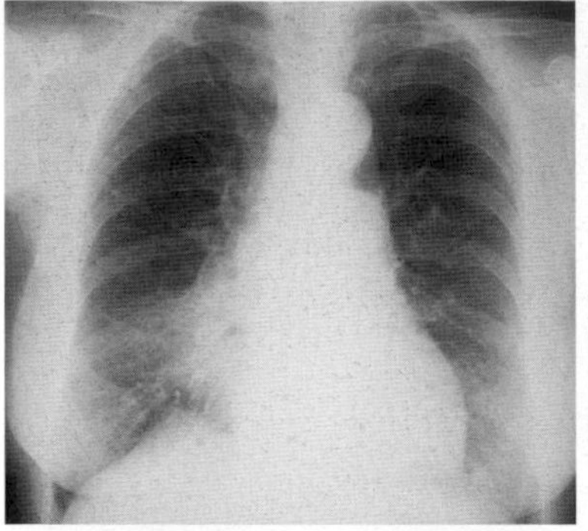

A

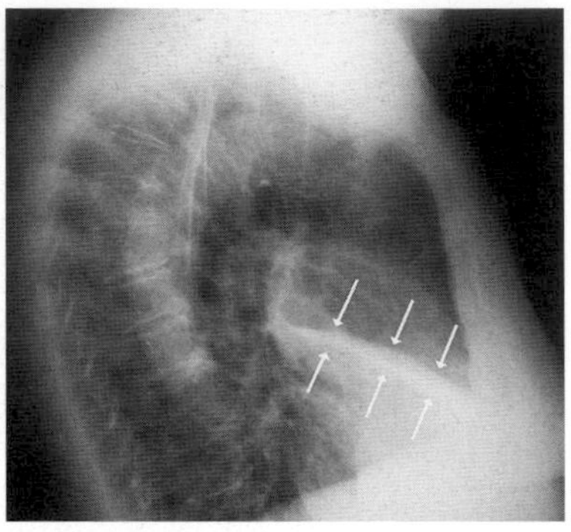

B

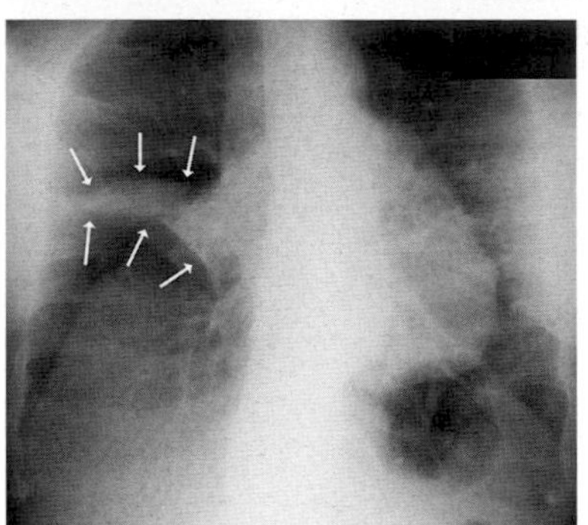

C

Fig. 9.7 *Series of films showing right middle lobe collapse.* ***A*** *PA film. Note the haze and poor definition around the right heart border.* ***B*** *Lateral view. Note the dense triangle of the opaque right middle lobe.* ***C*** *Radiologist's trick of the trade. A steep angled-up shot sharply defining the right middle lobe.*

Dissecting thoracic aorta

This dangerous condition, which usually occurs in hypertensive patients, may be associated with unequal pulses and blood pressure in the upper limbs. On the chest X-ray, look for:

- *Widening of the aorta* but take into account the degree of rotation.
- *Separation of intimal calcification from the outer wall* as the dissection progresses down the media.
- *A left pleural effusion.* This may track over the apex and form a veil of generalized increased density on the left side if the patient is supine, as the effusion sits behind the lung. If erect, the classic configuration should be seen.

Early progress to angiography, CT or MRI is usually indicated (Figs 9.10, 9.11).

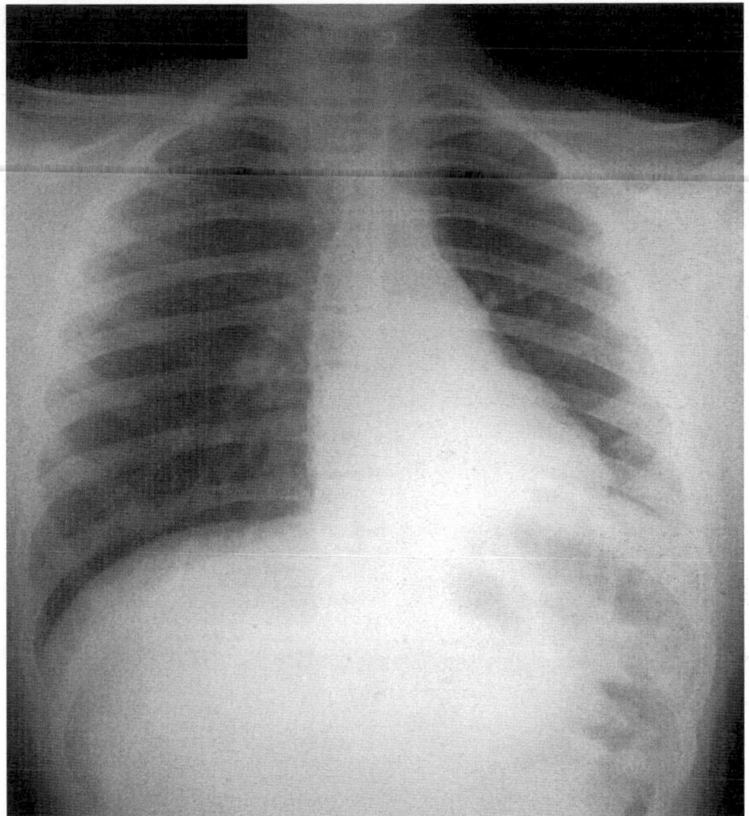

Fig. 9.8 A classic film! Left lower lobe collapse. You ***must*** be able to identify this condition, which often occurs with pneumonia, underlying bronchogenic carcinoma, following foreign body ingestion and postoperatively. Note these classic radiological signs: lower thoracic disc spaces visible – well penetrated, so you ***should*** be able to see through the heart; deviation of heart to left; deviation of trachea to left; crowding of ribs on left; elevation of left hemidiaphragm; markedly increased density behind heart = abnormal; top of left hemidiaphragm not visible medially; no vessels/ribs visible behind left side of heart medially; loss of lateral margin of descending thoracic aorta; depression of left hilum; increased radiolucency and paucity of stretched vessels in left lung. All the signs are present – definition of a classic case!

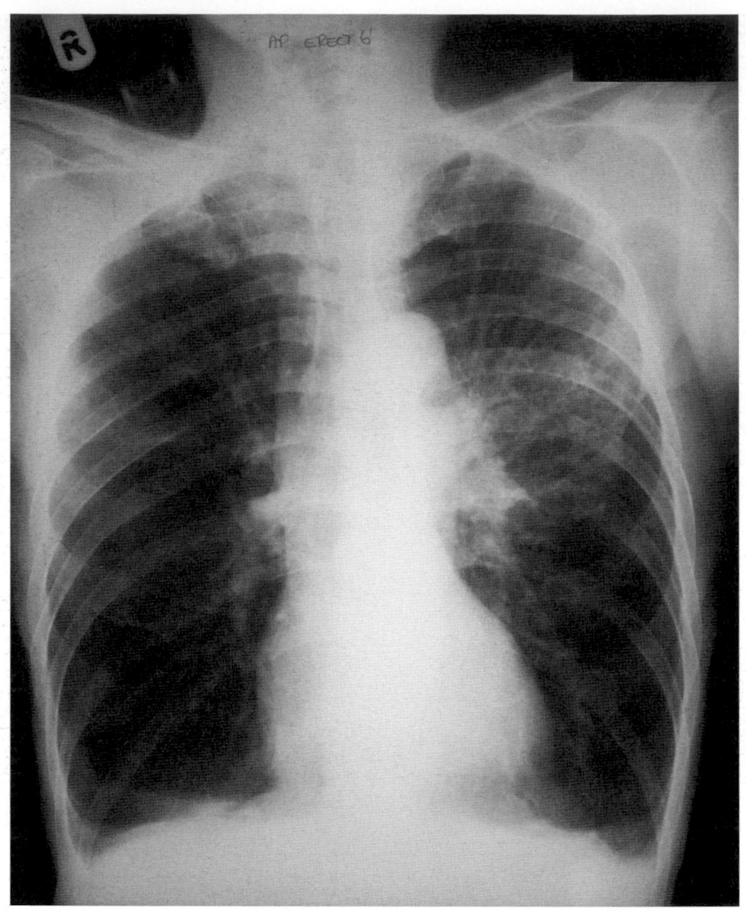

Fig. 9.9 *COPD with left upper lobe pneumonia. Note the barrel-shaped chest, low-set hemidiaphragms, chunky central pulmonary arteries and hyperlucent lung fields.*

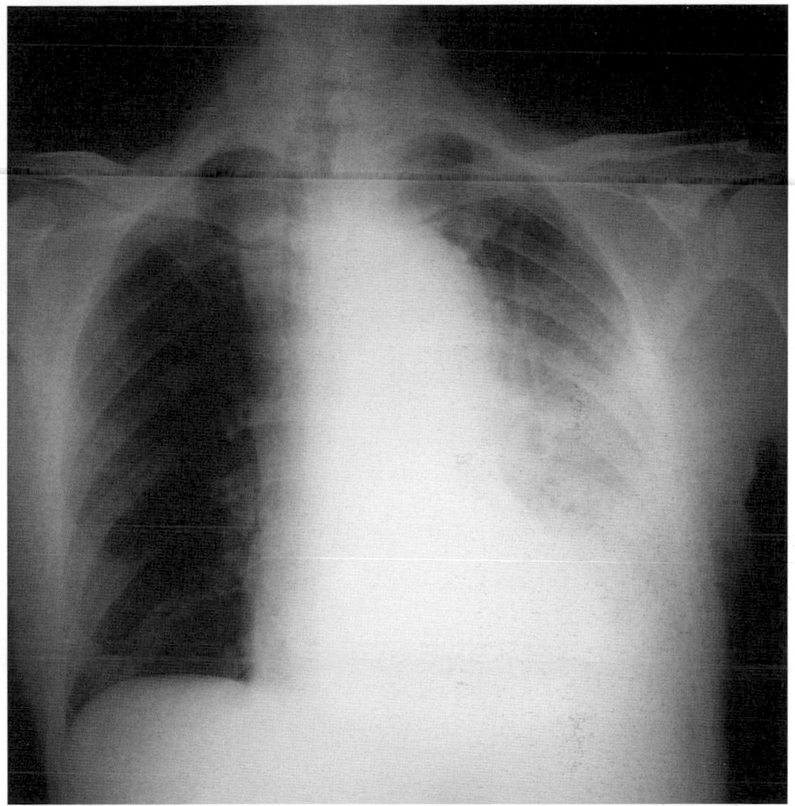

Fig. 9.10 *Dissecting aorta. Note the widened aorta and big pleural effusion. Indwelling nasogastric tubes can show increasing displacement to the right as the dissection progresses.*

Pericardial disease

A pericardial effusion may create a big cardiac silhouette. The heart becomes more symmetrical about the midline and bottle-shaped, with a sharp edge because the movement of the myocardium is masked and muffled by the fluid. An echocardiogram will confirm or exclude a pericardial effusion. Sometimes pericardial calcification is present – best seen on laterals or obliques.

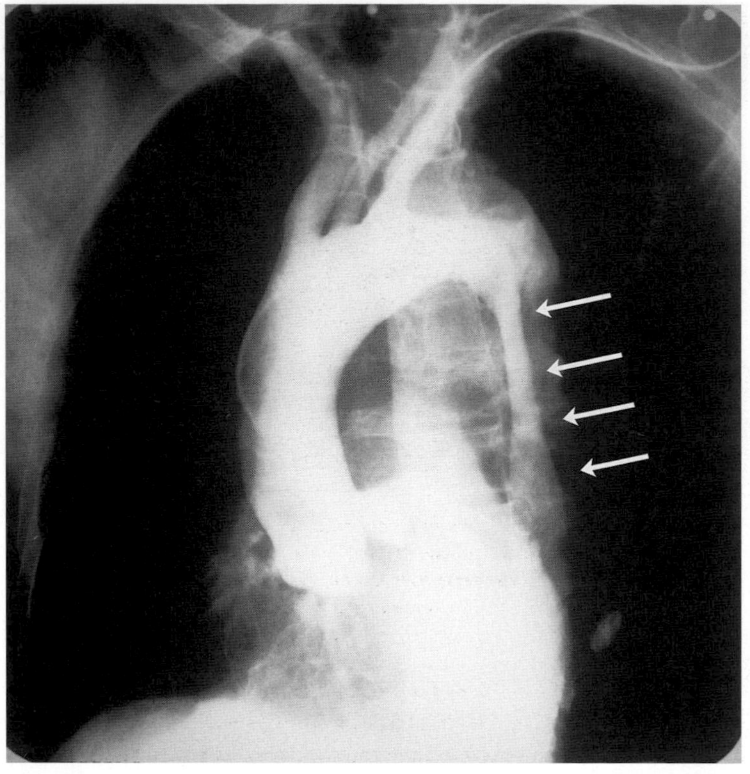

Fig. 9.11 *Angiogram on same patient (Fig. 9.10). The 'twisted tape' sign. CT or MRI may now be the first option of choice. Gold medal point: the catheter has been inserted up the brachial artery to avoid negotiating or exacerbating the dissection by a femoral approach.*

Inhaled foreign body (Fig. 9.12)

Beware of this as an underlying cause of consolidation and collapse, particularly in children, as no history may be offered. The classic scenario is the inhaled peanut, which, being made of vegetable matter, is non-opaque. The preferential route is down the right main bronchus. The peanut then impacts and creates a ball-valve effect.

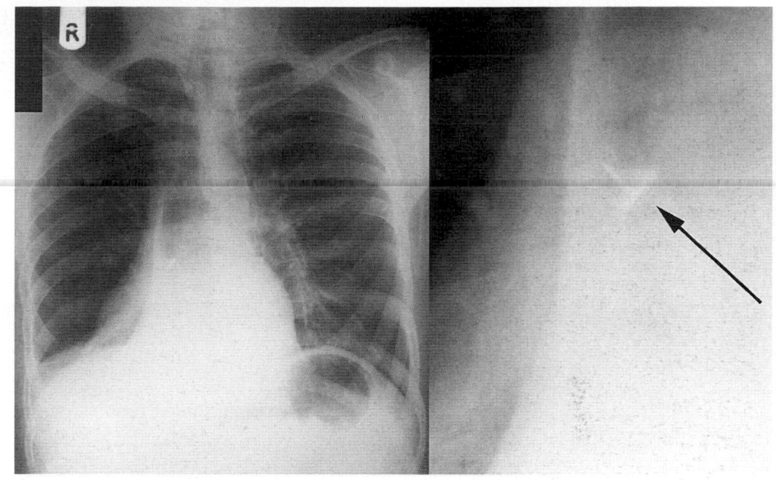

Fig. 9.12 ***A, B*** *Right lower lobe collapse. Detail of right lower bronchus. The patient had inhaled a drawing pin! Note: always suspect and look for underlying foreign bodies, especially in children. No amount of antibiotics will cure a patient whose bronchus remains occluded by a missed foreign body.*

NB Initially the inspiratory film looks normal. The expiratory film, which you need to ask for, is very abnormal. The obstructed bronchus allows air to enter but blocks its exit so the affected lung cannot empty on expiration. It therefore remains inflated and the mediastinum (heart) swings to the contralateral side on expiration. Later the obstructed lung may hyperinflate before ultimately collapsing.

NB If you strongly suspect a foreign body but cannot see it on the X-ray, refer the patient urgently for a bronchoscopy.

Spontaneous pneumothorax (i.e. non-traumatic)

While a pneumothorax complicating a rib fracture is the commonest cause of all pneumothoraces seen in A & E, a pneumothorax occurring out of the blue is an important differential of chest pain. Spontaneous pain and breathlessness will frequently be the presenting symptoms of this condition, associated with diminished breath sounds and increased resonance to percussion. Tracheal deviation should always be sought as well. Look for:

- A thin line representing the edge of the lung retracted from the inner chest wall, initially at the apex.
- A lack of lung markings beyond the lung edge.
- Evidence of tension developing (Fig. 9.13), e.g. mediastinal and tracheal displacement to opposite side. The lung can contract to a very small ball, as it is basically just like candy floss.

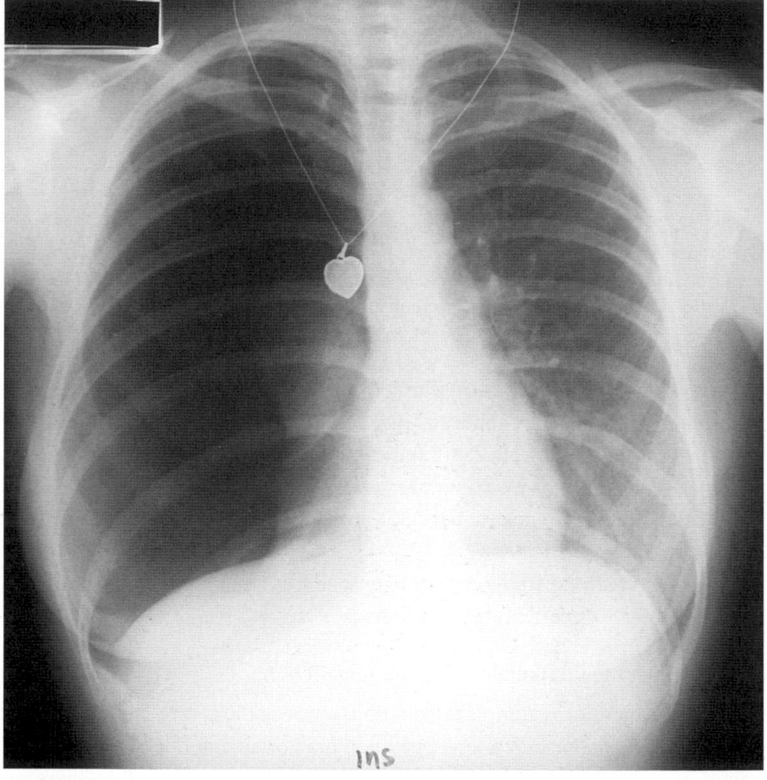

Fig. 9.13 *Lucy Locket's chest X-ray. Right-sided tension pneumothorax with total collapse of the right lung. So where is the heart?*

- Depression of the ipsilateral hemidiaphragm.
- Increased radiolucency on the affected side.
- Separation of ribs on the affected side.
- Any remaining bulla or bullae: the one which 'blew' will be gone.

Important point: A pneumothorax will always look bigger on an expiratory film, – as the lung recoils back towards the hilum a fact you can exploit. Angling to the apex may also make it easier to pick up a small pneumothorax. An inspiratory film will diminish your chances of picking up a small one, which will not do your ego any good. Current protocols, however, now encourage the inspiratory view alone as if the pneumothorax is small it shouldn't need a drain.

Causes of spontaneous pneumothorax

- Apical bulla.
- Complications of asthma/COPD.
- Chronic fibrotic lung disease.
- TB.
- Metastatic lung disease.
- Primary tumour.

Gold medal points:

- *Catamenial pneumothorax* (due to ectopic endometrial tissue) causing recurrent pneumothorax, usually on the right. Occurs in endometriosis.
- *Buffalo chest*. Patients who have had sternal splits may have pleural spaces that communicate, so a pneumothorax on one side automatically creates one on the other. The term springs from the buffalo, whose pleural spaces communicate normally. The Plains Indians knew if they could get an arrow into the chest, and then pull it out again, it would probably kill the buffalo.

NB

- Do not mistake the medial scapular border for a pneumothorax – and give the patient one from an unnecessary drain.
- Spurious pneumothoraces may be misdiagnosed due to *skin folds*, especially on the supine films of elderly or dehydrated patients and premature infants. These can normally be traced beyond the lung fields (Fig. 9.14).

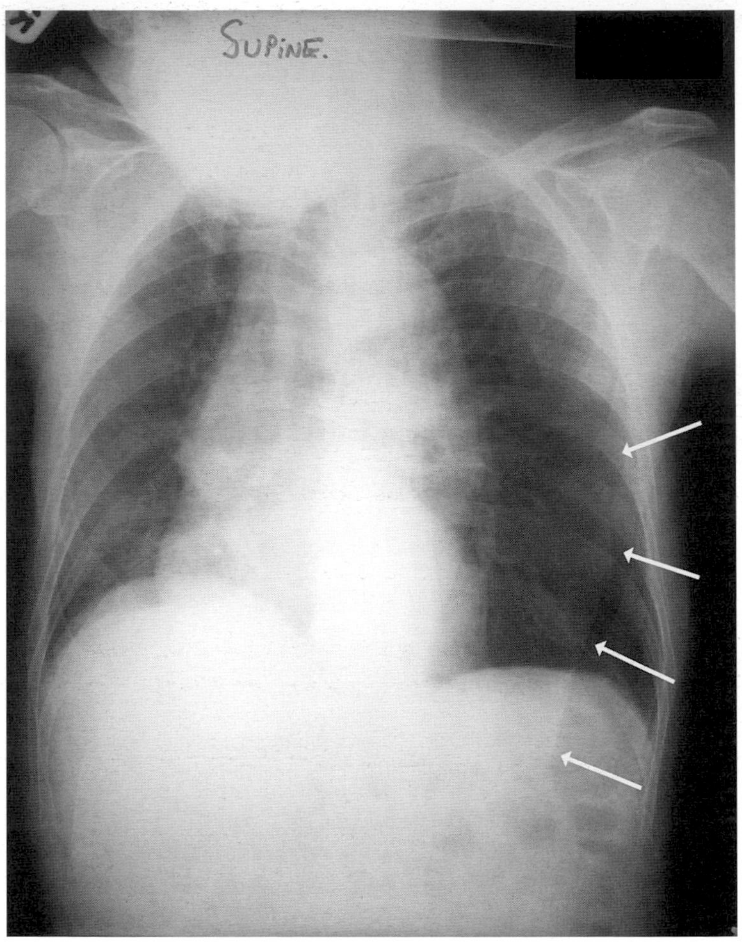

Fig. 9.14 *A trap for the unwary! A skin fold simulating a pneumothorax. Note the patient is supine, and the fold can be traced below the level of the lung field into the upper abdomen. Vessels were also visible beyond it; careful analysis will get you out of trouble. An erect film taken shortly afterwards showed this edge had gone.*

Chest trauma

Background

The RCR guidelines identify 'minor, moderate and major trauma'.

- *Minor trauma*, which may involve cracking a rib or two, apparently 'does not require X-ray', as the demonstration of a fracture will not alter management.
- *Moderate trauma* does require a 'frontal chest X-ray' to demonstrate the complications of rib fractures, e.g. pneumothorax, haemothorax or pulmonary contusions. (**NB** Defining the boundary between these 'minor and moderate' injuries must depend on clinical assessment and judgement.)
- *Major trauma*. These cases comprise manifestly dangerous injuries in patients who may have vascular instability and/or respiratory complications (Fig. 9.15). They may be multiply-injured or unconscious and the chest may form part of the routine screen on arrival, but **stabilizing the patient is always the prime concern before seeking X-rays**.
- Crucial point: When the patient is stabilized, CT may be urgently indicated to assess the aorta and mediastinum, etc.
- *A chest X-ray on arrival* is a vital adjunct, however, as it may confirm a known pneumothorax requiring immediate drainage, even if it is strongly suspected clinically.
- *Mediastinal widening* and loss of the aortic knuckle may indicate a vascular tear of the aorta, with a surrounding haematoma, but see p. 233.
- *Stab wounds*. These require urgent chest X-rays, preferably erect. Ultrasound may also help to localize a haemothorax; assess the heart and pericardium (echocardiogram) and abdomen, if that has been penetrated as well, for collections of blood.

Important point: A *haemopericardium* may cause *cardiac tamponade* – a life-threatening build-up of blood in the pericardial sac, causing cardiac embarrassment. Note how often this condition lends itself to medical dramas on television. The patient is at death's door but the doctor makes a really smart diagnosis. He then performs the heroic measure of a pericardiocentesis, clearly seen by the viewers. The patient immediately stages a genuine and miraculous recovery, sits up and asks the nurse out for a date. The doctor reaches hero-like

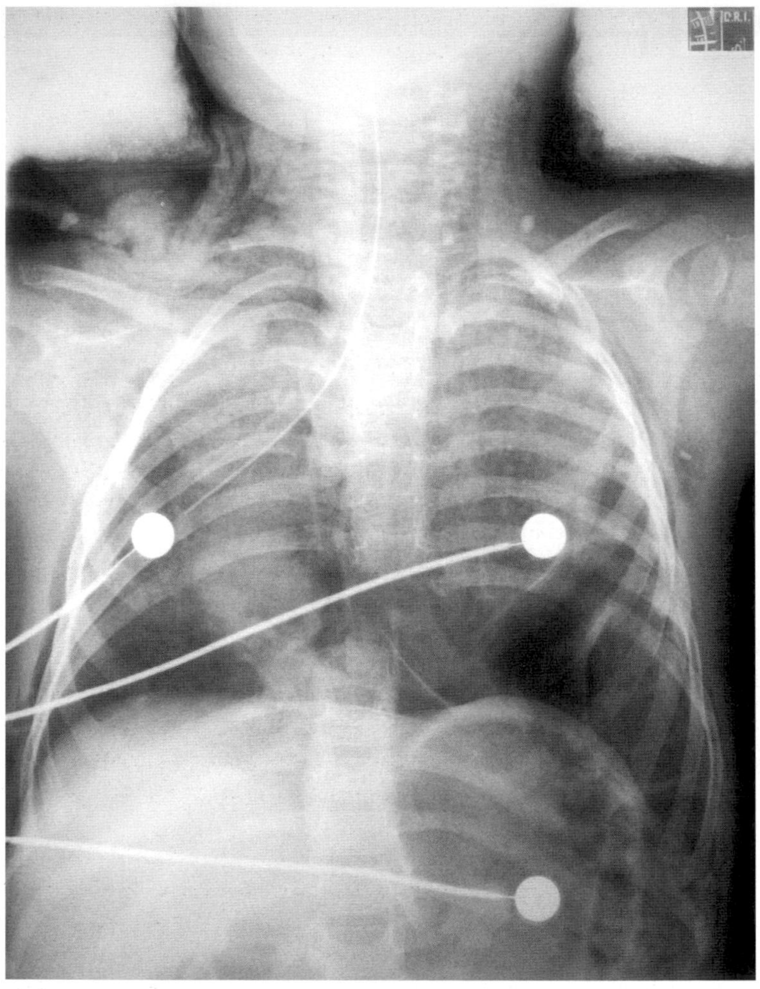

Fig. 9.15 *Multiple injuries. Devastating chest and spinal trauma (child thrown out of car on impact – not wearing a seatbelt). Note the transected and separated thoracic spine, the rupture of the left hemidiaphragm, and colon in the chest. There is also displacement of the heart to the right, a left pneumothorax, left upper rib fractures and extensive bilateral surgical emphysema. Note the sandbags stabilizing the head. The child died of these head and associated injuries.*

proportions in the nurse's mind, and gets the date himself instead of the patient. So make sure you don't miss the next one which comes along!

Sternum

Background

Because of its position, the sternum is inevitably susceptible to direct impact from the front, classically from hitting the steering column of a car in a road traffic accident.

Radiography

Oblique views are often attempted but a lateral which shows the bone in isolation gives the best results. Backward displacement and cortical breaks should be readily assessable, but it is important to achieve accurate 'coning' – this refers to the visible edges of the collimating devices which determine the field of view. If left wide open, the films may lack contrast or come out too black for technical reasons.

Fundamental principle: All X-rays should be as tightly coned as possible to *minimize radiation* and to *optimize contrast*.

Normal variants

Surprisingly little of the sternum is visible on chest X-rays. Usually only the manubrium is seen sticking out to the right in rotation, which the unfamiliar observer is likely to mistake for a mediastinal mass: more than one patient has been sent for a CT or mediastinoscopy on the strength of this normal appearance on unreported films.

Moral: Get your films reported!

An underdeveloped baby's sternum consists of a row of rounded bony blobs which may cause diagnostic confusion if seen in rotation (see Keats & Anderson 2001).

A radiolucent gap usually exists between the manubrium and the body of the sternum, i.e. the manubriosternal joint, and in young children (Fig. 9.16) unfused sternal segments appear as further lucent gaps simulating fractures.

NB Fractures of the sternum may be hard to see if heavily calcified costal cartilage is present and approaching from either side. Non-calcified and invisible costal cartilages make life much easier, but remember the first costal cartilage is calcified in everybody over the age of 25. Sometimes this structure causes

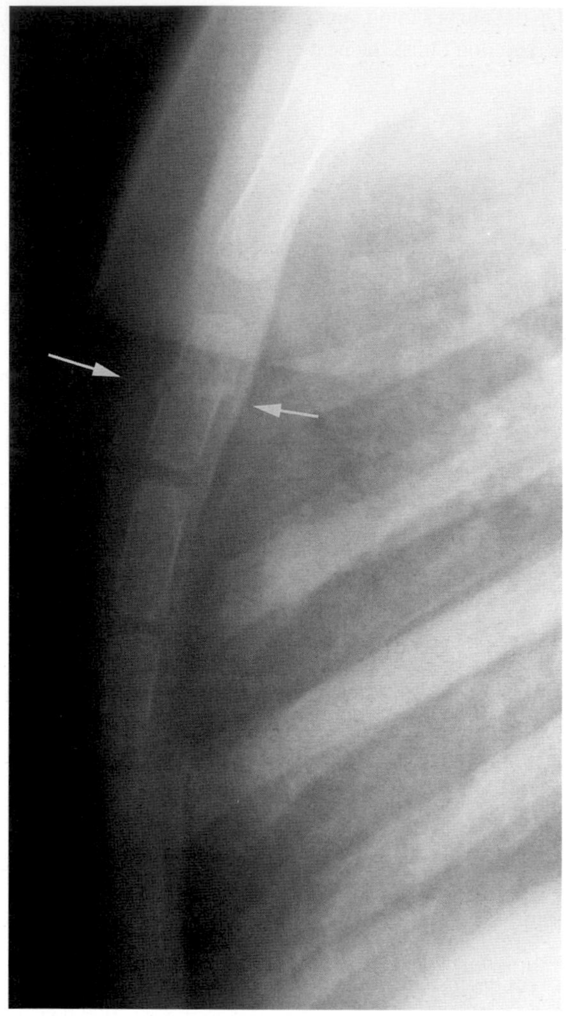

Fig. 9.16 *Fracture of sternum (arrows) (lateral view) in a child. Note the normal intersegmental cartilaginous components (dark) between the bones.*

concern about underlying masses or tuberculosis, necessitating further views to confirm its location unequivocally.

Danger of death

There is an increased risk of cardiac and aortic trauma in the presence of a sternal fracture. Make sure you get a chest X-ray to assess for associated rib fractures, their complications and widening of the mediastinum. Echocardiography and CT may be necessary as a follow-on. Remember uncalcified costal cartilage is invisible.

Hint: Sometimes a sternal fracture can be associated with a thoracic spinal injury and lead to a crippling kyphosis, so a baseline thoracic spine X-ray can be helpful.

Assessment of rib trauma

NB There can be no doubt that in the past the expiratory 'frontal chest X-ray' (PA or AP) combined with specific 'views for the ribs' optimized the chances of detecting *all* rib fractures that were present, plus their most important complication, the *pneumothorax*, which of course is why they evolved over decades (Fig. 9.17).

Recent concerns over minimizing the radiation dose to patients in the UK (IRMER Regulations 2000) have resulted in some centres restricting the initial assessment to an *inspiratory* PA or AP chest X-ray. The rationale for this is that it is not the fractured ribs that matter, so much as any complications which they may cause, and any pneumothorax big enough to need a drain ought to be visible. This single view may suffice **as long as the limitations of a solitary chest film are appreciated.**

Crucial point: The lowermost ribs do not appear routinely on conventional chest X-rays, being lost in the white-out of the upper abdomen, unless fortuitously visible through interposed colonic or gastric fundal gas. They should, however, be demonstrable by image manipulation with digital technology.

A fracture that is clearly visible on an oblique rib view may be entirely invisible on a straight chest X-ray, and vice versa; this depends heavily on its position and orientation relative to the X-ray beam.

Some hot tips for hunting out rib fractures (Figs 9.18, 9.19)

Few things are less productive than bestowing a vacant stare at a chest X-ray, waiting for something to happen. In addition, the uppermost four or five ribs,

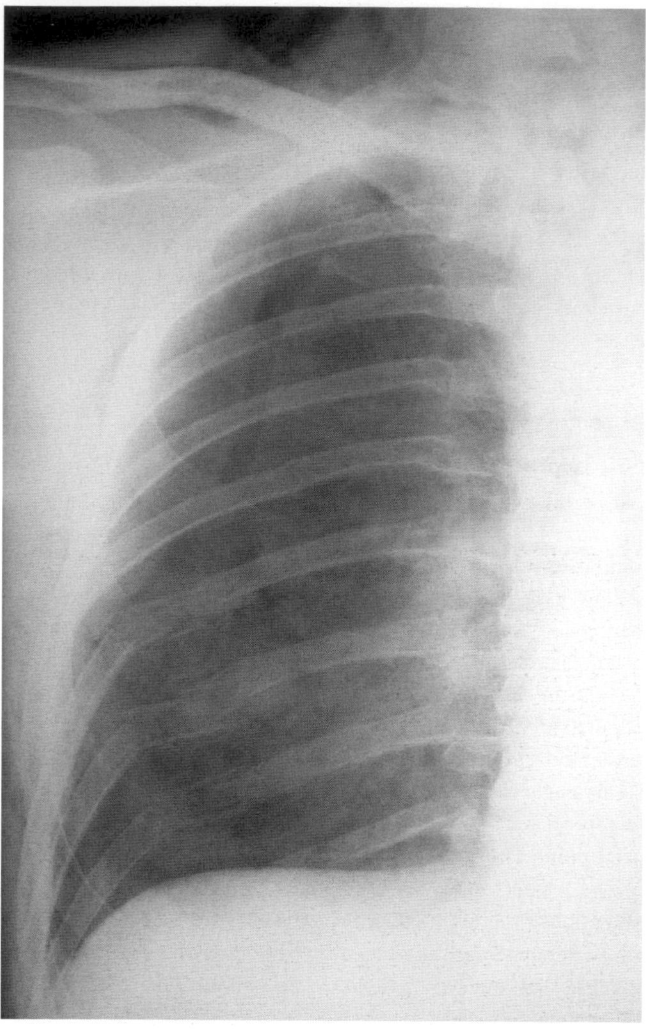

Fig. 9.17 *Multiple double fractures of right lower ribs. Note also the big right pneumothorax convex out the way, the medial margin of the scapula intruding into the lung field, convex in the way, and surgical emphysema extending up into the neck. Medial scapular margins are often flat or convex.*

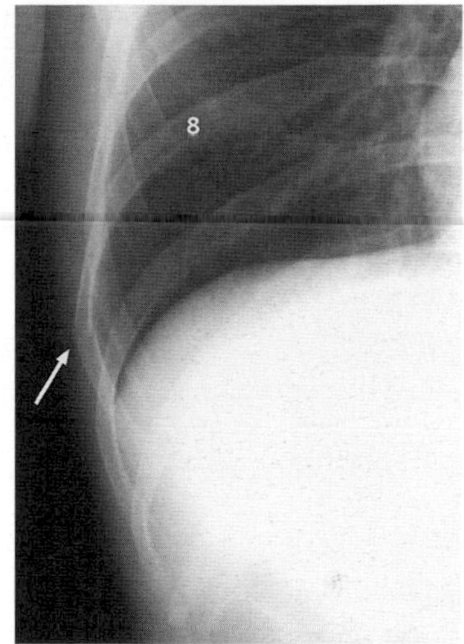

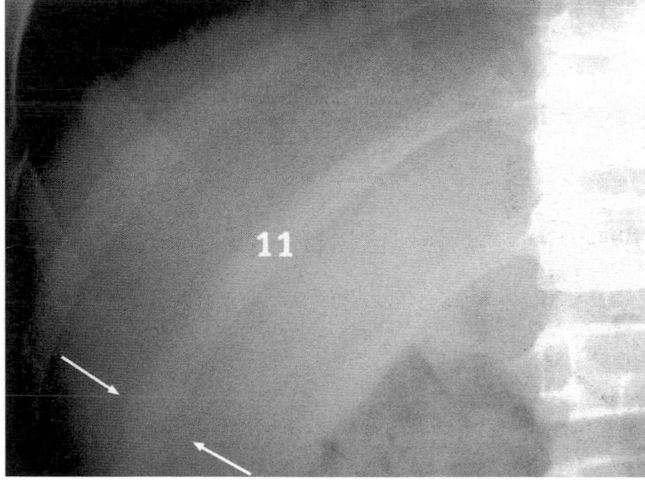

Fig. 9.18 **A** *Fracture visible in the lower right 8th rib at the axillary margin. Note how the lowermost ribs over the upper abdomen are 'whited out' and impossible to evaluate properly.* **B** *Penetrated AP view of the upper abdomen revealing a fracture in the 11th rib as well.*

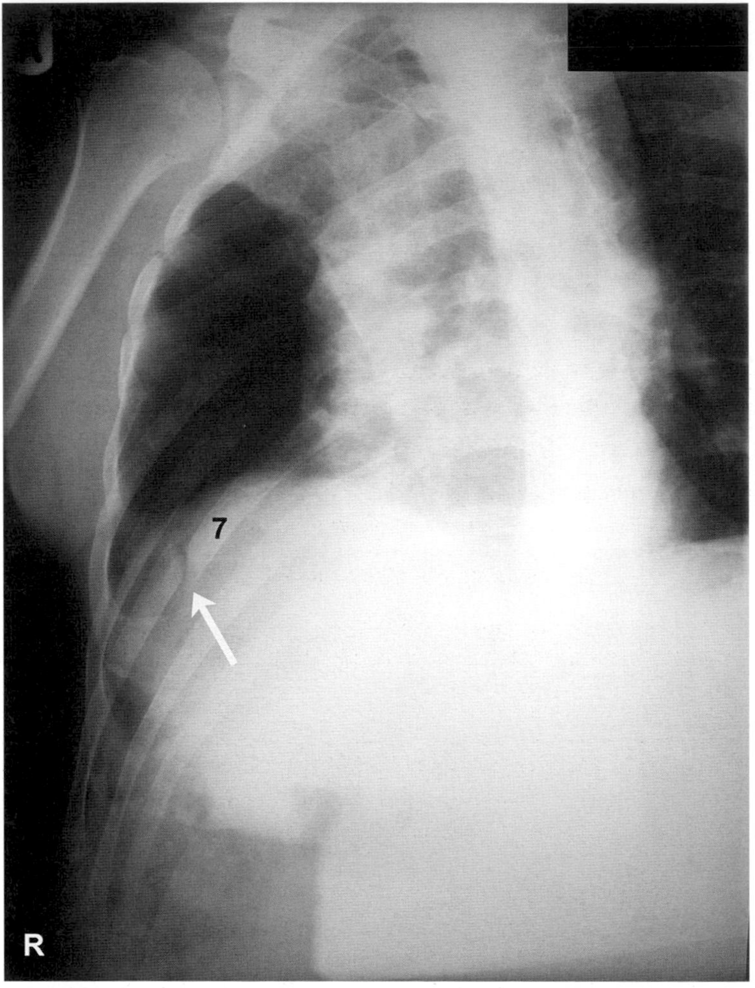

Fig. 9.19 *Typical oblique view of ribs showing a fracture in rib number 7. Don't mistake these steep oblique views for over-rotated chest films! Note: these projections are going out of fashion, which means more rib fractures will be missed.*

overlain by the clavicles, are hard to sort out, as the eyes keep slipping off one on to another; and it takes a great deal of practice to start seeing this jumble of bones individually on top of and through each other. In elderly kyphotic patients who are bent severely forwards you may actually have to step up from rib to rib initially, as the first and second ribs lie 'below' the third and fourth.

Again, unfortunately, in elderly kyphotic patients with thin gracile bones, multiple ribs may completely overlap each other and even if you do find a fracture you cannot be sure which rib it is in. In this situation, oblique views will separate out the ribs if you are seeking a cause of pain or its location.

What to do?

- You must look meticulously around every rib in turn and trace its course from back to front, including its upper and lower cortex. (This is laborious, but if you do not find it so, you are not doing it properly.)
- Put your thumb or finger against the rib you are looking at and *hold it there* until you have inspected all of the rib, from back to front.
- Then move your digit on to the next one, and so on.
- If the film is very dark, use a bright light to highlight each rib. If you have a digital system, use it to crisp up the bones by increasing the contrast and conspicuity of the ribs.
- Look for a small convex opacity on the inner aspect of a suspected rib fracture at the pleural margin: this may occur due to localized bleeding. Similarly, there may be a small haemothorax, with a curved top down at the costophrenic angle but beware of old preceding pleural thickening here – and check for previous films.
- A black line may appear across a rib alongside where a vessel crosses over it. This is the Mach effect again and not a sign of a fracture. Sometimes inferior rib margins appear to have defects in them – due to small flanges of bone.
- Do not just settle for one fracture in one rib. Make sure there are no more *in the same rib*. Multiple fractures in adjacent ribs causes flail segments and paradoxical motion (see p. 224).
- *'The Crystal Palace view'*. Turning the chest X-ray on its side will present the ribs as a series of hoops (like the Crystal Palace structure that burned down in

London in 1936). This will remove the overfamiliar view of the underlying vascular markings, which can be distracting, and allow you to look at the ribs in relative isolation. This is also something 'cool' you can do at a meeting! Incidentally, tilting films and looking at them obliquely increases the subjective contrast and visibility and improves your level of confidence in assessing subtle lung field and retrocardiac abnormalities, as well as allowing you to look extremely erudite.

Surgical emphysema

- If a fractured rib punctures a lung, as well as causing a pneumothorax, air may quite naturally escape and track into the chest wall between the muscle layers. Clinically this creates a crackling sensation on palpation, like brown paper under the skin, which you must learn to recognize. Radiologically, the equivalent finding is of intensely dark irregular black streaks of air travelling up and down the way – which may decompress up into the neck, into the arms or down into the abdominal wall.
- Always look for this after trauma. Finding it makes the presence of at least one rib fracture very likely.
- Do not mistake it for the normal bilateral symmetrical dark grey layers of fat between the chest wall muscles and those underlying trapezius in the root of the neck, which will be (1) symmetrical and (2) less dark.
- **NB** Surgical emphysema can also track down into the chest from fractured sinuses.
- When gross, surgical emphysema can reveal the exquisite unipennate or multipennate structure of muscles such as pectoralis major by 'negative contrast'.

NB Because of the dark streaks it produces, surgical emphysema can simulate as well as obscure both rib fractures and a pneumothorax.

Haemothorax

Bleeding may, of course, occur after trauma and create a haemothorax. This looks like a simple effusion, unless there is air above it (pneumothorax), in which case it will have a flat top (i.e. haemopneumothorax). You can therefore diagnose the presence of a pneumothorax from afar, even if you have not yet seen the edge of the lung, just from the way the fluid is behaving (Fig. 9.20).

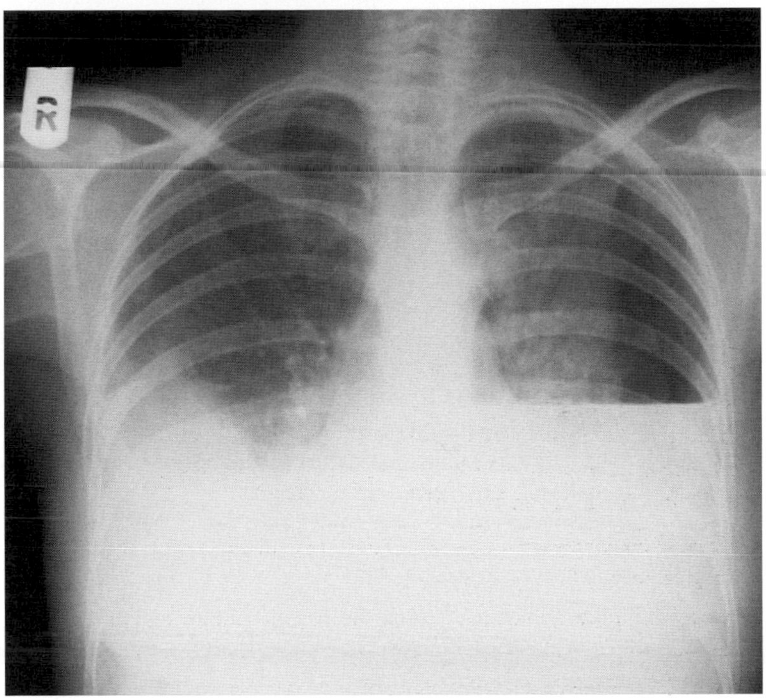

Fig. 9.20 *Fluid behaves differently when there is air above it. Note: the right pleural effusion with the hazy upper margin; the razor sharp left fluid collection, because this is a hydropneumothorax, i.e. there is air above it. Corollary: you can tell at a glance and from a distance that a patient must have a pneumothorax as well – even if you cannot see the edge of it. Note: you get extra points if you spot the 'air bronchogram' in the left lung as well = consolidation. (This patient had ovarian carcinoma and came to A & E with severe breathlessness. Her lung surface had ruptured due to a metastasis.) A normal lung shows soft tissue vessels contrasting with black air. Normally the thin-walled bronchi are invisible. In consolidation, the lung becomes opaque and the vessels disappear, but the air-containing bronchi are suddenly thrown into relief. This is an 'air bronchogram'. When supine an effusion just forms a veil of increased density on the affected side.*

Pulmonary contusions

Blunt or blast trauma may cause irregular opacifications in the lung fields and these can be due to parenchymal bruising. There are, however, other potential causes, of scattered changes on A & E chest films such as bronchopneumonia, aspiration of gastric contents, smoke inhalation, or drowning. The clinical context will give appropriate clues. Unconscious supine patients will tend to aspirate into the upper lobes. Conscious upright patients who aspirate will tend to do so into the lower lobes.

'Shock lung'

Damaged lung can become inflamed and consolidated. Associated with trauma, hypoxia and vascular occlusions lead to bronchospasm, pulmonary hypertension and respiratory failure. Extensive opacification of both lungs may be seen, leading to the formation of an air bronchogram.

Fat embolism

This may complicate fractures. Check the retina, sputum and urine for fat globules. Multiple small opacities may be seen on the chest X-ray and the patient may become confused.

Enter Madame Guillotine: a memorable patient

Look at Figure 9.21:

This is the chest film of one of two glaziers who were up a ladder helping to manoeuvre a very large pane of glass into a frame.

This man was in the lower position when a loud 'crack' was heard, followed by the sudden descent of a heavy razor sharp sliver of glass which had got out of kilter and sliced instantaneously through the major vessels in the left side of his neck.

Fortunately a first-aider dived on him and staunched the flow with pressure, cloths and whatever else was to hand, thus enabling him to survive the trip to A & E, with the help of the paramedics. The number one priority on arrival was stabilizing the patient – the multiple haemostats attached to the bleeding points tell their own story.

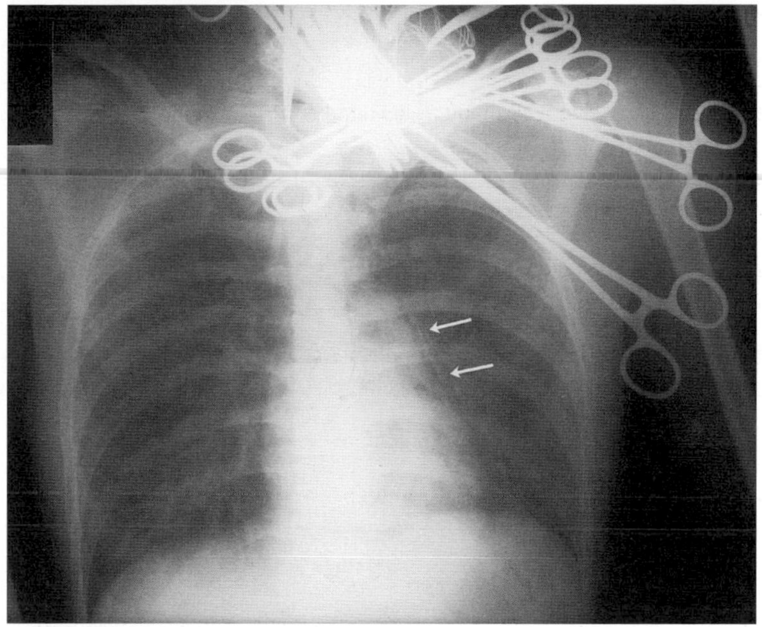

Fig. 9.21 *A case of near decapitation. Note the mediastinal emphysema (arrows).*

Note the irregular streaks of air in the neck and the clear-cut lucency around the left side of the heart with elevation of the pleura, because his trachea has been cut: this is mediastinal emphysema – a very important finding in chest radiology and A & E medicine.

Some causes of mediastinal emphysema

- Blunt trauma to the chest.
- Penetrating injury to the chest.
- Associated with a pneumothorax.
- Blast injury to the chest.

- Gunshot wound.
- Spontaneous rupture of the oesophagus (Fig. 9.22).
- Iatrogenic – ruptured oesophagus at endoscopy.
- Extension from facial fractures.
- Homicidal cutting of the throat.
- After hanging (suicide) – with, for example, rupture of the larynx.
- Diving accidents.

Learn to recognize this important finding. And finally – beware of congenital abnormalities (Fig. 9.23). These may well present in trauma patients, potentially causing gross misdiagnosis.

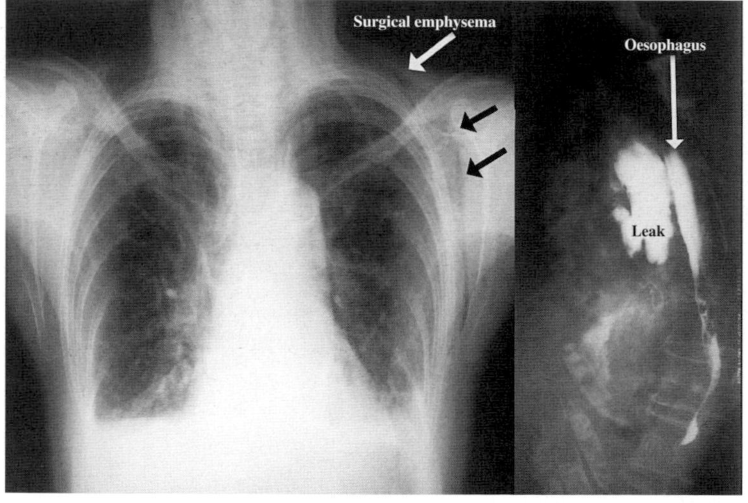

Fig. 9.22 *Spontaneous rupture of the oesophagus. Beware of other people's diagnostic labels. This patient was sent in as having a 'myocardial infarction'.* ***A*** *Surgical emphysema noted around left side of chest.* ***B*** *The contrast study confirmed a leaking oesophagus.*

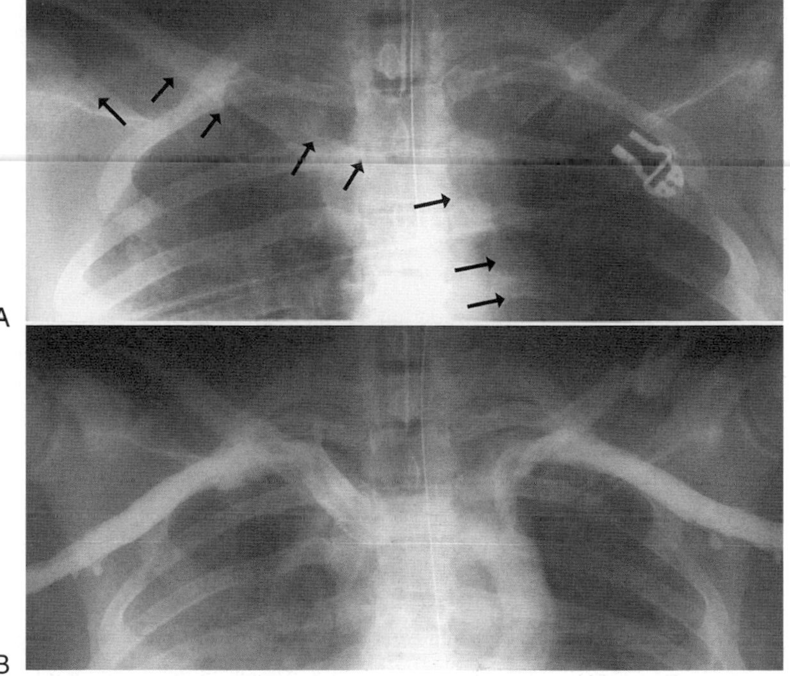

Fig. 9.23 *Beware of congenital anatomical abnormalities. This patient struck his sternum in a road traffic accident. The mediastinum was wide and the aortic knuckle not clearly defined. An arch aortogram was requested for further evaluation.* **A** *A very astute radiologist noticed, however, that the central venous line (arrows) entering from the right side was descending on the left.* **B** *He therefore decided to do a bilateral arm venogram (a lot less trouble than an arch aortogram) and confirmed a left-sided superior vena cava.*

Chapter 10

The abdomen

Background

Second only to the chest X-ray in importance is the plain abdominal X-ray, which is an altogether more taxing proposition because so many structures are lying on top of each other in an infinitely variable kaleidoscopic mixture of gas, solid organs, calcified opacities and colonic residue. Many junior doctors have never even tried to conquer the abdominal film: when confronted with one they simply gaze at it, wait for something to jump out, and, if nothing does, declare that it is 'normal'.

In addition, there is also a tendency in some circles to declare the abdominal X-ray as 'inappropriate in the following conditions…', which are then listed. This presupposes that the clinical diagnosis is always right, which is, of course, not true. Indeed, more than one horrified clinician who thought that he was dealing with a renal colic has been confronted with a leaking aortic aneurysm. So abdominal films are often asked for in order to 'see what is going on'. Abdominal films should not therefore be requested with preconceived fixed notions of what is wrong, but with an open mind as to what they might reveal.

Interestingly, recent radiological research has shown that simple unenhanced CT scanning in the acute abdomen can considerably improve the accuracy of diagnosis even from plain films, and as stated plain films themselves are not infrequently already at variance with the presumptive clinical diagnosis.

Radiography

The standard film is the AP supine, but two films are often needed to include all the anatomy from the hemidiaphragms to the inguinal canals.

Beware the pregnant female! You must do your utmost to exclude pregnancy in women before exposing them to X-rays. In some centres in the USA, patients are catheterized and their urine tested before X-rays for pelvic trauma are used – to avoid subsequent lawsuits.

What to do?

As with the chest, a systematic method of analysis is needed to give you a framework to work to when trying to interpret abdominal films.

- As always, check *the name of the patient* and that you are dealing with the *current film.*
- In acute cases check *the time.* The patient may get X-rayed again later the same day.
- Find the *left/right marker* and make sure you have *put the film up the correct way round.* It should automatically be correct on a digital on-screen system.
- *Check the bones.* These are important in major trauma and in malignant disease.
- *Check the outlines of the retroperitoneal landmarks,* i.e. the kidneys and psoas muscles, which normally contrast with the background retroperitoneal fat. Often only parts of the renal outlines are visible, and the psoas muscles may be obscured by overlying bowel gas. Their absence, however, may indicate a retroperitoneal mass or haematoma.
- *Look for the liver and spleen.* The lower edge and tip of the liver are often visible, but often the spleen is not. Enlargement can occur in trauma and disease.
- *Look for the bladder.* This presents as a round or oval mass in the pelvis. A big pelvic mass may be due to acute retention of urine in the bladder or a pelvic haematoma, e.g. with pelvic fractures. Pelvic haematomas can displace the bladder, which, if outlined by fat, may be seen on plain films. They also push small bowel up out of the pelvis. Most common is just a full bladder in a patient who has had to wait in A & E.
- *Check the gastrointestinal tract.* This consists of the hollow organs which contain gas, fluid (stomach and small bowel), and faecal residue (colon), in varying degrees.
- **NB** Parts of these hollow organs are all that is normally visible. Only when distended by gas and fluid is there extensive visible anatomical continuity with ileus and obstruction.

- **NB** Do not mistake the resting gastric fluid in the left upper quadrant for an abnormal mass (i.e. the normal round gastric pseudotumour).
- The small bowel shows as multiple small pockets of gas in the central abdomen and pelvis. To diagnose dilatation you need *three loops, each greater than 2.5 cm* in diameter, unless it is a localized sentinel loop.
- The large bowel tends to be peripheral and normally contains granular semi-liquid faecal residue on the right and formed faecal masses on the left. (These masses themselves contain small pockets of gas.) *The upper limit of normal for the colonic diameter is 6 cm.* The critical diameter for the caecum, above which perforation may be imminent, is 9 cm. **NB** Some patients have chronically distended bowel greater than this, often with constipation, and are not in immediate danger of perforation.
- Be aware of *normal calcified structures:*
  - Costal cartilages: can mimic renal and biliary calculi when punctate
  - Arteries: calcify with increasing age and early in diabetes
  - Lymph nodes: can simulate calculi and spinal metastases
  - Pelvic phleboliths: mimic urinary tract calculi.

Renal trauma

UK guidelines identify minor and major degrees of renal trauma. If a patient with blunt renal trauma has only microhaematuria, is haemodynamically stable and has no other injuries, imaging is not required.

With more severe trauma, ultrasound can be used to assess the kidneys, but if negative does not exclude renal injury. Plain films and intravenous urograms (IVUs) have been used in the past to assess renal injuries and to look for perirenal haematomas, with loss of renal and psoas outlines and extravasation of intravenous contrast, proceeding when indicated to renal angiography. With definite major trauma, plus or minus prior shock and with or without macrohaematuria, **multislice CT with dynamic enhancement is the imaging modality of choice.** This means with intravenous contrast fired in by pump (see Fig. 14.5, p. 312).

Gold medal point about CT: 'The patient must be studied both in the nephrographic (blushing) phase of contrast administration, and the pyelographic (or excretory phase), the latter to exclude any leakage from the collecting systems' (RCR guidelines).

Important points

- In any renal trauma patient, **it is crucial to establish the status or even presence of another functioning kidney before scheduling the patient for nephrectomy of the one and only kidney.**
- In exceptional circumstances it is possible for a patient to completely shear off a kidney from its pedicle (i.e. artery, vein and ureter) and have no haematuria on testing. If the patient survives, the vessels have probably gone into spasm, or the flow has been stemmed by the pressure of the haematoma.

Corollary: The absence of haematuria does not exclude significant renal trauma.

More generalized trauma

The liver, spleen and gut can also be assessed by CT for haematomas and ruptured viscera. Plain films may be useful after a stab wound to check for free gas in the abdomen or retroperitoneum.

Abdominal gunshot wounds ('red blanket' cases)

These patients are often best sent straight to CT if stable or when resuscitated. Abdominal films, with the entry wound marked, can be taken to locate a bullet if there is no visible exit wound. Some patients will, of course, be dead on arrival or 'bleed out' shortly after, but films might be required for forensic reasons.

Point of interest: In some cities of the world, gunshot wounds form the majority of acute abdominal cases.

The non-traumatized acute abdomen

See below for a list of common causes of the acute abdomen, the radiological signs to look for, a number of illustrative examples, and a note of the investigation(s) of choice, when indicated, to which you should rapidly move.

Radiological signs in the acute abdomen

Suspected conditions	Signs
Perforated viscus	Pneumoperitoneum. Gas under the diaphragm on erect chest films. Air also on outside of the bowel

	wall, increasing its clarity – *Rigler's* or *double-wall sign* (Fig. 10.1). May need water-soluble contrast swallow, but not barium! Absence of sub-diaphragmatic gas does not exclude a perforation.
Ruptured abdominal aortic aneurysm (or 'Triple A')	Expanded calcified aorta, usually to the left but not always, sometimes with loss of retroperitoneal landmarks. Small aneurysms can rupture as well.

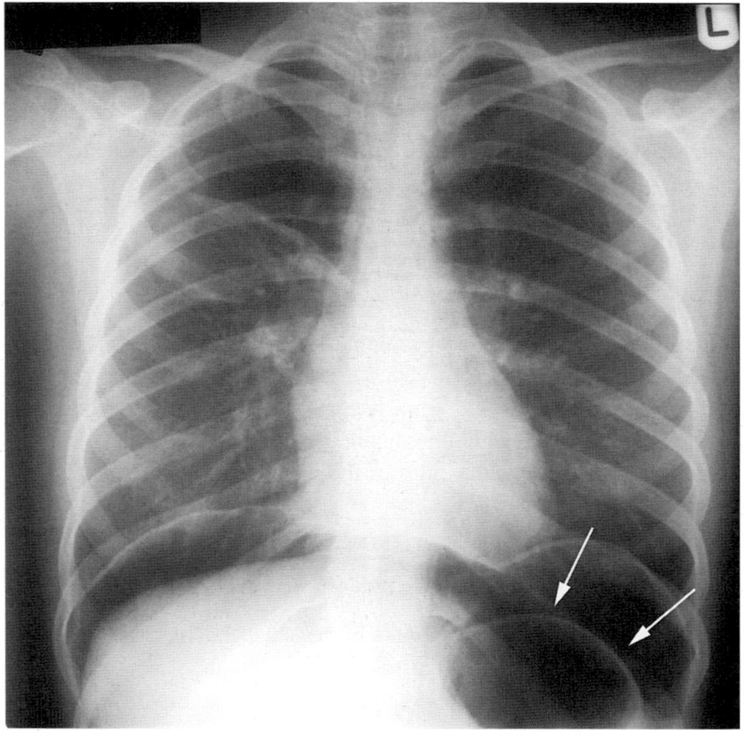

Fig. 10.1 *Massive bilateral pneumoperitoneum. This patient had a perforated duodenal ulcer. Note the positive Rigler's or double-wall sign, i.e. air on either side of the gastric fundal wall. Gold medal observation: incidental finding of absent spleen (previously removed).*

	Needs urgent CT if haemodynamically stable (Fig. 10.2).
Renal colic	Calculus/calculi in ureters (check also the kidneys and bladder. Needs ultrasound, IVU (Fig. 10.3), low dose CT or MRI (to show a 'standing column' of urine – obstruction).
Biliary colic	Stone in bile duct – rare as only 10% are visible. Needs ultrasound.
Cholecystitis	Stones in gallbladder, air in wall of gallbladder (emphysematous cholecystitis). Needs ultrasound or CT.
Pancreatitis	Ileus. Retroperitoneal gas. Occasional pancreatic calcification (with acute on chronic pancreatitis). Gallstones – as a predisposing factor. Needs ultrasound or (better) CT.
Appendicitis	Calcified faecoliths/sentinel loops. Mass or abscess in the right iliac fossa. Consider ultrasound or CT for further evidence.
Intestinal obstruction	Dilated multiple small/large bowel loops (Fig. 10.4). Maximum diameter of normal small bowel = 2.5 cm; maximum diameter of normal colon = 6 cm. Check for hernias at groins (causing obstruction). Fluid levels (if erect). Gas in bile duct and gallbladder in gallstone ileus. RCR guidelines now readvise *erect* abdominal films in 'doubtful' cases.
Diverticulitis	Localized pockets of gas. Possible abscess. ?Water-soluble contrast enema (not barium).
Sigmoid volvulus	Gross distension of sigmoid. 'Coffee bean sign'. Water-contrast enema if in doubt. **NB** Sometimes the caecum can also 'volve'.
Abscesses	Focal persistent gas collection. Fluid levels on erect films. Do ultrasound or CT.
Mesenteric occlusion	Localized ileus of small bowel. Gas in wall of bowel. Needs Doppler ultrasound/angiography/CT.
Ischaemic colitis	'Thumbprinting' due to oedema of mucosa in colon. (? Water-soluble contrast enema.)
Pyloric stenosis	Infants need ultrasound or barium meal.

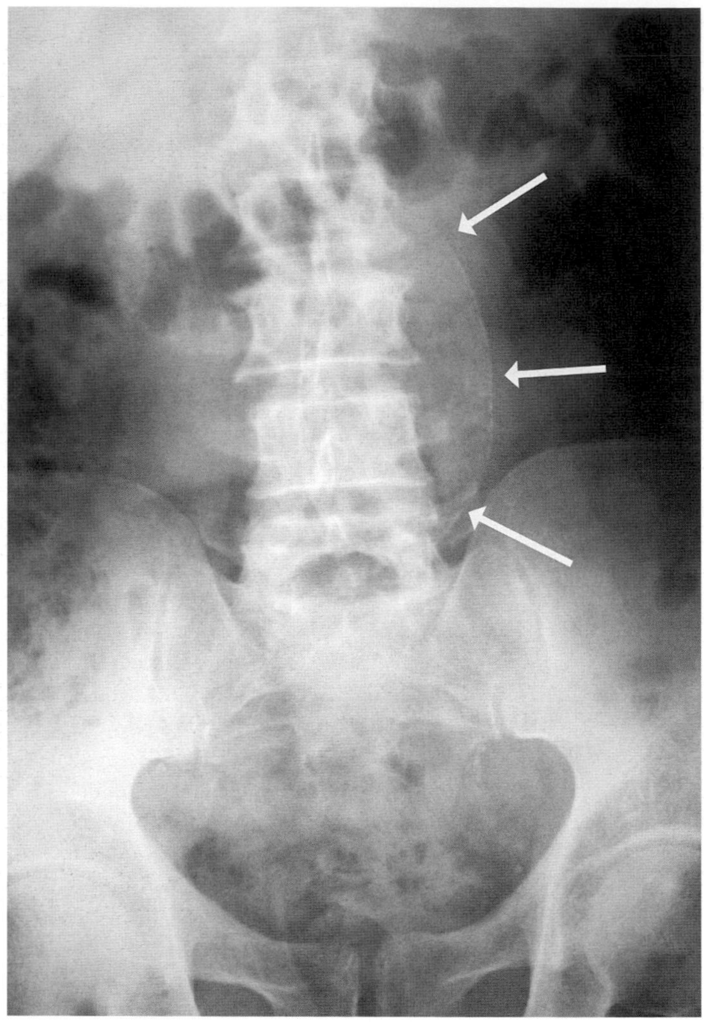

Fig. 10.2 *The old enemy! The abdominal aortic aneurysm or 'Triple A', bulging to the left. Look for these on every abdominal film on everyone over 40 years.*

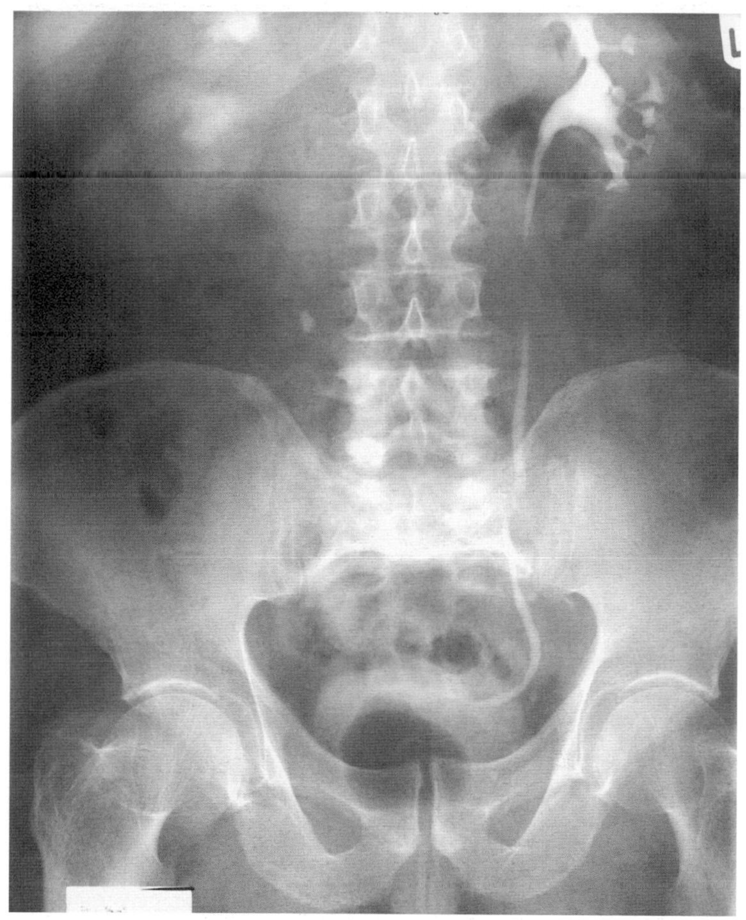

Fig. 10.3 *Right renal colic: an IVU showing delayed excretion and dilatation on the right due to a calculus to the right of L3.*

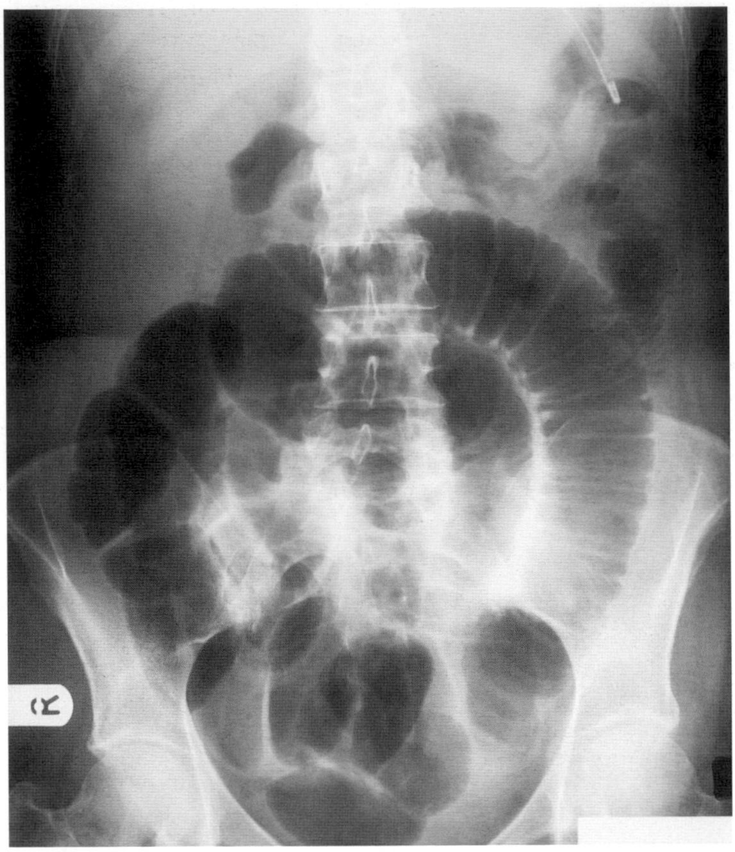

Fig. 10.4 *AP supine film. Distal small bowel obstruction. Note the dilated central loops and valvulae conniventes going right across the lumen (left side). Note: as the pockets of gas build up, eventually they begin to form a continuous column of gas in the lumen. The cause was adhesions.*

Intussusception	Gas in dilated colon outlining intussusception. ?Air/hydrostatic/barium enema reduction, under sedation. May require surgery.
Toxic dilatation of the colon	Dilatation of colon (i.e. > 6 cm). Oedema of mucosa with loss of haustral folds and pseudopolyp formation. Needs urgent surgery.
Necrotizing entercolitis	Affects infants. Gas in bowel wall. Usually very ill. May have gas in portal vein as antemortem event.
Massive constipation (occasional danger of perforation)	Gross faecal overload. Needs laxative regimens/ enemas/manual extraction or colectomy.
Suspected drugs mule	Multiple sachets of swallowed heroin inside the abdomen.
Gynaecological conditions	Plain films often not helpful. Need pelvic ultrasound. Do not forget to consider the differential of pregnancy, e.g. ruptured ectopic and pelvic inflammation.

NB Do not forget that the acute abdomen can be mimicked by **myocardial infarction, pulmonary embolism, dissecting thoracic aorta and basal pneumonias, etc., so you must request a chest X-ray (preferably erect) as well. Rarer medical causes also include acute hepatitis, porphyria, irritable bowel syndrome typhoid, sickle cell disease and diabetic ketoacidosis.**

Chapter 11

The pelvis

Background

Injuries to the pelvis are both dangerous and disabling. They usually occur in two main groups of people:

1. Young individuals with healthy bones who sustain high energy impacts or falls from a height.
2. Elderly patients with weakened osteoporotic bones who have sustained a fall – often from only standing height, e.g. after tripping over a paving stone.

The danger of these injuries lies in associated blood loss, and the potential complications of enforced immobility, particularly in the elderly (pneumonia, deep vein thrombosis, etc.). Their clinical assessment will frequently reveal inability to weight-bear, pain on lateral compression, evidence of blood loss from torn vessels and sometimes urethral bleeding or evidence of rectal injury.

Radiography

Inability to weight-bear after a fall or local pain and tenderness merit X-ray examination. The initial assessment is the standard AP supine film, which gives a great deal of information. Any suspected femoral neck fractures require lateral views of the hip. Steep angled up and down shots can emphasize separation of the pubic rami. In the past, steep oblique or Judet views to look at the hips and acetabula have been 'something clever to ask for' but any complex injury should now be assessed by multislice CT, preferably with 3D imaging.

Anatomy (back to the rings) (Fig. 11.1)

- The pelvis (and sacrum) form one big ring.

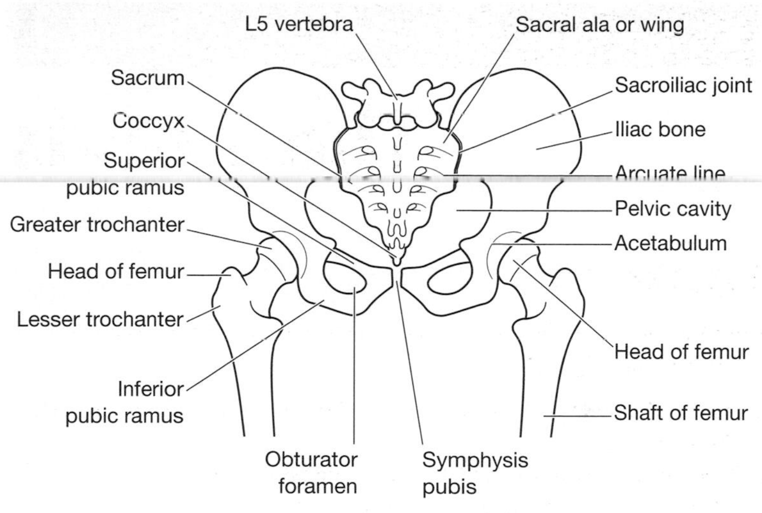

Fig. 11.1 *Anatomy of the pelvis.*

- The superior and inferior pubic rami form smaller secondary rings: together they simulate the appearance of a harlequin mask.
- Radiolucent cartilaginous components cushion the sacroiliac joints and pubic symphysis.

Important anatomical variants

NB These relate mainly to the developing pelvis (Fig. 11.2). Note:

- Slightly wide sacroiliac joints, typical of a young patient. These are not usually greater than 2 mm in an adult.
- The triradiate cartilage of the acetabulum. This forms three irregular gaps in the acetabular cups.
- The epiphyses of the proximal femora.
- Cartilaginous points of fusion at the inferior ischiopubic junctions. These are often asymmetrical, and it has been said they can even disconnect themselves

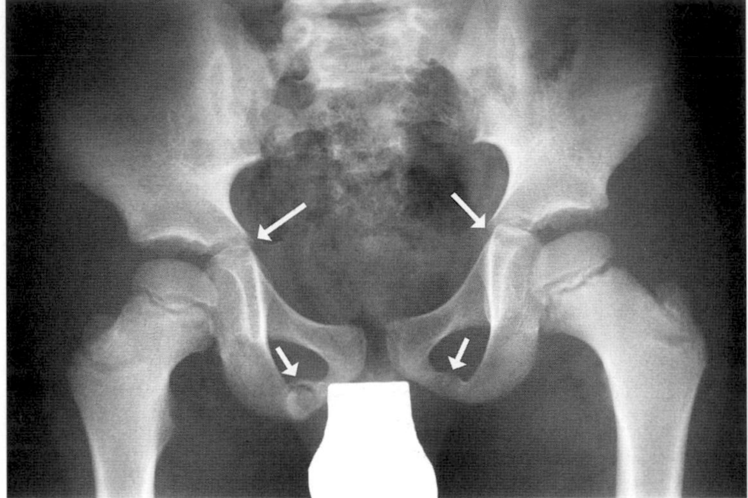

Fig. 11.2 *The juvenile pelvis. Note the two main sites of importance of developing cartilage (arrows). Note also the femoral neck and greater trochanter epiphyses. The lesses trochanters have some too but these have now fused (right) or are invisible (left) due to internal rotation.*

after fusion and undergo a second fusion. Try not to mistake these for healing fractures. They are usually seen between the ages of 5 and 7 years. In adults, sclerotic Y-shaped nutrient and vascular channels may be seen in the iliac blades.

- **NB** Be aware of the epiphyses of the iliac crests – these may not fuse until the early twenties. They form a dense line over the top of the crests with irregular lucent (cartilaginous) inferior margins.
- The configuration of the sacrum, which has already been discussed, under the spine. Note particularly the arcuate lines surrounding the sacral foramina. You are more likely to miss a fracture than find one in the sacrum. Use CT.
- **NB** Bowel gas often severely restricts your view of the sacrum.

- The symmetrical symphysis pubis. This can be out of alignment in postpartum women, presumably due to ligamentous laxity in pregnancy. Osteophytes can also disturb its symmetry and should not be mistaken for trauma.

Fractures of the pelvis

- In falls, the pelvis may undergo lateral or frontal compressive forces, as well as unilateral shearing effects or combinations of all of these. In addition to suffering sudden impacts, the pelvis may also be incrementally compressed to the point of fracture, e.g. by falling masonry in an earthquake.

- Because it is a ring structure, any one fracture identified should be assumed to indicate the presence of another and carefully sought by meticulous inspection right round the coastline of the pelvis. So keep your eyes open. This is your opportunity to be 'Lord of the Rings'!

Crucial point: Disruption of either sacroiliac joint (>2 mm) or symphysis pubis (>2.5 mm) in an adult also counts as 'failure of the ring' and, if found, should be accepted as a second fracture rendering the pelvis unstable.

Types of fracture

- Lateral compressive forces may crumple the iliac blades and disrupt the sacroiliac and hip joints.

- Vertical shearing displacing forces may cause fractures and dislocations through the sacrum, the sacroiliac joints, the pelvis proper or the symphysis pubis.

- Severe AP compressive forces, e.g. getting crushed by a fork-lift truck against a wall, may disrupt the sacroiliac joints and symphysis pubis and flatten out the iliac blades – the so-called 'open-book fracture' (Fig. 11.3).

Fractures of the pubic rami

- If broken in two places, these can be unstable. If both pubic rami break on both sides (*Malgaigne's fractures*) the central components become flail. In the elderly this may stop patients mobilizing and such patients often do not do well (Fig. 11.4). Pubic ramus fractures are initially often occult on X-ray, only being confirmed by subsequent callus formation.

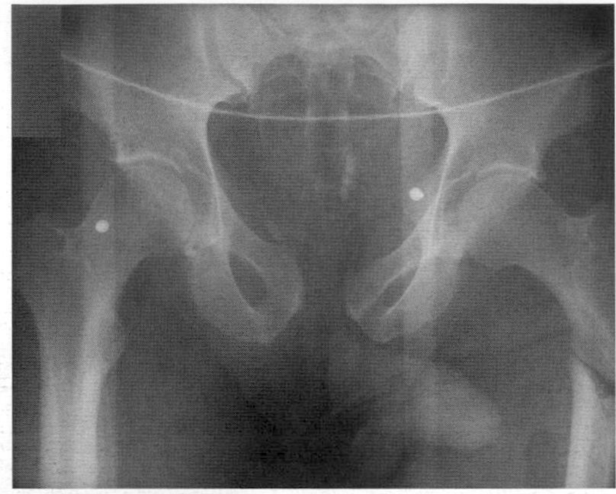

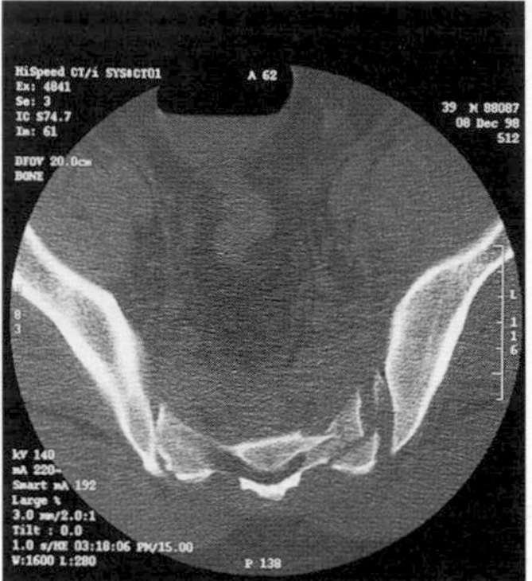

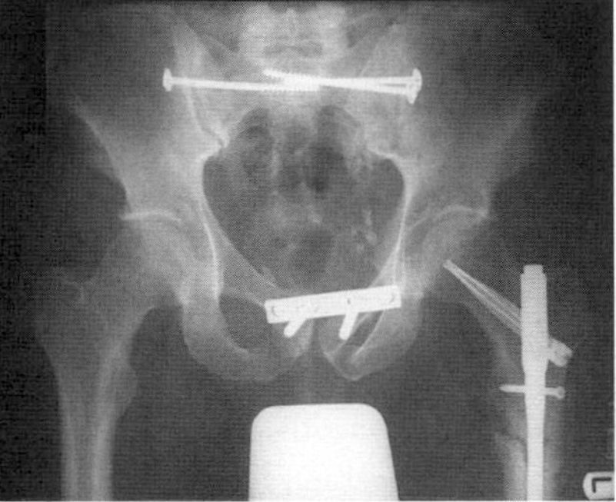

Fig. 11.3 ***A*** *Plain film,* ***B*** *CT scan and* ***C*** *postoperative appearances of an 'open book' fracture of the pelvis. Note the fracture of the sacrum and separation of the left sacroiliac joint, along with the diastasis of the symphysis pubis and fracture of the left femur. Bleeding tends to stop when the ring is closed again.*

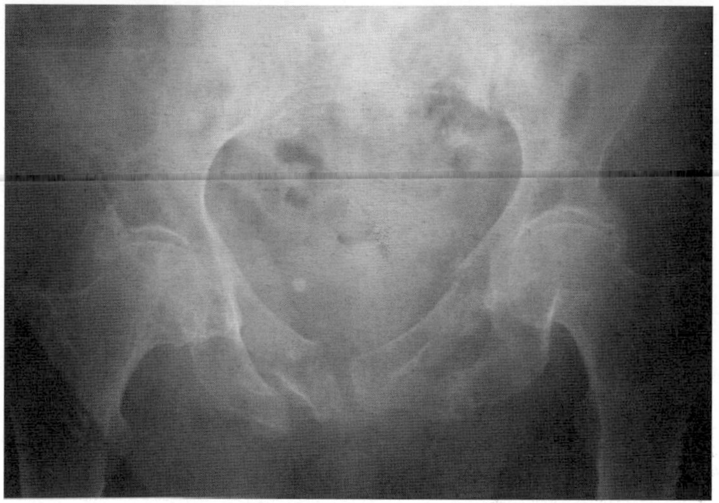

Fig. 11.4 *Bilateral fractures of superior and inferior pubic rami.*

- Stress fractures (e.g. in military recruits) and insufficiency fractures may also affect the pelvis.
- Beware *crack fractures in the iliac blade,* which may be missed if the film is very dark. A dangerous scenario is the '?neck of femur' referred in by a family practitioner. No fracture is found in the hip but there is a crack, which is missed, in the iliac blade. More than one such patient has quietly bled into the retroperitoneal space after being discharged, only to be found dead in bed back home in the morning. So make sure you examine the dark areas with a bright light.

Moral: Check meticulously all of the pelvis in any patient in whom a fractured neck of femur is suspected but not found, especially if your mind-set is primarily joint orientated. Any patient with a crack fracture should be admitted for observation. You should be checking the rest of the pelvis anyway.

Avulsion injuries These can occur from various locations, such as the adductor tubercles, ischial tuberosities and anterior superior iliac spines, usually in the context of sports injuries.

Appearance of pelvic fractures

In common with depressed fractures of the skull, these can be dense if crumpled or lucent if separated. Disruption of the trabecular pattern may be a further subtle sign.

Summary

The pelvis is a dangerous area and is therefore automatically included in every major trauma protocol. If a patient is shocked, always consider bleeding from the pelvis as a potential source, and assume it if the pelvis is disrupted. Check for signs of urethral bleeding, and if necessary request a contrast study of the urethra. This may be done as a follow-on from contrast-enhanced CT by voiding.

Crucial point: Make early contact with the interventional radiologist if you have the services of one. He or she may be able to arrest torrential bleeding early by embolization with coils, etc., thus stabilizing the patient and avoiding all the dangers of excessive transfusion (e.g. respiratory failure) that are otherwise necessary before theatre. **Always consider the patient as a whole, however, and do not forget about head, chest and upper abdominal injuries in your triage.**

Further crucial point: Survival is improved by stabilizing the skeleton.

Chapter 12
The hip

The acetabulum

The acetabulum or cup which articulates with the femoral head is an inextricably integral part of both the pelvis and the hip joint, but merits special mention. The basic problems are that, following trauma, conventional films underestimate both the extent of any fractures and the degree of malalignment of any fragments around the articular surface, so this is a job for CT. Untreated malalignment of fragments will inevitably lead to premature osteoarthritis in the joint.

If a dried hemipelvis is viewed from the side, the extension to the superior pubic ramus lies anteriorly and that to the inferior pubic ramus lies posteriorly. Esoteric classifications have therefore been constructed in relation to *anterior column* and *posterior column fractures*, when the cracks appear in relation to these structures. Your job as an A & E doctor is to identify any fractures which involve or extend down into the acetabulum and ensure that the patient is sent for a CT (Fig. 12.1).

Dislocations

Look at Figure 12.2. This patient's car hit a motorway bridge while he was being pursued by the police. Note the increased density of the right thigh due to the degree of soft tissue injury. This is a superior dislocation of the right hip.

- This film shows obvious upward displacement of the right femoral head, which has been driven right out of its socket. Shenton's line is grossly interrupted and the lateral view showed the femoral head to be lying posteriorly in relation to the pelvic bone. High levels of violence are usually needed to produce this injury, often caused by the knee hitting the dashboard in a high-speed impact, as in this case, with the force of the blow being transmitted up the femur. This is the commonest form of dislocation at the hip.

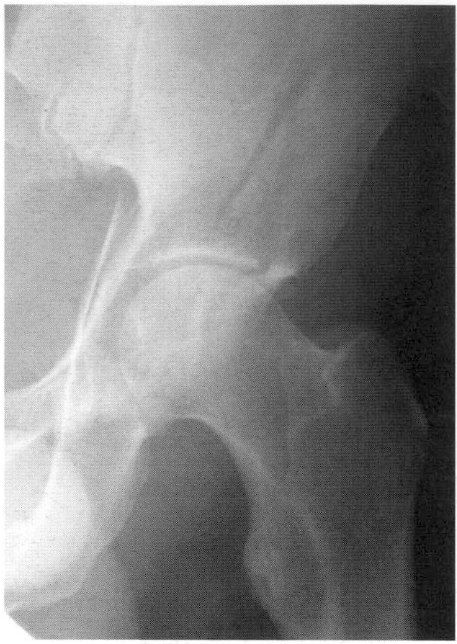

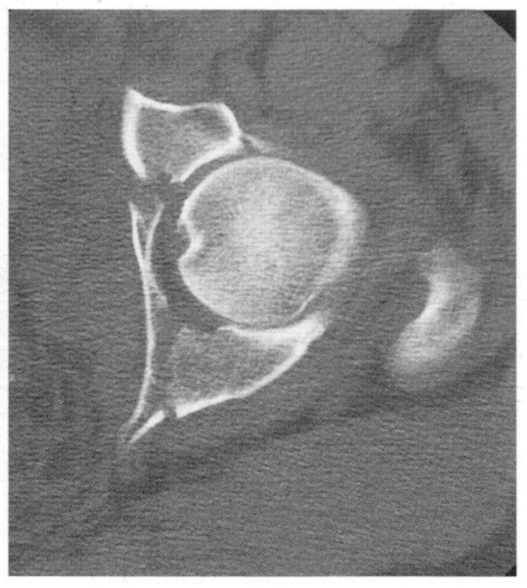

Fig. 12.1 *Conventional film showing fractures and splinters around the acetabulum. Insert shows CT scan of same patient. Note how much better the involvement of the articular surface can be appreciated. 3D images will give even more spatial information if required.*

- *Inferomedial dislocation* may also occur. Note that it is much less common than in the shoulder, and it may be associated with a compression fracture of the femoral head when it impacts against the inferior acetabular rim.
- *Central dislocation of the hip*. This is a **devastating injury**, usually caused by a compressive force. The femoral head smashes its way through the acetabulum into the pelvis, with associated splintering of the acetabulum. **NB** Any film showing a hip dislocation must be inspected very carefully to confirm or exclude any evidence of an associated fracture of the acetabulum or pelvis, and if such a fracture is found, the patient should have an **urgent CT scan**. Initially, transverse slices can be taken; however, the best appreciation will come from 3D reconstruction with surface rendering for the optimum elucidation of any obvious or coexistent unsuspected injury.

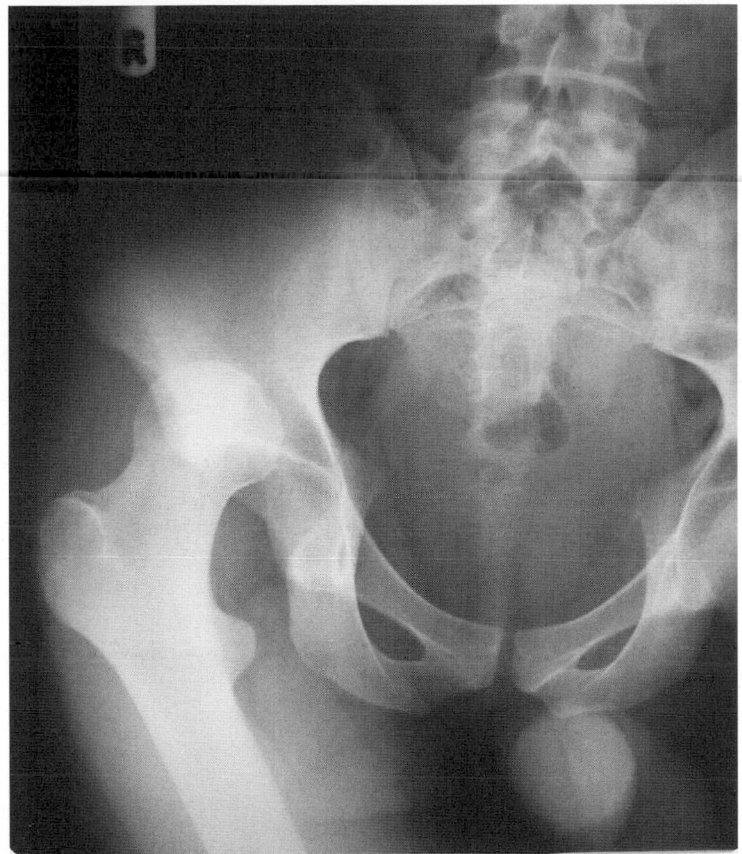

Fig. 12.2 *Superior dislocation of the hip. These tend to go backwards as well and can knock a fragment off the acetabulum. Sciatic nerve damage and avascular necrosis of the femoral head can also occur.*

Prosthetic hips

You must also be aware that prosthetic hips can dislocate and will then also require reduction. The delicate subject of the resumption of sexual activity by women who have been given prosthetic hips may also have to be addressed, as significant abduction of such a hip can predispose to spontaneous dislocation.

Shake, rattle and roll!'

A recent case in the *British Medical Journal* described a dislocation of the hip with no predisposing factors during Scottish country dancing. So rock and rollers beware! It is interesting to speculate how 'Elvis the Pelvis' managed to avoid dislocating his hips – not to mention his knees.

The hip

Background: danger of death

For those who have never experienced it, the sudden uncontrolled violence with which the floor comes up to hit you when you have a fall has to be experienced to be believed. Either a loud crack on impact or excruciating pain at the first attempt to move will indicate that your 'hip has gone' and the precise location where you hit the deck will determine how long you lie there – unless of course you can reach the phone or have a community alarm. For some of the osteoporotic elderly this is the beginning of a 3-day ordeal on the kitchen floor until they are discovered – often suffering from dehydration, deep venous thrombosis, hypothermia – and even then, for an unfortunate third of them, it is a death sentence.

NB Any middle-aged or older female patient who sustains a Colles' fracture should alert you to the possibility of osteoporosis and the need for bone densitometry. 'Hip protectors' (specially designed cushions for the greater trochanters) may prevent fractures in the elderly who suffer falls, and do not forget that some men may get osteoporosis too; many of these patients are walking around with bones like eggshells.

Anatomy

The hip is a simple ball and socket joint, the components of which are set more deeply than the shoulder, which gives it increased stability but reduced manoeuvrability. It therefore requires much more force than to a shoulder to dislocate it, and if normally mineralized, considerably more force to break it.

Another crucial fact to understand is that, if you follow the curve of the inferior margin of the superior pubic ring round, it will describe a graceful and continuous arc on to the curve of the femoral neck. This is known as *Shenton's line*. If this line is interrupted in the acute setting, this will usually be due to a fracture or dislocation of the hip. (**NB** This relationship also obtains in infants with congenital dislocation of the hip but ultrasound, not X-rays, should be used to investigate this nowadays.)

Intraosseous anatomy Note the arcing lines of the trabeculae in the femur, which can be traced on into the acetabulum, that you see every day. Interruption of these lines also means trauma has occurred. These structures indicate the lines of stress.

Normal variation: the juvenile hip (see Fig. 11.2)

Note the unfused triradiate cartilages of the acetabula. These appearances should not be mistaken for fractures.

Radiography

As with the pelvis and sacrum, inability to weight-bear after a fall triggers the indication for X-ray films under current RCR guidelines.

Appropriate views are the full AP pelvis plus a lateral of the symptomatic hip, so that any associated or purely pelvic fractures may be identified in a patient who has been referred in as a 'neck of femur'. Be very careful in this context to check left and right, and to put the films up the correct way.

Important radiographic anatomy

The AP film

Because the femoral necks point upwards, medially and forwards in the supine position, in external rotation the necks are severely foreshortened on AP views and the lesser trochanters are very prominent. As the hips are progressively internally rotated, the femoral necks present more and more of their long axes to the oncoming AP beam, and more and more of the arches of the femoral necks appear until ultimately they lie parallel to the table top on full internal rotation. Simultaneously, the lesser trochanters become less and less obvious and in some cases disappear completely from view (Fig. 12.3). The importance of knowing this is that an immediate inspection of the lesser trochanters will tell you how far

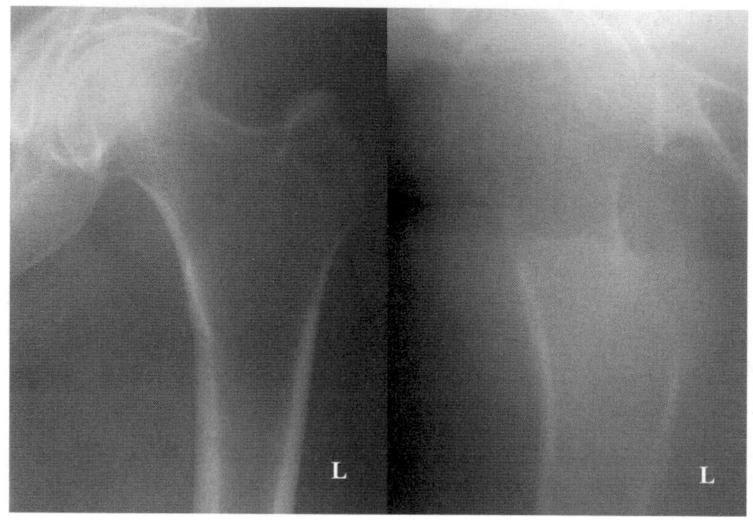

Fig. 12.3 ***A*** *AP and* ***B*** *lateral views of the left hip. Note the sweeping arc of the femoral neck is optimally demonstrated when the lesser trochanter is almost out of sight. Note how the central axis of the neck bisects the head symmetrically on both projections.*

the femur is internally or externally rotated. To put it another way, **the less you see of the lesser trochanters, the more you see of the femoral necks, and you want the best possible view of the neck before you decide it is not fractured.** When completely shorn from its head at the neck, the distal femur goes into external rotation and is often shortened as well, creating the classic clinical signs of the out-turned shortened leg.

Crucial point: Never assume that the film you have been given is the best one humanly possible. Like family snapshots, they all have imperfections but each one will normally be a trade-off between what is reasonably achievable in the circumstances and the state of a patient in a great deal of pain.

The lateral view

Many texts will seek to illustrate a perfectly positioned and exposed lateral hip film in the presence of a fracture to show what can be achieved in favourable circumstances, but for many technical reasons such a film is often far from what you get. The human thigh at the level of the hip is a large block of tissue that generates a lot of X-ray scatter, reducing contrast, so that you may feel you are peering through so much Scotch mist. If the patient is portly, the difficulties of radiography are greatly compounded. Sometimes the films can come out very dark (X-rays by moonlight). So get that bright light on, or start interrogating on your workstation.

The detection of fractures

Fractures of the hip will vary in appearance, from ones you could see galloping past on a horse, to extremely subtle (even when you know what you're looking for), to literally invisible, even when later confirmed to be present (e.g. by bone scan or MRI).

Golden rule: Know what you're looking for!

To find a fracture

- Look right round the edge of every bone for cortical discontinuities, and check the whole of the pelvis.
- Use a bright light on any dark areas (i.e. the iliac blade).
- Look for dark lines in the bones (separations).
- Look for dense bands in the bones (impactions) (Fig. 12.4).
- Follow the arcing trabeculae in the femoral neck through the head and over into the adjacent pelvis (malalignment = a fracture).
- Establish the eccentric position (if present) of the femoral head relative to the extended centre line of the neck when margins are hard to see = displacement and fracture even if you can't see the fracture itself.

NB 'Invisibility' may be largely due to technical limitations, but even with two optimum films some fractures are indeed 'radio-occult'.

Crucial point: You must therefore be guided by the state of the patient. If there is excruciating pain, but you cannot see a fracture, admit the patient anyway. Follow-up with an isotope bone scan; CT or MRI will usually resolve the matter.

Classification of hip fractures (by position)

- Subcapital (Fig. 12.5) – head broken off at junction with neck.

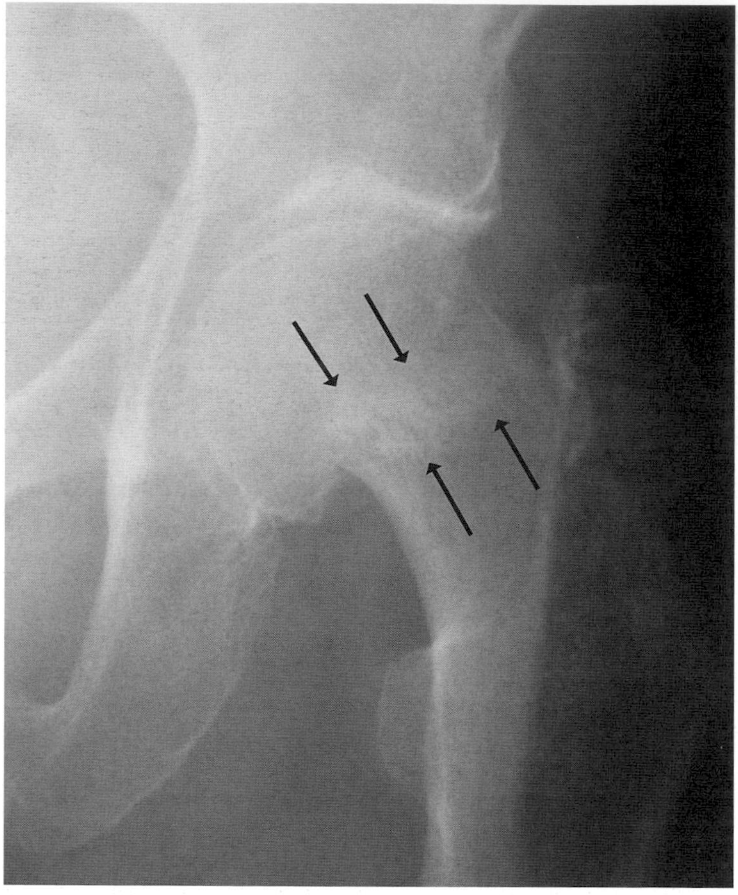

Fig. 12.4 *Impacted fracture neck of femur. Note the cortical discontinuity and irregular dense band where the impaction has occurred (arrows). Some patients will walk on these!*

- Transcervical – across the neck.
- Basicervical – across the lower neck.
- Pertrochanteric – right through both trochanters.

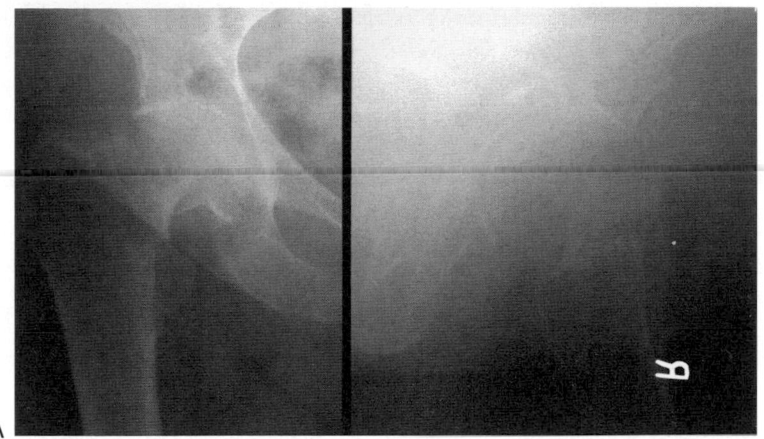

Fig. 12.5 ***A*** *AP and* ***B*** *lateral views of subcapital fracture neck of femur. Note how the head remains in the acetabulum but the neck has been completely shorn off.*

- Intertrochanteric – between the trochanters.
- Subtrochanteric – under the trochanters. Often pathological, e.g. 'the banana fracture'.
- Isolated avulsion of greater or lesser trochanter.

More important is the distinction between *intracapsular* and *extracapsular* fractures.

The hip joint capsule inserts circumferentially on to the lower femoral neck and brings with it the main blood supply to the femoral head. About 10% enters through the ligamentum teres into the fovea (a small crater on the medial femoral head), which should not be mistaken for an injury. Fractures above the capsular insertion therefore put the head at risk of an avascular necrosis of the femoral head, which will rapidly lead to degeneration and osteoarthritis. Displacement at the fracture site is also a bad sign and care must be taken not to convert an undisplaced fracture to a displaced one in the A & E or X-ray departments, or even during surgery.

The orthopaedic surgeon therefore has to make a decision as to whether or not to replace the femoral head at the initial operation, to save doing a second operation later on, or simply to internally fixate the bone with dynamic screws or plating, etc., depending on the precise position. The more fragments that are present, the greater the instability of the fracture. The degree of any preceding arthritis that may already be present must also be entered into the equation.

Point of interest: It has been said the best thing you can do with an osteoarthritic hip in the UK is to fracture it – that way you may save yourself another 2 years of pain on the waiting list.

X-ray appearances that may mimic hip fractures

There are quite a lot of these and you need to become familiar with them. They include:

- The normal developing epiphyseal lines in the juvenile femur (see Fig. 11.2).
- Soft tissue folds, fat lines and creases causing black lines over the femoral necks. These can usually be traced beyond the bones. Beware of surgical emphysema.
- 'Vacuum phenomena' – dark crescents of temporary gas in the joint simulating fractures, but they always lie in the joint between and parallel to the articular cartilages.
- The anterior and posterior acetabular margins. These can cause dense bands across the femoral necks from their edges, but careful inspection should reveal what they are. Their density may simulate impactions, but their edges extend beyond the neck. Dark Mach bands may also be associated with them.
- A fringe of osteophytes on the femoral heads. These can simulate the dense bands of an impacted fracture, but are visible just beyond the neck. Look for other signs of osteoarthritis – joint space narrowing and cyst formation.
- The 'scar' of the position of the closed epiphysis in an adult.
- Calcified arteries. Do not mistake these irregularly calcified objects for impacted fractures where they cross the femoral head. They usually extend both proximally and distally from the pelvis to the thigh.

Spontaneous pain in the hip

Patients will on occasion be brought into A & E complaining of pain in the hip without any history of preceding trauma; they are usually (but not always) young children.

NB Infants should already have been screened for congenital dislocations and dysplastic hips. Consider:

- *Infectious arthritis.* A high index of suspicion must always be maintained for this, as the joint can rapidly be destroyed, and early needle aspiration to exclude it should be carried out. Consider ultrasound.
- *Irritable hip.* Pain and stiffness plus or minus effusion but negative tap.
- *Perthes' disease.* Usually in the preschool or primary school age group. Look for fragmentation of the femoral head (although there are many other causes for this). Refer to orthopaedics.

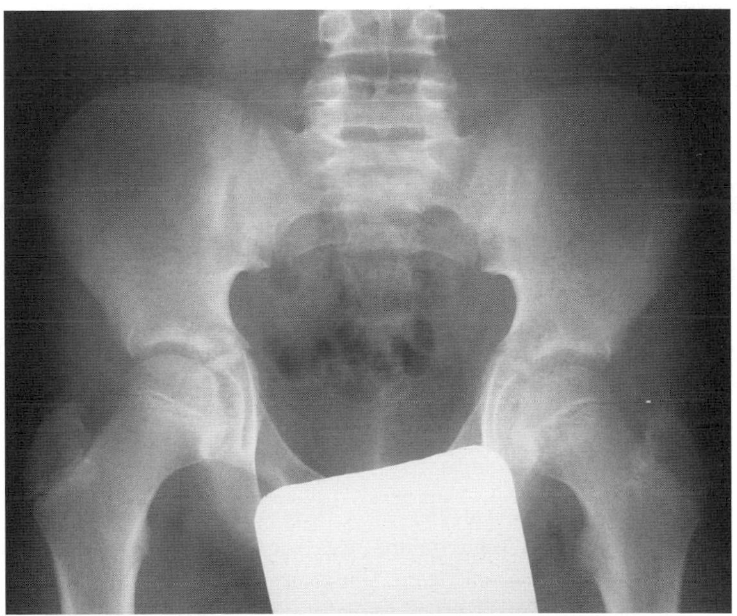

Fig. 12.6 *Slipped epiphysis. AP film – looks normal? See Figure 12.7.*

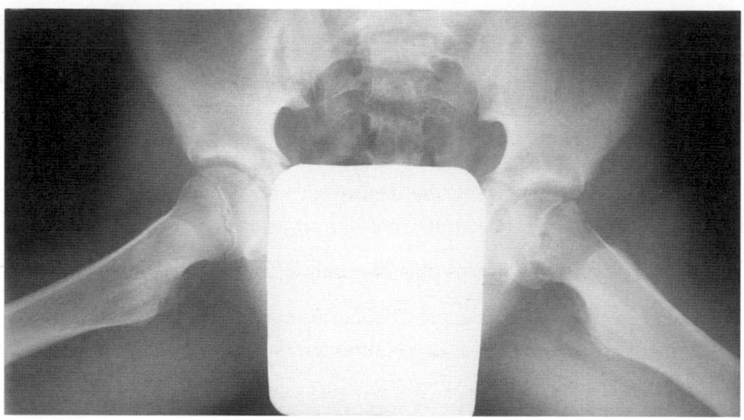

Fig. 12.7 *'Cossack dancer's view' (abducted lateral). The left femoral epiphysis has slipped posteriorly and medially. Moral: never settle for an AP view alone if you suspect this condition. Note the gonadal shield (no trauma). There should be no shield for the first film after trauma.*

- *Slipped femoral epiphysis.* This occurs in adolescents, often overweight children, especially boys. The crucial film is the 'Cossack dancer's' or 'frog's leg lateral', as the AP will often be incorrectly interpreted as normal (Figs 12.6, 12.7). Look for the epiphysis going backwards and medially (great multiple choice question). Refer to orthopaedics.

Crucial point: Hip pain may be referred to the knee, so remember to X-ray the hip if necessary, even if the presenting complaint is knee pain.

In older patients, consider:

- *Exacerbations of known arthritis.*

- *Avascular necrosis of the head of the femur.* There are many medical and surgical causes of this apart from trauma, e.g. arteritis, steroids, postoperative, radiation, which you should learn. This is also a great subject to test you on trauma, paediatrics, orthopaedics, medicine, surgery, oncology, etc., and if you have it at your command, you have a great chance to shine.

- *Transient osteoporosis of the hip.* This is a very painful but self-limiting condition, usually occurring in pregnant women and middle-aged men. The femoral head can be so painful it feels like a red-hot cinder! Bloods and X-rays are usually normal. A bone scan or MRI will be very abnormal. By definition, this ultimately resolves spontaneously in 3–9 months.

A number of avulsion injuries may sometimes be seen around the pelvis, for example:

- Avulsion of anterior superior, and inferior iliac spines, due to sudden contraction of the rectus femoris or sartorius muscles.
- Avulsion of the ischial tuberosity ('weaver's bottom'), due to excessive contraction of the hamstring muscles.
- Avulsion of the iliac crest, often due to running.

Goldenrule: Never forget to consider pregnancy in females of reproductive age before requesting X-rays of the pelvis. Failure to do so may initiate a lawsuit.

Chapter 13

The lower limb

Fractures of the femoral shaft

Background

Main femoral shaft fractures tend to occur in young adults as a result of high-impact sporting or road traffic accident injuries. These are dangerous because of the associated blood loss – manifested by the enormous soft tissue swelling, both clinically and on X-ray.

Crucial point: Half of your blood volume may exsanguinate into your thigh from an open fractured femur and, by logic, all of it from bilateral femoral shaft fractures. By contrast, losing just two drops of blood would cause a sparrow to go into shock! **NB** This degree of blood loss can lead to *deoxygenation*.

Radiography

The aim is to obtain optimum full length AP and lateral films to provide the most accurate assessment of displacement and angulation – often difficult in a multiply-injured patient in splints. It is easy to misjudge a rotational injury and angulation without the joints above and below (i.e. the hip and knee) being visible on each film.

Normal variants

The main variant is that of the nutrient canal 'fleeing' from the knee, i.e. entering the outer cortex more distal to the point of entry to the medulla, but the clinical setting of a fractured femur will leave little doubt as to whether it is broken or not. This is usually a clear-cut situation.

Fracture types

- Open or closed.
- Spiral.
- Comminuted.
- Supracondylar.
- Pathological.

Beware of coexistent vascular injury to the femoral artery and vein. Fat embolism is another potential complication, symptoms of which may include confusion, retrosternal discomfort and dyspnoea. Check the fundi for fat globules in the retinal arteries (if possible) as well as the sputum and urine. Oxygen may protect against fat embolism.

The knee

Background

- Knee injuries are commonest in adolescents and young adults, from games like rugby and football, fast contact sports, skiing, road traffic accidents and falls. Bound both internally and externally by powerful ligaments, the knee is a big sturdy joint, moving in one plane and cushioned by cartilaginous menisci between both articular surfaces of the femur and tibia.
- It is important to understand that fractures around the knee can be associated with serious intra-articular cartilaginous and ligamentous injuries and also that a severe internal derangement of the knee can occur *without* any visible fracture, but other indirect signs of trauma may be present on the plain X-rays. MRI is playing an increasing role here in assessing such soft tissue injuries and occult bony trauma.

Crucial point: A totally comprehensive and accurate diagnosis is unlikely to come from clinical examination alone.

When blunt trauma or a fall is the mechanism of injury, RCR guidelines recommend plain X-rays for patients between 12 and 50 years of age if they cannot walk more than four weight-bearing steps. X-rays are not therefore indicated in lesser degrees of injury.

Radiographic assessment

Virtually all major knee trauma assessments in the UK will start with straight AP and cross-table lateral or 'shoot-through' views. These will provide a global overview of what has happened to the knee, may provide direct or indirect evidence of trauma, and dictate what further views, if any, are required.

Further views/investigations may include:

- *Skyline views of the patella* (Fig. 13.1) if a fracture is strongly suspected clinically but invisible on AP/lateral views.
- *Intercondylar or 'open-joint' views* to show the posterior condylar surfaces, for loose bodies, osteochondritis, etc.

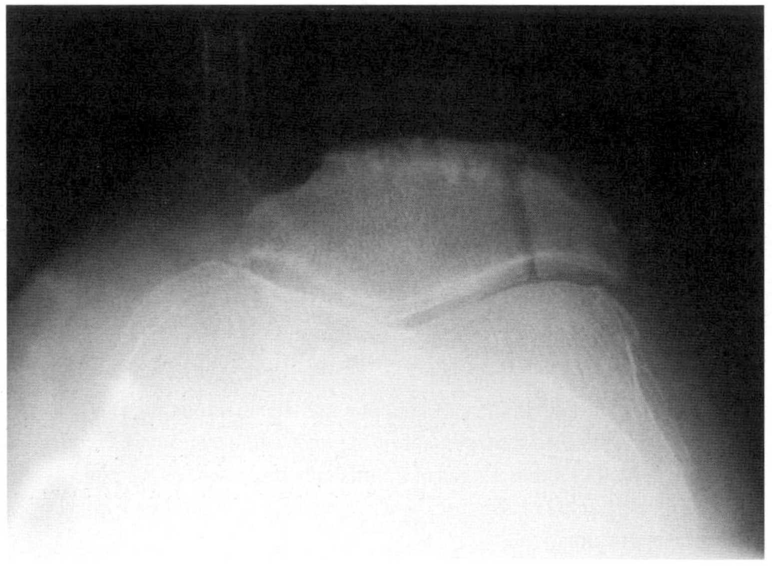

Fig. 13.1 *A skyline view of the patella – useful for finding occult fractures (as here) and evaluating the aetiology of lateral dislocations. The long shallow component is the lateral side. Point of interest: If you must fracture your patella do it vertically. If you transect it horizontally, the pieces will fly apart and you will lose the extension mechanism of your knee.*

- *Oblique views* for fractures of the articular surfaces of the tibia and tracking fracture lines in oblique planes. These are routine in some places but not in the UK.

Follow-up after A & E which you need to know about includes:

- *CT scanning*, plus or minus 3D reconstructions, for evaluating complex fractures and intra-articular fragments.
- *MRI scanning*. This will provide optimal information concerning cartilaginous damage associated with fractures on to joint surfaces (which is common), internal and external ligamentous injuries, and 'bone bruises'.
- *Radioisotope bone scanning*. For delayed assessment of occult fractures, and other suspect pathology presenting in A & E, e.g. if no CT/MRI is available.
- *Conventional CT or magnetic resonance angiography* may be used to assess concomitant vascular injuries, as clinically indicated.

Anatomy (Fig. 13.2)

The areas behind the quadriceps and patellar tendons are usually dark due to fat contrasting with the tendons and rendering them visible. Fluid collections like blood or pus will tend to cause these edges to disappear.

Normal variants

- *Bipartite patella*. An apparently separate bony fragment nearly always located in the upper outer quadrant on an AP view. A crucial observation is that, if you try to 'put it together again', it will not create a normal patella (because of the intervening cartilage), so it looks too big. Its margins will be sclerotic and it is usually bilateral so an X-ray of the opposite knee helps to clinch the diagnosis (Fig. 13.3).
- *Tripartite/multipartite patella*. Even rarer variants of the above. Apart from even more fragments, the same observations apply.
- *Naughty patella*. The patella will on occasions break the rules and show *incomplete fusions* inferiorly or elsewhere. Occasionally *fissures* will appear anteriorly on skyline views, or even spiky anterior crenellations known as *patellar teeth*. The list is endless.

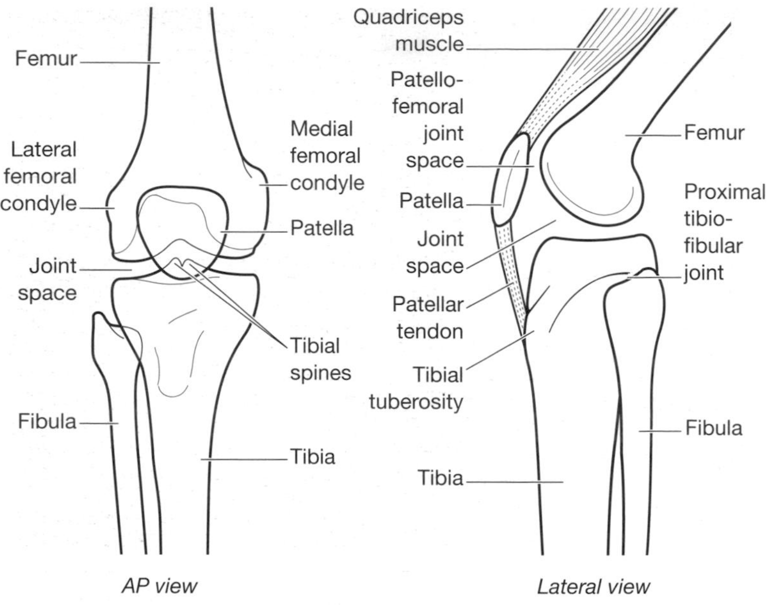

Fig. 13.2 *Anatomy of the knee.* ***A*** *AP;* ***B*** *lateral.*

- *The juvenile knee with its developing epiphyses.* This is notorious for all manner of femoral condylar irregularities and rough edges (see Keats & Anderson (2001) for multiple examples). Articular grooves can also cause apparent sudden steps here too, simulating fractures. Metaphyseal irregularities may also simulate non-accidental injury.
- *Fabella.* A small smooth ossicle lying laterally behind the knee. The mnemonic is 'L' as in 'fabella' lying on the Lateral side. This can also be duplicated, triangular, bifid or not-so-smooth!
- *Cyamella.* Another small normal variant bone.

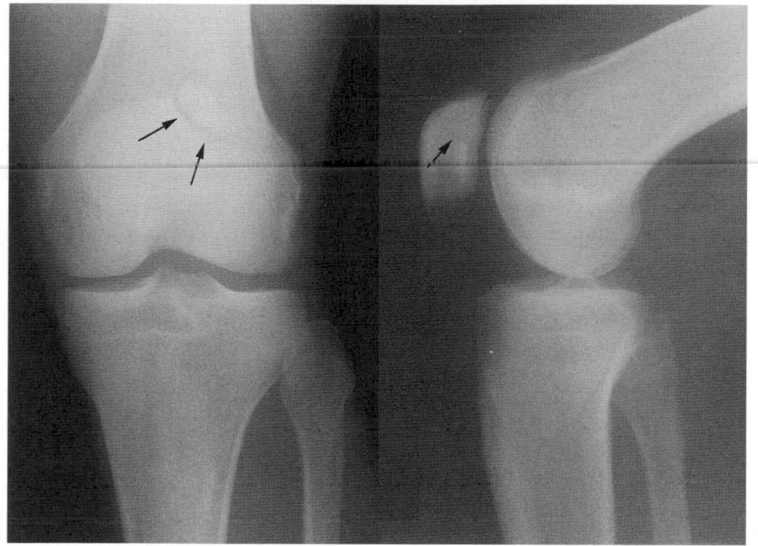

Fig. 13.3 ***A*** *AP and* ***B*** *lateral views showing a bipartite patella. Involvement of the upper outer quadrant is typical. Note: this phenomenon is almost invariably bilateral.*

Fractures of the lower femur

Lower femoral fractures at the knee are sometimes classified as supracondylar, condylar or intercondylar and may present as cracks, cracks with displacement or comminutions.

Paediatric fractures may of course go through the epiphyses and cause breaks in classic Salter–Harris style (see Fig. 13.9 p. 289).

Fractures of the tibia

Fractures at the knee tend to be due to sideways impacts, e.g. from cars, hence the term 'bumper' or 'fender' fractures, the effects of falls (vertical shearing forces) or combinations of forces.

Lateral blows tend to cause sudden severe abduction, with consequent stretching or snapping of the ligaments on the medial side, and the lateral femoral condyle being driven down to impact on the tibial articular surface, which will either crack or crumple or a piece will fly off the far side of it (Fig. 13.4). Inevitably, internal damage to the articular cartilages and menisci, as well as damage to the cruciate ligaments, can occur in these violent situations. Mirror-image injuries may occur from impacts to the medial side, but articular collapse tends to be less severe here, due to the presence of the underlying fibula.

NB Depression of more than 8 mm will usually be regarded as an indication for surgical intervention.

Confounding factor

These observations presuppose a previously normal joint. As part of osteoporotic and arthritic changes, elderly patients may already have narrowed joint spaces, deeply cupped upper tibial plateaux and multiple tiny fragments littering their joints, and may even already have swellings due to effusions. Indeed, there is a vast army of middle-aged individuals who already have advanced arthritic changes – just ask any family doctor.

Hint: Many such patients will have previous films. Try and obtain them or call them up on your picture archiving system.

Segond fracture

Beware this seemingly small fracture from the lateral aspect of the upper tibia which is due to varus strain of the flexed knee. This will also have been likely to have 'taken out' (i.e. traumatized) the lateral capsular ligament and the anterior cruciate ligament, and torn the lateral meniscus.

NB Splits and avulsions from the intercondylar eminence of the tibial articular surface especially the anterior cruciate ligament from the medial tibial spine, may indicate serious ligamentous damage. As stated above, oblique X-ray views may help to clarify and demonstrate these initially. This is important because serious avulsions will require operative reduction. Fractures of the lateral tibial spine do not, however, involve cruciate avulsions.

Indirect signs of trauma

Any wrenching or impacting injury to the knee can result in an effusion, even without a fracture. This can be identified on a lateral knee X-ray by bulging in the suprapatellar pouch and effacement of the normal fat here (Fig. 13.5).

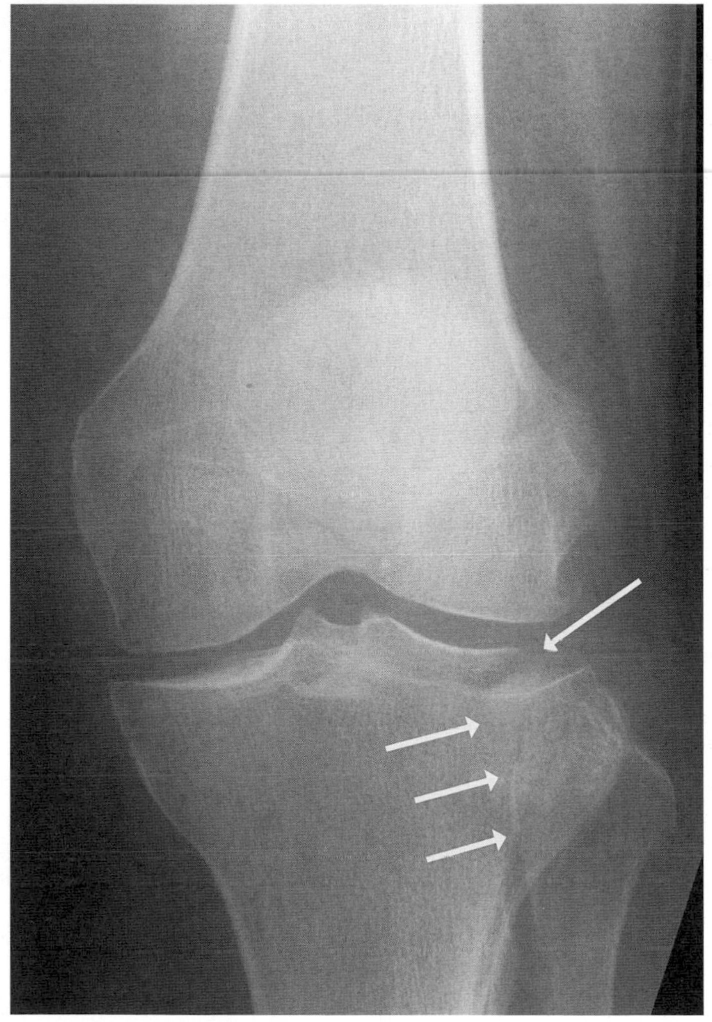

Fig. 13.4 *A depressed fracture of the lateral tibial plateau (arrows).*

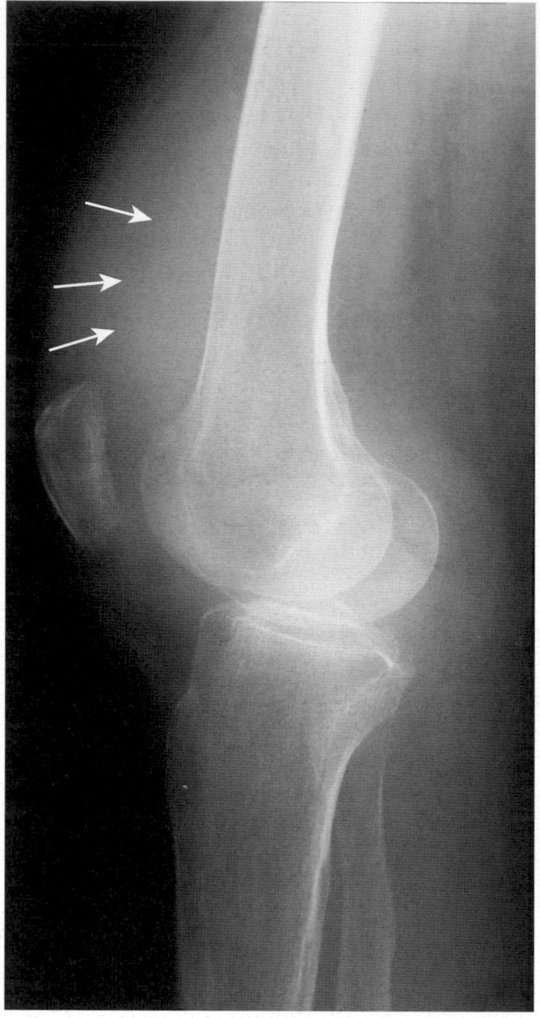

Fig. 13.5 *A big knee effusion. Note the anticlockwise and forward canting of the patella. Pus and haemarthrosis would look the same. Note: blood is sticky, causing adhesions, and should be aspirated. Sometimes air can get into a joint – a pneumarthrosis.*

Even more important is a *lipohaemarthrosis*. This is a collection of marrow fat forming a sharp interface, floating on top of a blood collection (Fig. 13.6), within the joint and providing indirect proof that an intra-articular fracture has occurred **even if you cannot see it**. This radiological sign requires a shoot-through lateral with the patient supine for its optimum demonstration and the knee extended.

NB Do not mistake the back of the quadriceps tendon on a non-shoot-through film of the knee for a lipohaemarthrosis. Big mistake!

Knee trauma: some further important considerations (Fig. 13.7)

If an adolescent child presents, for example, a couple of weeks or so after being kicked in the knee and still complaining of pain, periosteal reaction may be visible around the lower femur, with some underlying calcification. This may be due to a subperiosteal haematoma, a post-traumatic phenomenon that will resolve spontaneously. Look very carefully at the underlying bone, however, and it may show an abnormal texture, with sclerosis and 'sunray spicules'. You will then be dealing with an *osteogenic sarcoma*. **NB** Differentiation may be difficult so get a senior opinion before breaking the bad news.

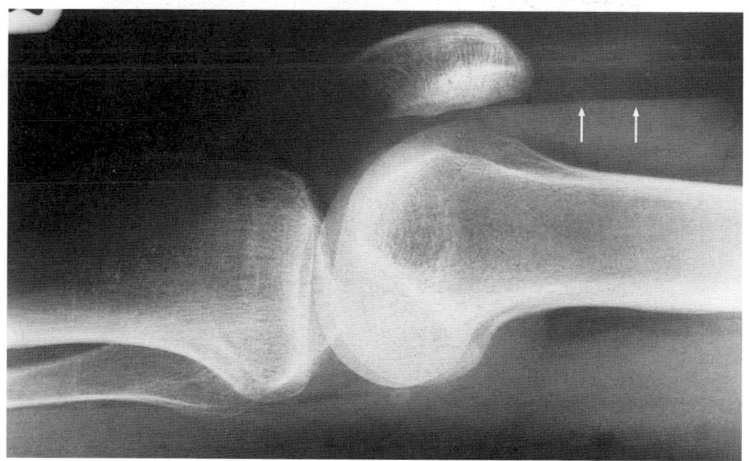

Fig. 13.6 *The 'FBI' (fat–blood interface) sign (arrows). A lipohaemarthrosis shown by a 'shoot through' lateral. The lucent fat floats on top of the denser, more opaque blood. Note the full extension used for this examination.*

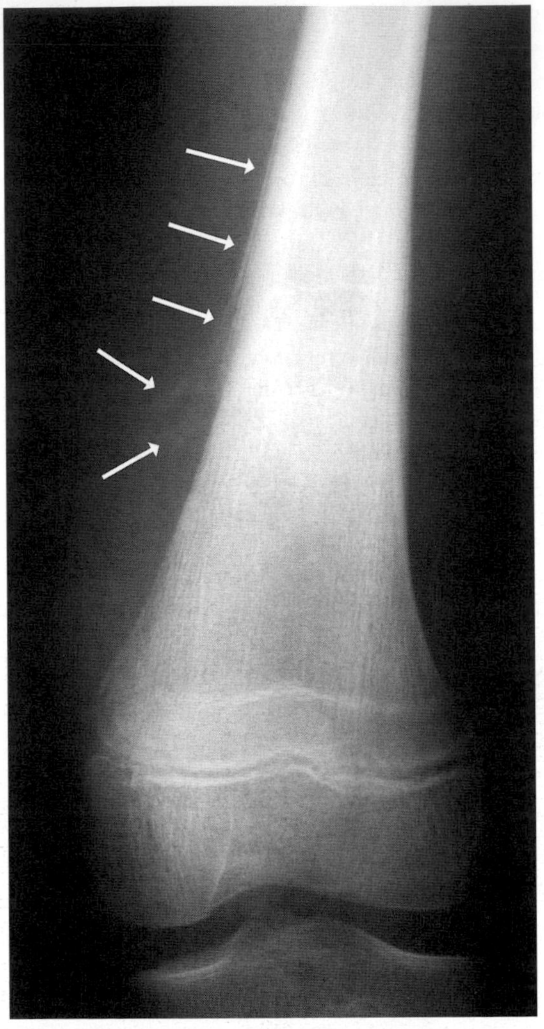

Fig. 13.7 *Periosteal reaction on the lower femur (arrows). The main differentials are: (1) trauma, (2) infection and (3) malignancy (as here). Note: occasionally, following a kick, an osteogenic sarcoma will present in A & E like this. Take a careful history – some pain may have preceded the injury.*

Gold medal point: Beware of microscopically visible bone callus following a fracture, as it can look pretty wild and resemble malignancy. Some children have actually suffered amputations as a result of this mistake as a tumour was wrongly suspected.

What about spontaneous pain in the knee?

This is an important topic and here are some important differentials:

- *Infective arthritis* – especially in children (Fig. 13.8). Always maintain a high index of suspicion for infection in any painful joint and look for early evidence of bone destruction.
- *Referred from hip* (slipped upper femoral epiphysis/Perthes' disease) – needs hip X-rays.

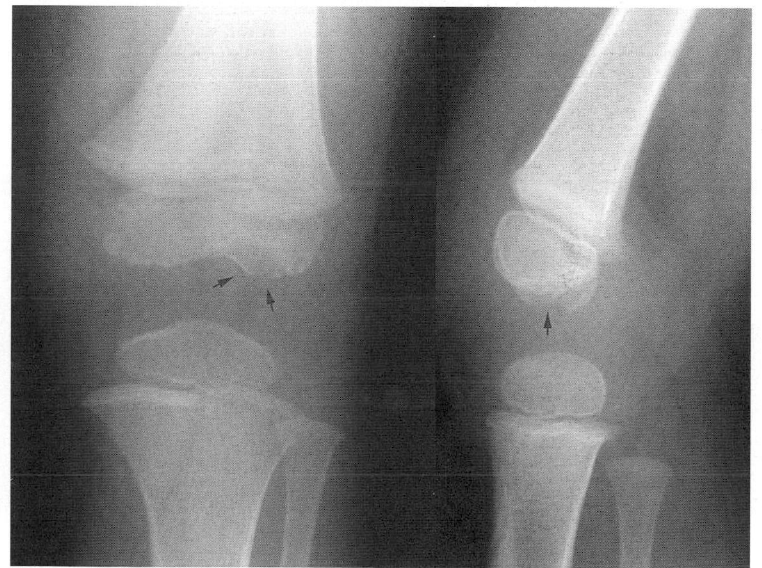

Fig. 13.8 ***A*** *AP and* ***B*** *lateral views showing infective arthritis (arrows) of the knee in a child. The critical observation is incipient destruction of the medial femoral condyle. Urgent aspiration of the joint revealed pus.*

- *Swollen, painful tibial tuberosity* – Osgood–Schlatter's disease (Fig. 13.9).
- *Osteochondritis dissecans* in the knee.
- *Osteoarthritis/rheumatoid arthritis* – exacerbations in adults.
- *Spontaneous haemarthrosis* – haemophiliac, patients on warfarin, etc.

Gold medal point: *Hypertrophic pulmonary osteoarthropathy:* effusion in joint, periosteal reaction around femur, tibia and fibula. A rare manifestation of carcinoma of the lung. These patients need a chest X-ray. May also present at the wrist and ankles.

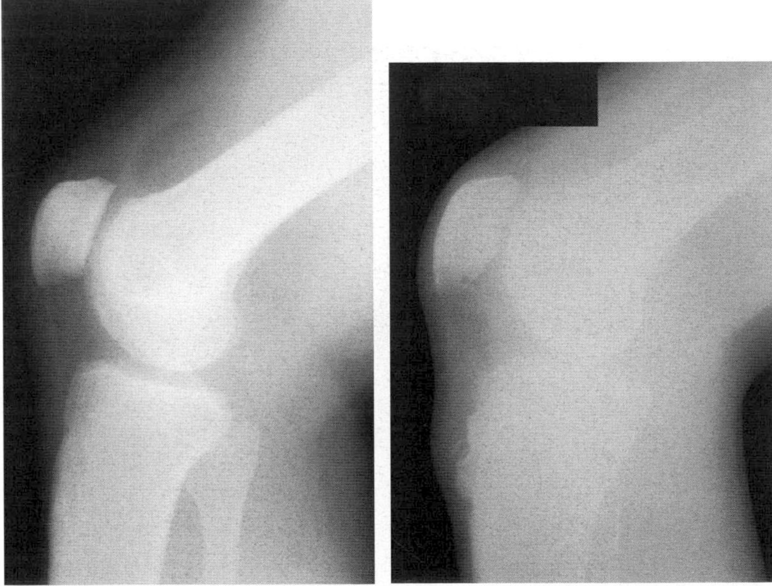

Fig. 13.9 ***A** Normal and **B** involved knee in Osgood–Schlatter's disease. Note the fragmentation of the right tibial tuberosity, overlying swelling and blunting of the inferior angle of fat in the affected joint. When the lower pole of the patella is involved, this is called Sindig–Larsen disease. Both are most likely traction injury effects.*

Fractures of the patella (Fig. 13.10)

These are usually due to direct impact and can take a cracked or stellate form. When complete, the extensor mechanism of the knee is lost and the fragments will have to be wired together.

Dislocations of the patella

These will virtually always go laterally because of the relatively shallow inclinations of the anterior surface of the lateral femoral condyle and retropatellar facet. They are usually obvious clinically. Do not however, misdiagnose a dislocated patella on an AP X-ray film just because it is not straight.

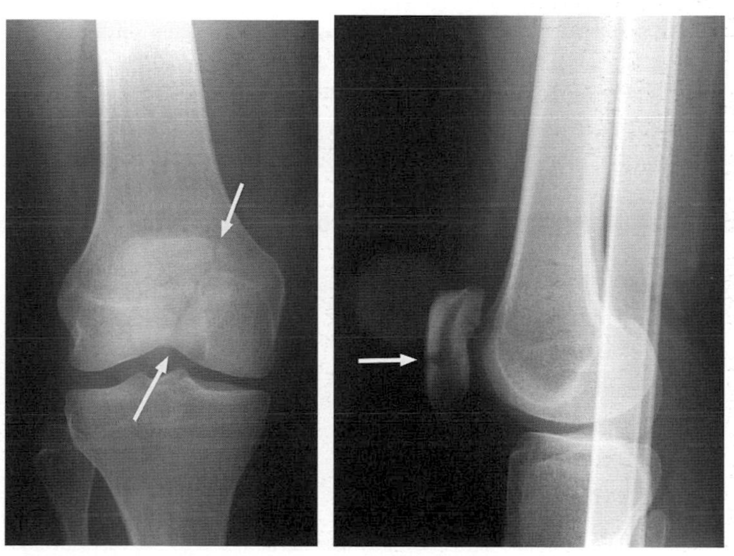

Fig. 13.10 ***A*** *AP and* ***B*** *lateral views showing a fracture of the patella.*

The tibia and fibula

Background

Being long bones, these are vulnerable to all manner of impacts, falls and twists from road traffic accidents and sporting injuries, either singly or together (Fig. 13.11). However, just like the radius and ulna, they form a ring of bone and need to be thought of in the same way whenever trauma occurs, usually breaking together obliquely or in spiral fashion. Often severe tibial and fibular fractures are open and prone to delayed union. Closed fractures here may be dangerous due to soft tissue swelling leading to 'compartment syndrome', which compresses the vessels and requires a fasciotomy for its release.

Radiography

Good AP s and laterals with the knees and ankles included on the films will answer most questions about fractures, i.e. presence or absence, angulation, alignment, comminution. etc. Sometimes only suboptimal films can be obtained so be conscious of the limitations of 'running obliques', i.e. neither true APs nor laterals. On occasion, if the films are inadequate you may not realize that the distal components are rotated 90° to the proximal ones, and may even mistake AP for lateral views and vice versa – it has been done!

Anatomy

This is straightforward (see Knee, above, and Ankle, below).

Normal variants

Nutrient canals and irregularities may appear in these long bones.

Fractures

The diagnosis of fractures here is usually easy. In addition to the vascular injuries referred to above, injuries to the nerves, e.g. the peroneal at the neck of the fibula, must be sought or excluded.

Stress fractures

With the great jogging ethic endemic throughout the world increasing, pain below the knee due to a stress fracture may often be found. A band of increased

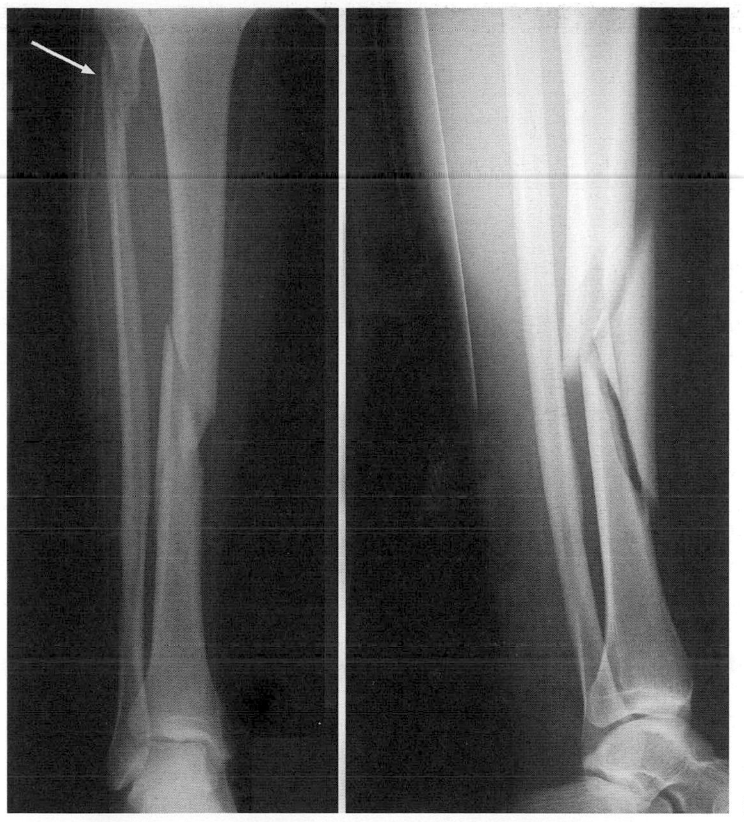

Fig. 13.11 ***A*** *AP and* ***B*** *lateral views of a butterfly (spiral) fracture of the tibia and fibula. The term butterfly refers to the central fragment.*

density and periosteal reaction may duly appear (Fig. 13.12) if the diagnosis has not already been established by a bone scan or MRI.

Toddler's fracture

This is a spiral fracture of the distal tibia. It may present with pain in the ankle or foot and refusal to walk. Check what you can see of the tibia carefully on ankle and foot films; if not satisfied, request formal views of the tibia and fibula as well.

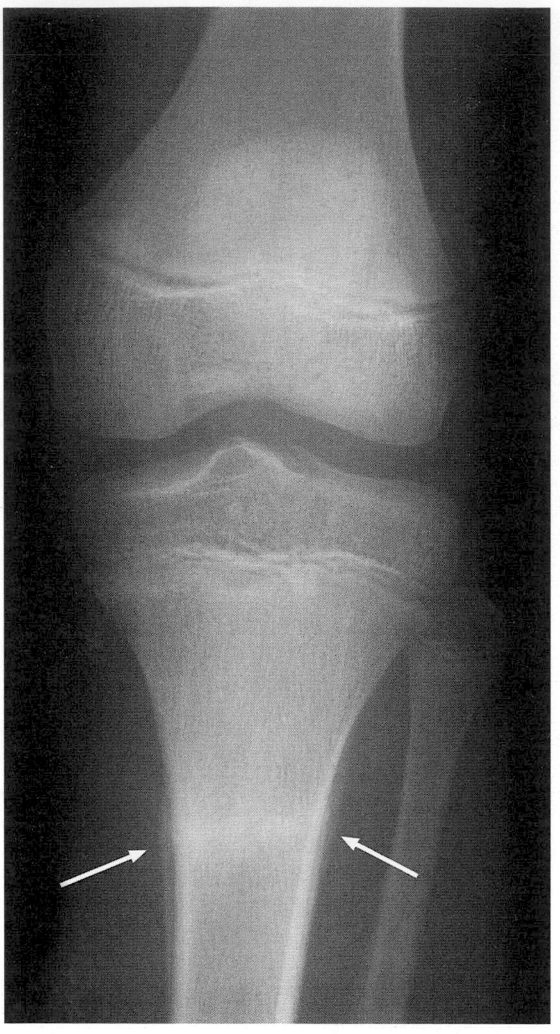

Fig. 13.12 *A stress fracture (arrows) of the tibia. Note the periosteal reaction and normal developing epiphyses in this teenager.*

Pilon fracture

This is a comminuted fracture of the distal tibia involving the articular surface, usually caused by a fall – e.g. off an electricity pylon!

Maisonneuve fracture

This is a nasty fracture with an eversion component at the ankle, lateral displacement of the distal fibula and an oblique fracture in the fibular neck – the sort of thing you could get if you fell off the roof of a maisonette!

The ankle (fractures and dislocations)

Background

Injuries to the ankle are extremely common usually due to twisting forces causing inversion or eversion, neither of which this joint is designed to perform. Crushing or direct blows are other potential mechanisms of injury. It is sometimes hard for the patient to localize the source of pain in this area, and marked soft tissue swelling can also make it difficult to assess clinically.

Radiography

Current guidelines advise ankle X-rays if there is inability to weight bear, or pain at or around the medial or lateral malleoli. Under the so-called Ottawa Rules, using point tenderness at the tips or within 6 cm of the tips along the posterior margins of the distal tibia and fibula as indications for X-ray has resulted in a 15% reduction in unnecessary ankle films being achieved. A foot X-ray should also be taken if there is tenderness in the midfoot, and particularly at the navicular or base of the 5th metatarsal.

Look at Figure 13.13. In the UK the standard views that are taken after trauma are the AP and lateral. To get the lower fibula off the tibia and talus a further film with 10° of internal rotation is also often taken – the so called 'mortice' view.

Stress views If you request one of these to be taken under sedation to check for ligamentous laxity, expect to be called to come and do it yourself. Do not expect the X-ray staff to collect all the radiation themselves.

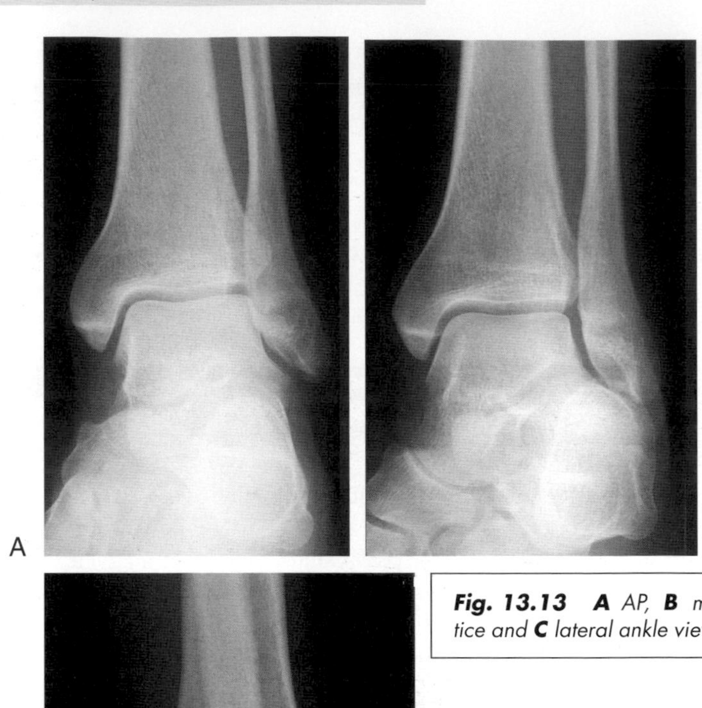

Fig. 13.13 **A** *AP,* **B** *mortice and* **C** *lateral ankle views.*

Anatomy (Figure 13.14)

The bony anatomy of the adult ankle consists of the distal tibial articular surface and the superior articular surface of the dome of the talus (which together form the ankle 'mortice') and the inner aspects of the medial and lateral malleoli. The bones of the ankle are stabilized and bound together to each other and the hindfoot by powerful ligaments, particularly on the medial and lateral sides, and also the lower parts of the interosseous membrane and distal anterior tibiofibular ligament.

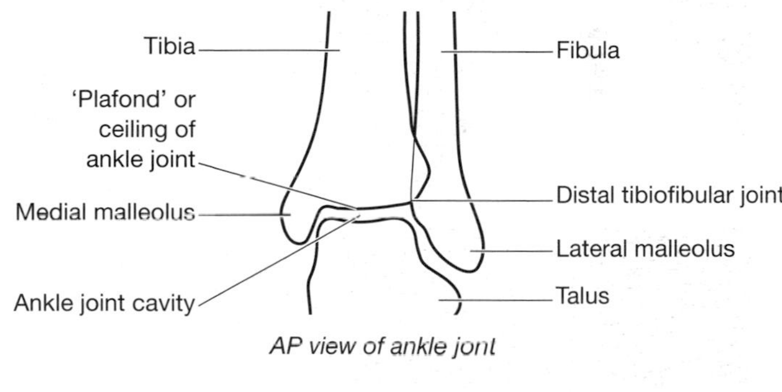

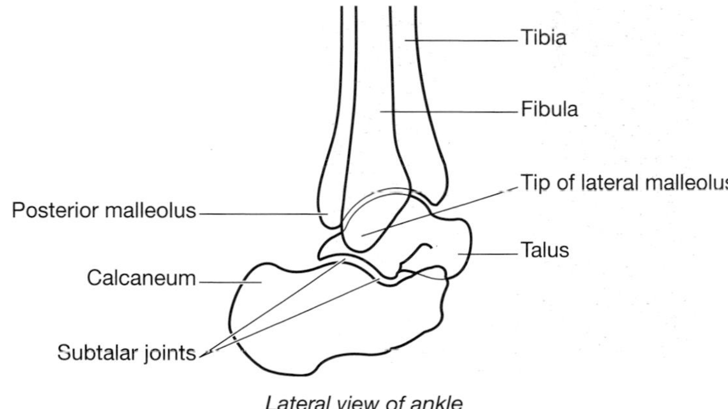

Fig. 13.14 *Anatomy of the ankle joint.* **A** *AP;* **B** *lateral.*

The simple implications of this are that when the ankle 'comes apart', either the bones or the ligaments have given way, and, by implication, if the ankle is disrupted but no fracture is present, a significant ligamentous injury must have occurred. Because the ligaments are invisible on X-rays, the diagnosis of a tear must therefore be indirect, either through separation of the bones or marked soft tissue swelling, although obviously mixed fractures of the bones and ligamentous injuries can occur around the ankle as a result of a single incident. The paediatric or developing ankle is a special case. Comminuted fractures, cartilaginous and ligamentous injuries and instability problems can be investigated by CT and MRI.

Important principle (Fig. 13.15)

This shows a completely normal AP view but an oblique fracture with slight separation in the lower fibula on the lateral view. This is the simplest example of the radiological aphorism that in cases of trauma 'one view is no view'. Everything hinges on the relationship between the direction of the X-ray beam and the main axis of the fracture line, which of course is in the lap of the gods. Sometimes an ankle fracture will only be visible on a third oblique projection.

Crucial point: If there is a conflict between clinical findings and X-ray findings, **treat the patient not the X-ray.**

Because inversion injuries in particular are so common and ankle injuries may be complex in their aetiology, make sure the whole calcaneum and base of the 5th metatarsal are on the lateral view, otherwise injuries here may be missed. The peroneus brevis muscle or lateral plantar aponeurosis may avulse the base of the 5th metatarsal following inversion injury, so you need to *see* it.

Normal variants

These include:

- Normal developing epiphyses (lucent).
- Scar at site of closure of epiphyses (dense).
- Harris growth lines (Fig. 13.16): reflect periods of interrupted growth in childhood (dense).

These should not be mistaken for cracks or impacted fractures. Also:

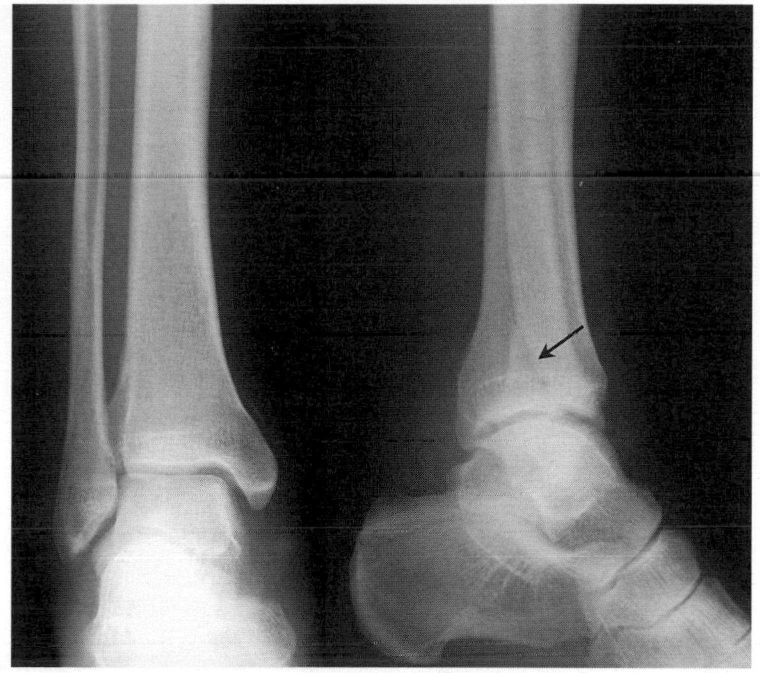

Fig. 13.15 ***A*** *AP and* ***B*** *lateral ankle. The fracture of the distal fibula (arrow) is only visible on the lateral view.*

- Accessory ossicles at tips of medial and lateral malleoli (e.g. os subfibulare; Fig. 13.17). These are usually corticated and smooth (see Keats and Anderson 2001).
- Sometimes old, small, and ununited and undocumented fractures may be seen as particles of bone around the malleoli but, again, these are usually smooth.
- Os trigonum. A smooth extra bone at the posterior aspect of the ankle joint.

Fractures of the ankle

When sufficient adduction, abduction, rotational or upward compression forces are applied to the ankle, the medial, lateral or posterior malleoli may break, in

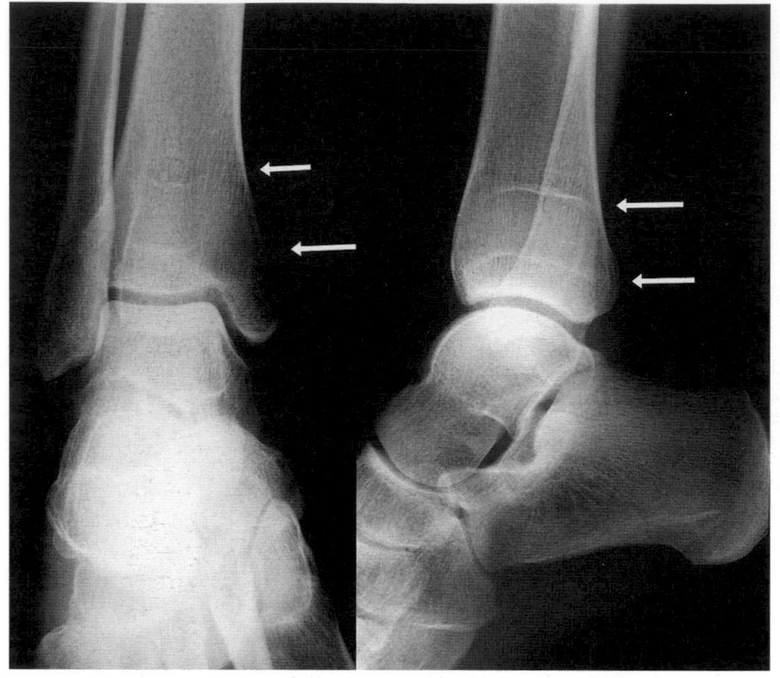

Fig. 13.16 ***A*** *AP and* ***B*** *lateral ankle showing Harris growth lines (arrows).*

various combinations along with the ligaments that hold them together. Careful inspection right round all the edges of the malleoli will render most fractures visible.

With severe displacements where the fractures are obvious, it is usually easy to picture the direction from which the major force has come and carried the fragments and talus with it. One film alone can be very misleading (Fig. 13.18).

Ligamentous injuries may occur alone and will usually be manifest by soft tissue swelling. **NB If a malleolus has broken, that usually means its ligament is intact.** The aims of treatment are to reconstitute the joint in a stable position, via referral if necessary to orthopaedics.

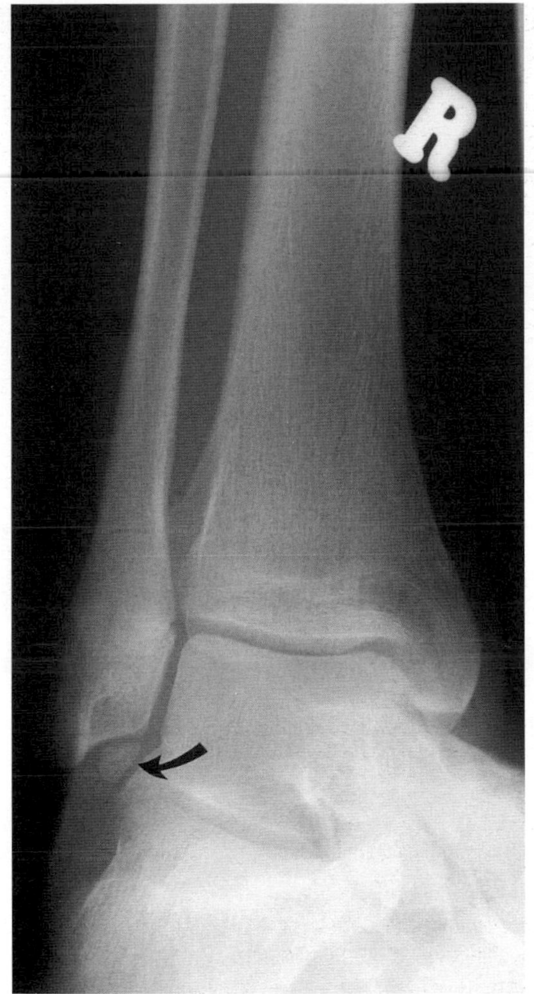

Fig. 13.17 *Os subfibulare (arrow).*

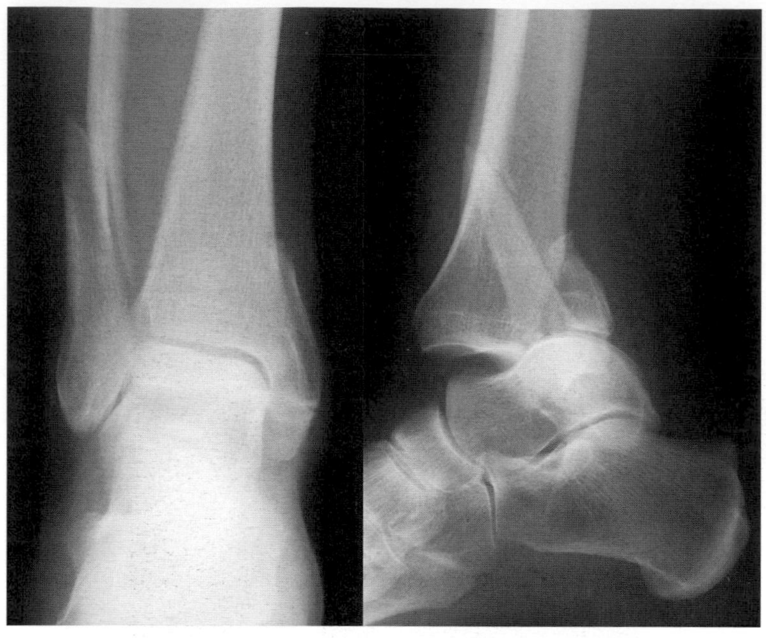

Fig. 13.18 *Caught in a rabbit hole! Fracture of ankle with posterior dislocation of the talus. Note how the talus appears in normal position on the AP film (**A**). Moral: you need laterals (**B**) to see dislocations.*

Fractures of the talus

- The talus appears on every ankle X-ray where the lower leg meets the foot.
- Ankle X-rays are most commonly taken for twisting injuries when the talus gets jammed against the underside of the distal tibial articular surface or *plafond* (French: ceiling), making it susceptible to compression injuries of greater or lesser degree, in either inversion or eversion (Fig. 13.19).
- Because the cartilage is sandwiched between the bones when a break occurs, this is referred to as an osteochondral fracture of the dome of the talus, and MRI is required to assess it fully.
- A fracture of the neck of the talus can lead to avascular necrosis of the dome, analogous to the scaphoid.

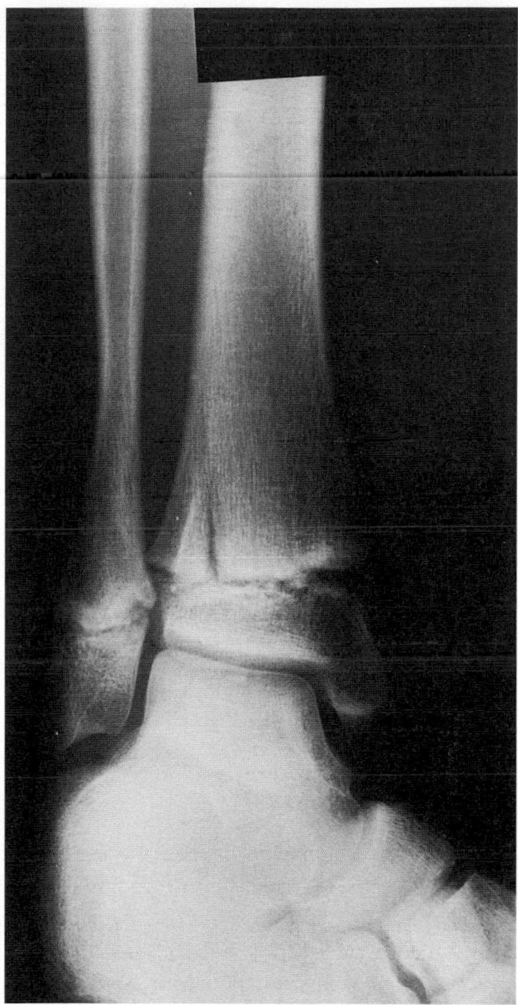

Fig. 13.19 *An abduction injury in a juvenile patient. Note the widening of the medial part of the distal tibial epiphysis, angulation and fracture of the distal tibia. Salter–Harris type 2.*

The foot

Background

Because it exists for weight-bearing, any injury to the foot is likely to lead to immediate loss of function and locomotion – witness the little boy hopping into A & E, as only little boys can, with the 'wounded soldier' routine!

Injuries vary from a simple stubbing of the toe to violent fractures and dislocations or total mangling of a foot, e.g. in a road traffic accident or an aviation accident due to a heavy landing. Pilots will tell you 'any landing you walk away from is a good one' but the 'aviator's astragulus' (a nasty fracture dislocation of the talus) will usually require the intrepid 'stick and rudder man' to be hauled from the wreckage! Aviation aphorism: 'The only certainty about flight is descent!'

Radiography

Current indications include inability to weight-bear and focal tenderness.

- The conventional views of the foot in the UK are the dorsiplantar and dorsiplantar oblique (Fig. 13.20), usually referred to as AP and AP obliques, because the dorsum of the foot is anterior (not posterior like the hand) in the anatomical position.
- Further views include the true lateral, special axial views of the calcaneum (Fig. 13.21) and views for the subtalar joints, although the subtalar views are rarely used these days.
- As soon as it becomes apparent that the injury is severe or that the calcaneum or subtalar joints are involved, an early request for CT will frequently be made to give a complete and 3D assessment of the fragments and degree of comminution, for an unrivalled display of the relevant anatomy. Future developments may take these patients straight to MRI. Recent innovations include a C-arm facility with 3D images generated in the operating room, without having to resort to CT.

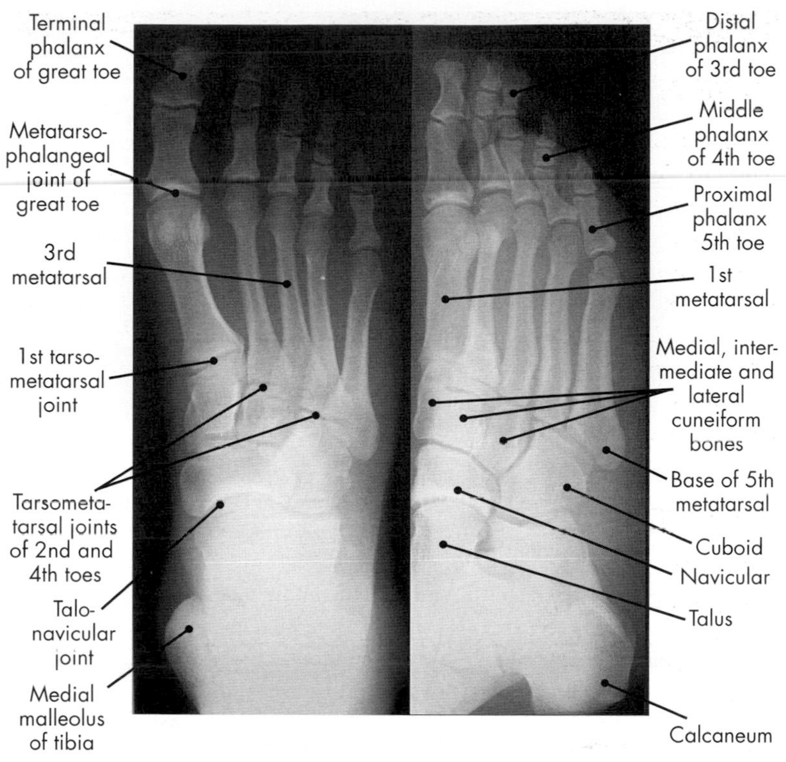

Fig. 13.20 ***A*** *AP and* ***B*** *AP oblique views of a normal foot. Each of the 1st, 2nd and 3rd metatarsals elegantly rests its base on its own individual 1st, 2nd and 3rd cuneiform bone (or medial, intermediate and lateral). The 4th and 5th metatarsal bases each share the cuboid bone, with the base of the 5th metatarsal overhanging the cuboid bone laterally.*

Anatomy (Fig. 13.20)

It is a sad fact that audible groans may almost be guaranteed from many senior medical students and junior doctors when asked to point out and name the bones of the foot. Long-forgotten anatomy is understandably hard to dredge up,

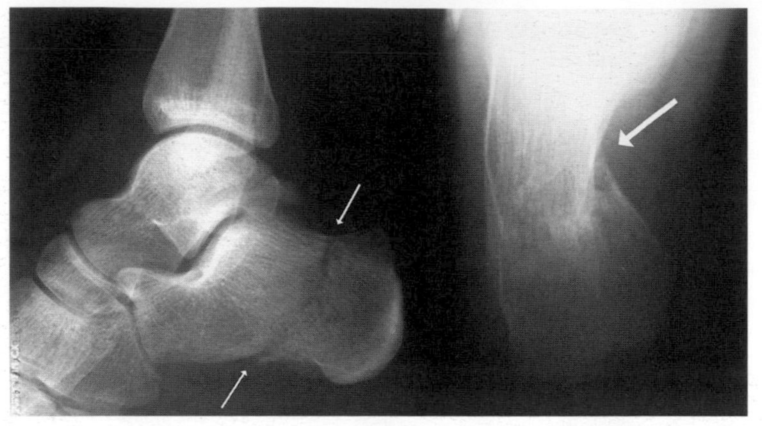

Fig. 13.21 **A** *Lateral view showing fracture of calcaneum (arrows).* **B** *Axial view; the arrow points to the fracture on the concave or medial side.*

although the words 'metatarsals' and 'phalanges' may eventually be uttered as the long bones receive their proper nomenclature. The round bones of the hindfoot (talus and calcaneum) and the midfoot, i.e. the three cuneiform (or 'wedge-shaped' bones-after Babylonic cuneiform writing), cuboid and navicular bones frequently require revision and reinforcement: a sustained effort to learn them (unless you are one of the lucky ones who already knows) is advised, and the same of course applies to the bones of the hands, before you begin your stint in A & E. Once you can point them all out effortlessly, put yourself down for a silver star.

Demonstrating you are less than totally familiar with bony anatomy after you missed something in A & E would be an easy way for an astute lawyer to undermine your credibility in a legal case. Remember F. E. Smith (see p. 137).

What about a mnemonic?

Try CCTV – 3, as in Closed Circuit TeleVision – 3:

- **C**alcaneum → **C**uboid (articulation sequence on lateral side).
- **T**alus → **na**V**icular** (articulation sequence on medial side).

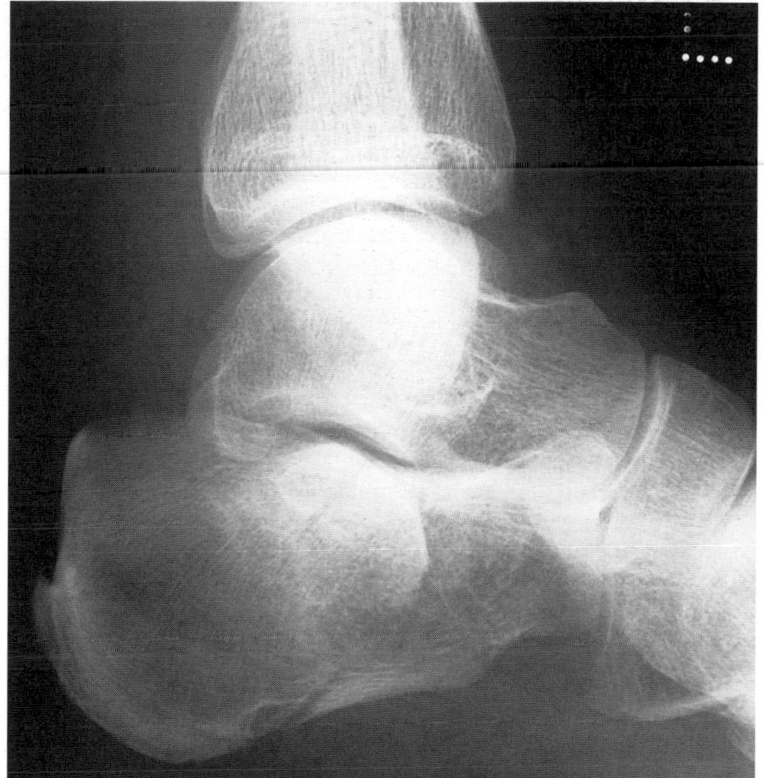

Fig. 13.22 *Fractured calcaneum with loss of Böhler's angle. The whole bone is virtually in a straight line and has lost its boomerang shape.*

This indicates the two hindfoot bones and the midfoot bones they articulate with. Then it's just the three medial, intermediate and lateral cuneiform bones. Then it's easy. Just metatarsals, and phalanges, proximal, middle and distal, or in the big toe, and sometimes the other toes too, just proximal and distal.

Fractures and dislocations

The calcaneum

Most injuries to this bone result from falls, landing on the feet with the inevitable impact driving the talus like a hammer through the anvil of the calcaneum, causing it to fracture, crumple or collapse; inevitably the trauma is frequently bilateral. It is important to remember that the force of the impact on concrete will be transmitted up to higher levels, causing associated fractures, e.g. in the pelvis, but particularly in the thoracolumbar spine, in around 10% of patients.

Radiography

NB There are no AP views of the calcaneum. Because of its positional anatomy the calcaneum cannot be demonstrated in the AP projection. It is therefore assessed by lateral and (when indicated) axial views (Figs 13.21, 13.22, pp. 292, 293). These are taken with 45° angulation to the supine patient with the feet in the air and 'stretch' the calcaneum into a thick crescentic shape, confirming any fractures and making them easier to see.

Moral: Tell radiographers what you want to see, e.g. 'left calcaneum', instead of trying to teach them their job and requesting things you do not fully understand.

Anatomy (Fig. 13.23)

Apart from looking like Australia, the most important radiographic anatomy is seen on the lateral view, when the lines joining the points indicated normally intersect at angles between 28 and 40°. Anything less than 28° is taken as evidence of compression, but the question is: 'What if it was 40° to start with, and after a fall (and an X-ray) is now seen to be only 28°?' Obviously compression has occurred, but the rule has let you down.

Answer? Treat the patient not the X-ray. Careful clinical assessment (e.g. excruciating pain), an axial view and, if necessary, CT scanning should be carried out for further evaluation, to assess comminution and see if the subtalar joints are involved, etc.

Axial view anatomy Puzzled looks are often seen on the faces of junior doctors handed an axial view of the calcaneum – a mental fugue is obviously in progress.

Question: Which is the medial side and which is the lateral side on an axial view?
Answer: The concave side is the medial side (Fig. 13.21B).

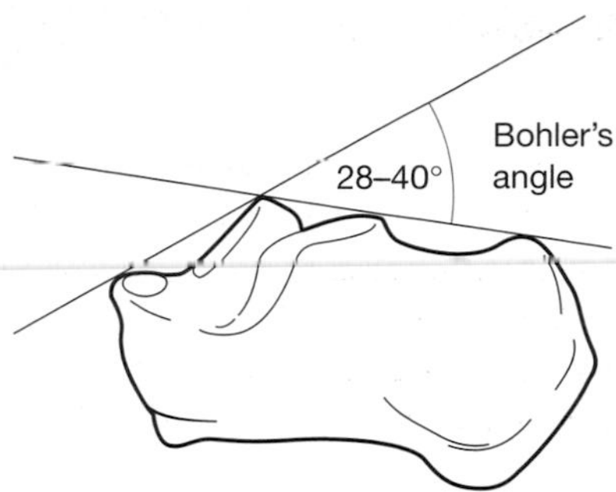

Fig. 13.23 *Böhler's angle.*

Normal variants In the juvenile patient the posterior calcaneal epiphysis can appear as a separated, fragmented, hyperdense irregular structure like a fractured crescent moon, yet be quite normal (Fig. 13.24). The contralateral side will look similar but one look at Keats & Anderson (2001) will demonstrate the startling range of normal variation. Do not mistake it for an injury or osteochondritis.

Important point: The body of the calcaneum may show a huge black hole in its centre (like Fig. 13.24). These have variously been described as normal variants, 'calcaneal cysts' and more recently as 'intraosseous lipomas' based on their CT numbers. The absence of normal trabeculae weakens the calcaneum and makes it more susceptible to trauma.

Fractures These are usually compression or shearing injuries with comminution. A so-called *beak fracture* occurs when sudden traction from the Achilles tendon 'rips' the calcaneum apart.

Important point: A horse-shoe configuration of bruising around the heel is typical of a fracture of the calcaneum and should lead to the review of any radiographs previously thought to be 'negative'.

Other tarsal fractures

- Other tarsal bones may sustain fractures either in isolation or in combination with the more commonly affected bones.

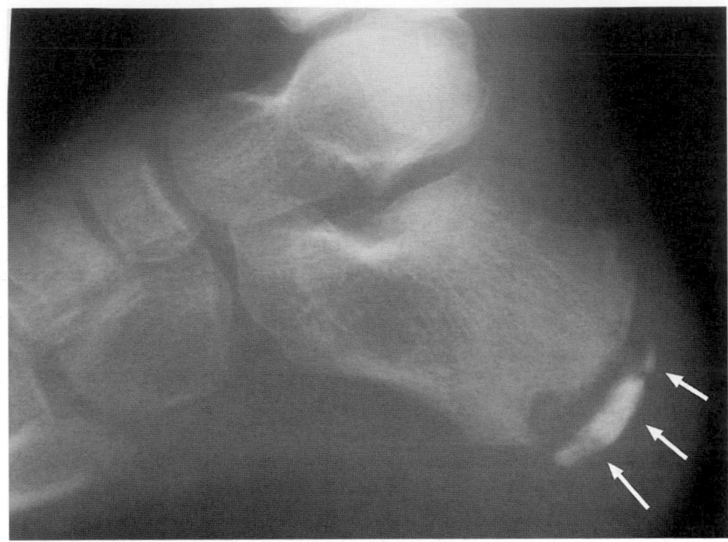

Fig. 13.24 *Normal developing calcaneal epiphysis.*

- Close attention to detail and looking right round the edge of every bone, then through its trabecular structure for lucent or sclerotic lines, are as ever the necessary prerequisites for not missing a fracture. CT and MRI remain as options and will on occasion inevitably uncover fractures invisible on plain films.

What about the paediatric foot? As in the hand and elbow, not every bone has formed in the very young child. Check the films of any such patients against your department's skeletal development chart. The calcaneum and talus are usually the first to appear. If truly perplexed, a comparative view of the opposite side will help.

The tarsometatarsal junction (an important area)

NB Five or ten minutes given to the study of the normal anatomy of the tarsometatarsal junctions (Fig. 13.20) is time exceptionally well spent. The crucial facts are:

1. Each of the 1st, 2nd and 3rd metatarsals articulates with its own 'private' cuneiform bone (i.e. the medial, intermediate and lateral).
2. The 4th and 5th metatarsals each share the same podium, namely the cuboid bone, although the base of the 5th metatarsal overhangs it laterally.

The medial margin of each 1st–4th metatarsal is normally in line on its medial side with the edge of the proximal bone. Unfortunately, depending on the precise lie of the land, some of these actual joint spaces may not be visible on individual foot X-rays and appear to have fused, but this is an illusion. Look carefully at the second film and usually between the two films you will see all of them. Make sure you get all these crucial facts into your head.

Caution! This is one of those areas like the hand where the eye tends to roam but does not see!

The Lisfranc injury

When the foot sustains a sudden forced flexion after landing on its tip (e.g. in a parachute jump), is jammed under a foot-pedal in a car accident, is run over, or is furiously wrenched by a runaway horse when the rider has been thrown off, but his foot is still caught in the stirrup, the tarsometatarsal joints may be ripped out and dislocated from their ligamentous attachments. This is called a *Lisfranc injury* (Fig. 13.25), and is usually missed by inexperienced observers.

A coexistent fracture at the base of the 2nd metatarsal may occur if only the oblique ligament around this position holds, i.e. the one between the medial cuneiform and the base of the 2nd metatarsal, known not surprisingly as the *Lisfranc ligament*.

On X-ray it looks as if the base of each metatarsal has been shunted along one or more spaces – as indeed they have. **The critical observation is that the medial margin of the 2nd metatarsal is out of alignment with the medial edge of the intermediate (middle) cuneiform bone.** Further refinements include medial displacement of the 1st metatarsal – a 'divergent Lisfranc injury' – if you are after the gold medal.

Normal anatomical variants

- *The base of the 5th metatarsal.* The most important common one is the unfused epiphysis at the base of the 5th metatarsal, which simulates a fracture. Many doctors have a fugue when confronted with this and cannot remember which way the epiphysis normally lies, i.e. in the long axis or transverse axis of the bone.

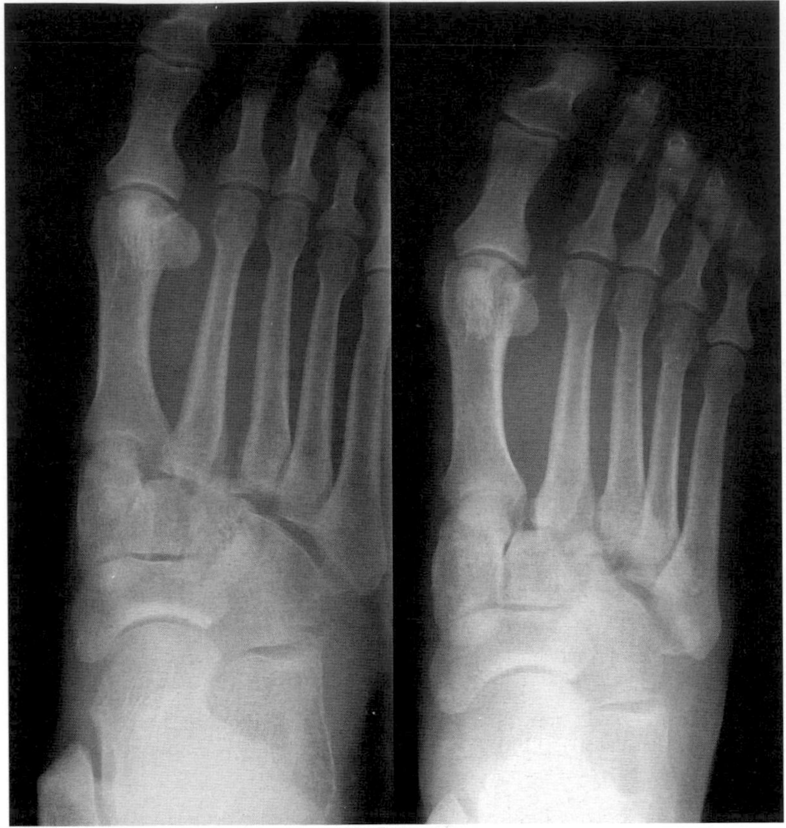

Fig. 13.25 ***A**, **B** A Lisfranc fracture dislocation. Note the lateral shunting of the 1st–5th metatarsals and separation of the proximal 2nd and 3rd metatarsals.*

- *Mnemonic.* Imagine you are breaking a small bone between your thumb and index finger. The break (i.e. fracture) will occur at right angles to the long axis – and so it does at the base of the 5th metatarsal. The epiphyseal line therefore runs longitudinally, or obliquely. Figure 13.26 shows a fracture and an epiphysis. Sod's law often makes these cases occur in the developing age group after an inversion injury to the ankle, so differentiation is important.

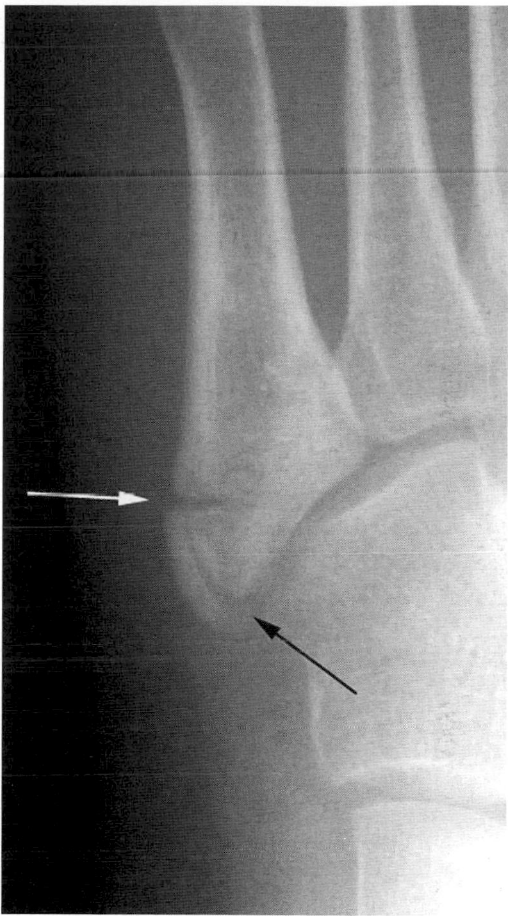

Fig. 13.26 *Injury to the base of the 5th metatarsal in a juvenile patient. The white arrow points to the fracture. The black arrow points to the epiphysis. The fracture is caused by an avulsion by the peroneus brevis due to sudden inversion of the foot. People often get confused with the Jones fracture and a 'base of 5th metatarsal fracture'. A Jones fracture occurs at least 2.5 cm distal to the base. This is important as such fractures tend to undergo non-union. True fractures at the base heal very quickly.*

- *Os tibiale externum.* This looks dramatic and is sometimes seen medially behind a large curved component of the navicular bone. Its well-corticated margin, however, indicates it is of long standing and is seen on the medial side. It may occasionally be associated with symptoms.
- *Talar beak.* A small spur on the upper surface of the talus, sometimes with a lucent cartilaginous base. It has been known for a patient with one of these to be diagnosed as having a fracture, be put in a plaster, suffer a deep vein thrombosis and a pulmonary embolus, and then die. Do not make the same mistake.
- *Bifid sesamoid bones* (under the head of the 1st metatarsal).
- *Other variants.* A host of other interesting normal variants can exist in the foot.

The metatarsals

Background

Metatarsal injuries are relatively common, often due to heavy weights being dropped accidentally on the foot or kicking against something too hard, i.e. the ground instead of the ball.

The 5th metatarsal base is a special case, as described above, usually avulsed due to inversion injury of the ankle.

Important normal variants

Crucial point: The developing epiphysis of the 1st metatarsal is at its base, i.e. *proximally.* The epiphyses of the 2nd to 5th metatarsals are at their necks, i.e. *distally.* So try not to mistake these for fractures.

- Various clefts, notches and spicules can be found at the proximal ends of the metatarsals. The more foot X-rays you see, the more familiar you will become with them.
- Nutrient arterial canals are sometimes seen passing obliquely through the cortices.

Stress fractures (Fig. 13.27)

These are important injuries commonly affecting joggers, army recruits and sports people, with symptoms coming on without a specific history of injury as they are due to repeated stress. An initial X-ray is often negative but will show a cloud of callus around the injury at a second X-ray examination after 10–14 days.

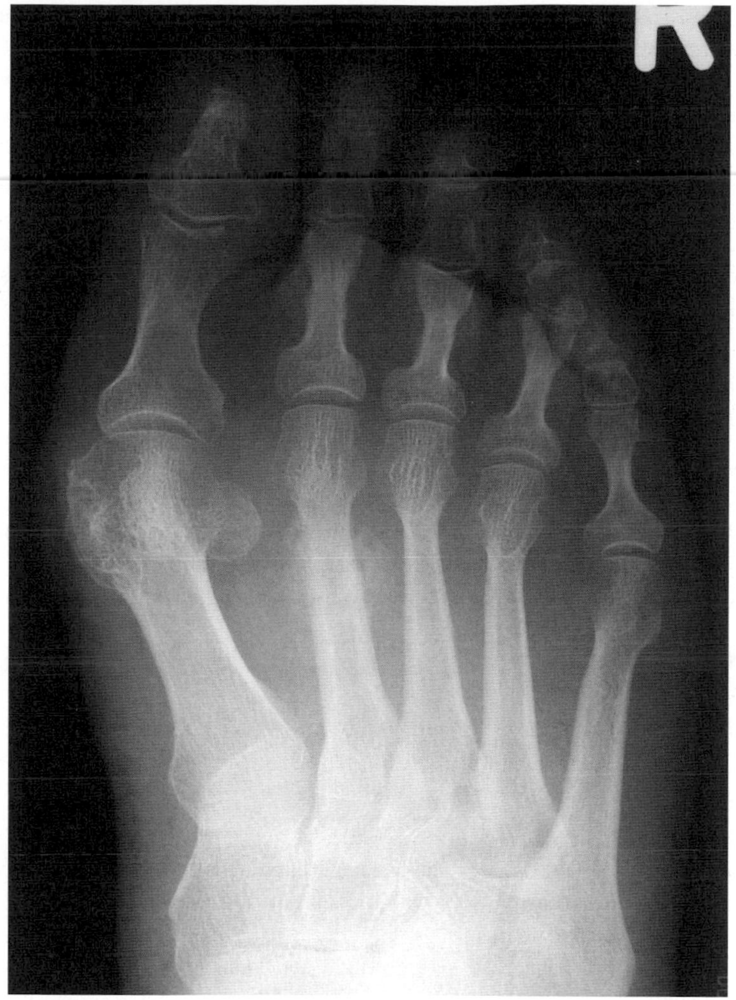

Fig. 13.27 *A stress fracture of the 2nd metatarsal.*

A bone scan will be rapidly positive after a day or two, following osteoblastic recruitment, and MRI is very sensitive here, as with any fracture.

'Important' individuals will tend to be diagnosed earlier, e.g. professional footballers – witness 'Beckham's break' – a reference to the then English football Captain's foot which had the UK tabloid newspapers in a spin for many weeks in the summer of 2002 over his fractured metatarsal. What had hitherto been regarded as a pretty clear-cut piece of medical knowledge, i.e. how long it would take a metatarsal bone to heal, suddenly became the subject of the most feverish, heated and speculative medical opinion! More recently (May 2003) Beckham staged his next break – of the scaphoid (p. 174).

Phalanges (Fig. 13.28)

Fractures of the phalanges of the feet are usually due to heavy objects being dropped on them, or stubbing toes. Traumatic dislocations at the metatarso-phalangeal and interphalangeal joints may also, of course, occur; however, exercise caution here because of the number of hallux valgus and hammer toe deformities caused by footwear, as well as patients presenting with preceding disease, e.g. rheumatoid arthritis, which causes subluxations without trauma.

Normal variants

- A bifid epiphysis at the base of the proximal phalanx of the great toe.
- Bifid sesamoid bones under the head of the 1st metatarsal.
- Beware the black bands of the distal edge of the soft tissues of the forefoot crossing the phalanges and simulating fractures.

Golden rule: If you see a black line crossing a bone, always look to see if you can trace it beyond the bone. If so, it will probably be a fat line, soft tissue edge or other pseudofracture or artefact.

NB You will often need a bright light and lots of patience to look right round the edge of every toe – unless you can see in the dark. They are often curled, and foreshortened, overlapping and distorted. At least with a workstation you will be able to brighten them up.

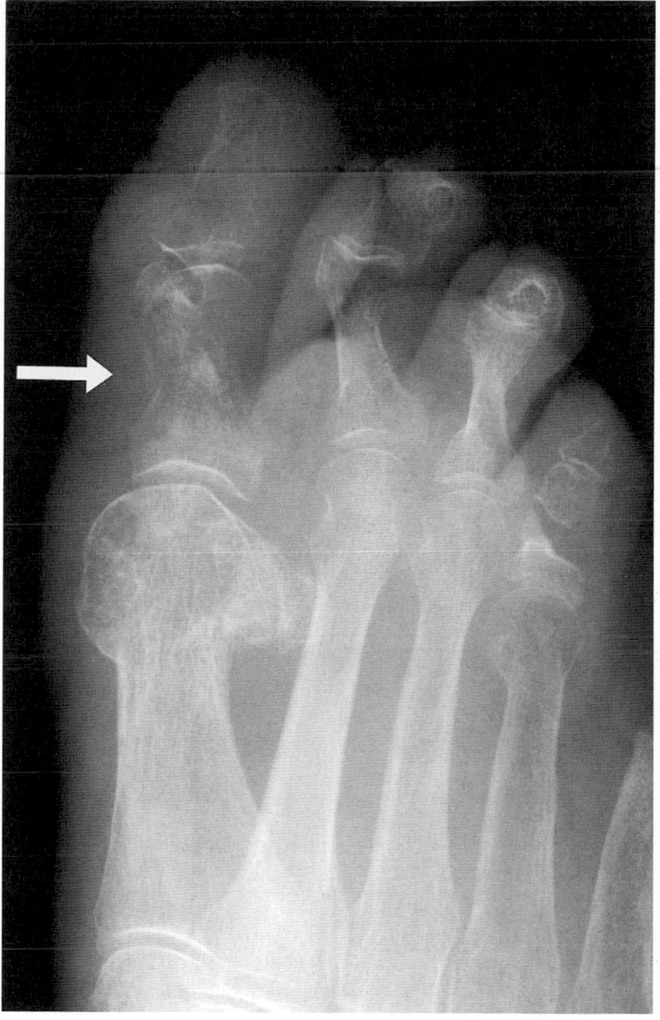

Fig. 13.28 *Fracture of the proximal phalanx of the great toe ('dropped a frozen turkey on his foot').*

Chapter 14

Foreign bodies and penetrating injuries

Foreign bodies: ingested or inserted

Background

Foreign bodies in the upper airway have already been discussed (p. 189). With regard to the gastrointestinal tract, some salient points are worth making:

- Things ingested from the top are usually taken by children.
- Things inserted at the other end are usually put there by adults.
- The history concerning the top end is likely to be true.
- The history concerning the lower end is likely to be bogus.
- Most ingested objects which negotiate the oesophagus will pass freely.
- Many put in at the lower end are now stuck.
- There is usually little embarrassment about the upper end.
- There is usually intense embarrassment about the lower end.

However, a decision needs to be made as to whether or not an X-ray is necessary. Smooth, swallowed objects like coins and marbles will usually pass spontaneously. An open safety pin or toy soldier is almost guaranteed to stick, so these need to be X-rayed. Some batteries are poisonous and need to be located. Regarding penetrating injuries, all glass is opaque but not necessarily easy to see, so remove the bandages, etc, if in a limb before taking the films. Wood, being vegetable matter, is radiolucent unless painted.

Danger of death

NB Make sure any X-rays are sufficiently penetrated, i.e. dark, for the lower intervertebral discs in the thoracic spine on chest films to be visible. Many an object impacted in the oesophagus has been missed because an excessively pale film was accepted (Fig. 14.1). These can erode through the oesophagus and cause mediastinitis and death if overlooked. The neck should be included on a child's chest film. To save radiation if something has been swallowed, an abdominal film can usefully be taken first; if negative, do the chest and neck.

Important points

- Beware of patients moving objects (e.g. medallions) between exposures. ('Oh! I'd better shift this out of the way!'). This may make it appear to be inside the body when it isn't – and this has happened. Hopefully the radiographer will already have removed it.

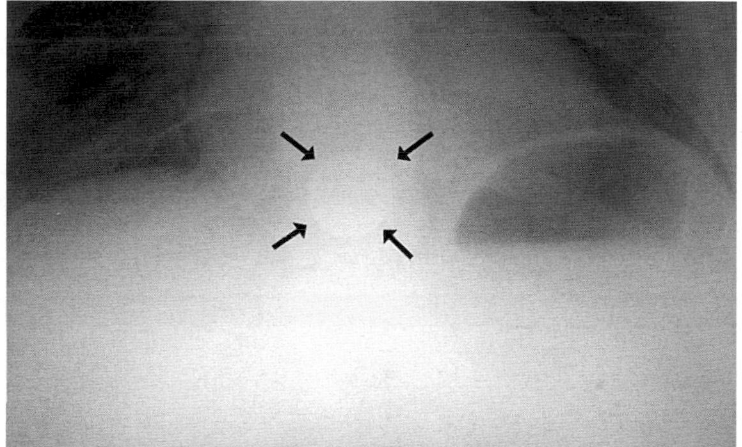

Fig. 14.1 *The typical location for an obstructed coin to be missed (as this one was) due to a film being underpenetrated for the retrocardiac position.*

- **Beware of a second or other foreign bodies.** Coins have been removed endoscopically when their rims have been glimpsed, leaving untouched a second, smaller coin behind and beneath in the oedematous mucosa, when a lateral X-ray would have shown two coins. The newer UK coins, minted later than 1992, contain ferrous metals and may potentially be removed successfully by magnets.

Some lateral thinking Some children will stick beads, ball bearings or stones not just up their own noses, or in their own ears, but into those of other children as well. So ask about friends and siblings.

Rectal foreign bodies (Fig. 14.2)

These are usually inserted for sexual gratification or as a perversion. The list of foreign bodies removed from the rectum is endless. Decisions need to be made as to whether or not these can be extracted manually or whether manipulation or surgery will be required. In some patients psychiatric assessment may also be appropriate.

Hints: With a rectal foreign body try to:

- Be sensitive to the patient's embarrassment and distress.
- Do not argue the toss about how it got there.
- Control the inevitable mirth in the department.

Point of interest: 'The vibrating umbilicus syndrome' is due to a vibrator stuck in the rectum or vagina, causing the umbilicus to be seen to move on inspection of the abdomen.

Penetrating injuries

Background

These can vary from the most minor of events, such as a splinter under the nail, to the devastating trauma of a gunshot wound to the head, chest or abdomen. In the latter, patients who survive the emergency dash to hospital must undergo, rapid triage, and vigorous resuscitation must be initiated or continued at the point of transfer from the paramedics. The site and degree of trauma will

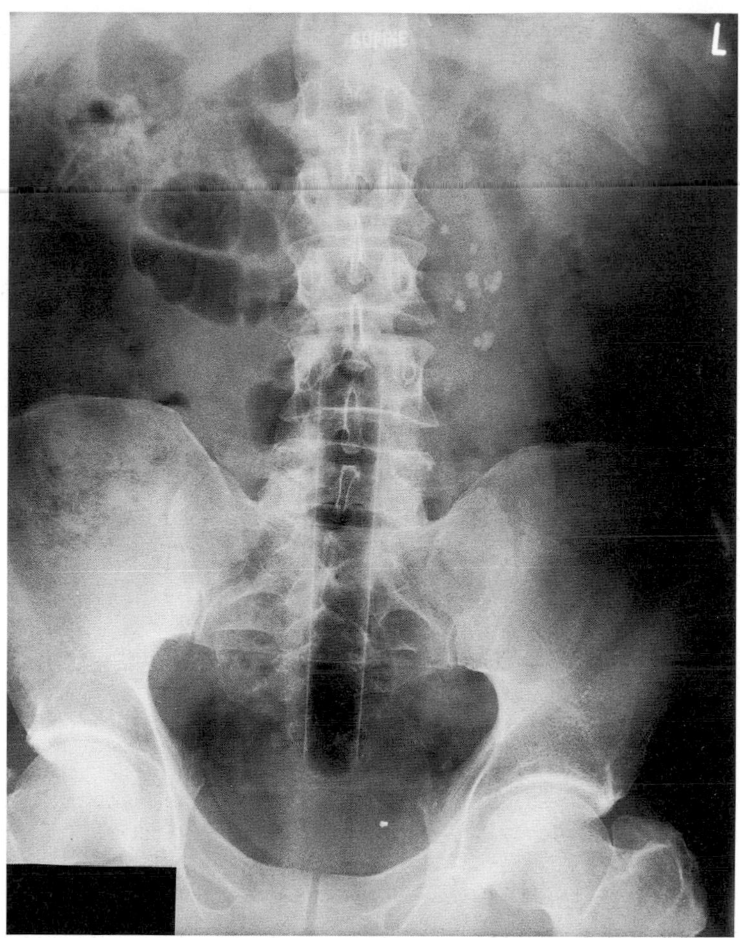

Fig. 14.2 *Rubber truncheon stuck in the sigmoid.*

inevitably determine the immediate outcome, and the longer term prognosis for those who survive the initial stages will depend on the complications (such as infection) that are likely to follow. Once stabilized, conventional X-rays may be taken to look for such things as the following:

In the head

- The position of a bullet and its trail of metal particles, if there is no exit wound, and if the patient cannot make it to CT.
- Air in the head.
- The position of shrapnel fragments following a blast injury.
- Glass in the head or scalp.
- Gravel in the scalp.

In the chest

- The effects of, for example a stab wound, or the position of a bullet in relation to vital structures and its attendant complications of haemothorax, pneumothorax, etc.
- Glass.
- Bomb fragments.

In the abdomen

- Pneumoperitoneum.
- Haemoperitoneum.
- Bullets (if no exit wound), with entry wound marked.
- Position of knife blades, machetes, airgun pellets.
- Glass.
- Bomb fragments.

In the limbs

- Buckshot.
- Bullets.
- Blades.
- Glass.
- Shrapnel.
- Gravel.

Air in the soft tissues

This may be surgical emphysema and may simply follow a penetrating injury. However, beware of rounded bubbles of gas and liquefaction with small fluid levels. This may indicate gas-forming organisms, e.g. *Clostridium welchii*, causing gas gangrene which is an acute medical/surgical emergency and potentially fatal.

NB In patients who are haemodynamically stable, optimum imaging assessment is often best provided by CT of the head, neck, chest, abdomen and pelvis, which gives 3D information and identifies missile tracks, trailed particles, haematomas, gas bubbles, lacerated gut and disruption of solid organs.

With intravenous, oral and rectal contrast, i.e. 'triple contrast', CT is the current state of the art for picking up evidence of:

- Torn gut.
- Vascular injury.
- Pneumoperitoneum.
- Haemoperitoneum.
- Rupture of the urinary tract.
- Damage to the liver and spleen, e.g. 'bear-claw' lacerations of the liver.

Gold medal points: CT may help in assessing a patient's haemodynamic status by showing the state of collapse or distension of the *inferior vena cava and renal veins*, should the patient be shocked or overtransfused – a sort of visual central venous line monitor.

Victims of explosions will inevitably sustain multisystem injuries, such as intracerebral haematomas, ruptured ear drums, pneumothoraces, pneumoperitoneum and haematoma formation, not just from the shock-waves of the blast but from being ripped apart by the flying shrapnel and glass if they are fortunate enough to survive. Often pools of blood and body parts are all that is left at the scene.

Emergency ultrasound of the chest or abdomen in A & E, and echocardiography of the heart, can give useful information. Colour Doppler ultrasound may be used in the emergency assessment of vascular flow or occlusion in the abdomen and limbs following trauma.

A selection of penetrating injuries is now illustrated (Figs 14.3–14.8). Each injury will generate its own constellation of problems.

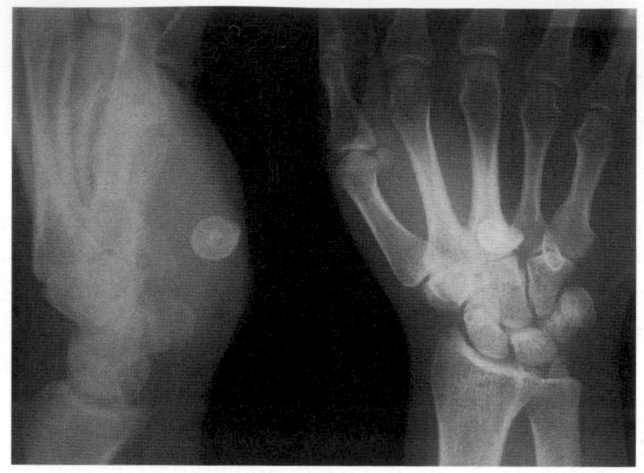

Fig. 14.3 *Cockleshell hero?* ***A*** *Lateral and* ***B*** *PA views showing a seashell embedded in the muscles of the palm.*

'Cockles and muscles': a memorable patient (Fig. 14.3)

History Slipped while jogging on the shore. This patient, who was trying to keep fit, fell over when out running, courtesy of a piece of seaweed. The inevitable 'fall on the outstretched hand' (the famous FOOSH) led to this penetrating seashell injury into the muscles of the palmar aspect of his hand.

X-ray findings

Lateral film This shows a rounded opacity on the anterior aspect of the soft tissues of the hand, with associated soft tissue swelling.

PA film A rounded opacity over the base of the 3rd metacarpal, oval in shape and of varied calcific density.

Potential misinterpretation: the lateral film

- Part of normal carpus – the pisiform bone often stands alone on a slightly oblique lateral.
- An accessory ossicle.

Potential misinterpretation: the PA film

- Opacity not perceived at all, among the jumble of carpal bones.
- Suspected dislocated carpal bone.
- Accessory ossicle of carpus.
- Fracture of base of 3rd metacarpal.

The history here is everything, so that the referring doctor knew what he was looking for. The finding of a seashell inside the hand is most unusual and most doctors would fail to recognize it for what it was without the relevant clinical information. The seashell even has a dense outer cortex, increasing its similarity to a round bone of the carpus, but its true identity is obvious once the history is known, usually to the accompaniment of 'oohs' and 'aahhs'!

Moral: Clinical histories can completely alter the interpretation of an X-ray, which itself is unchanged after the relevant information is given.

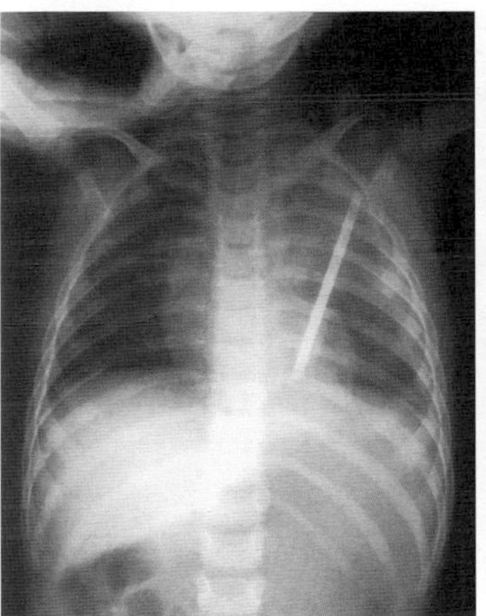
A

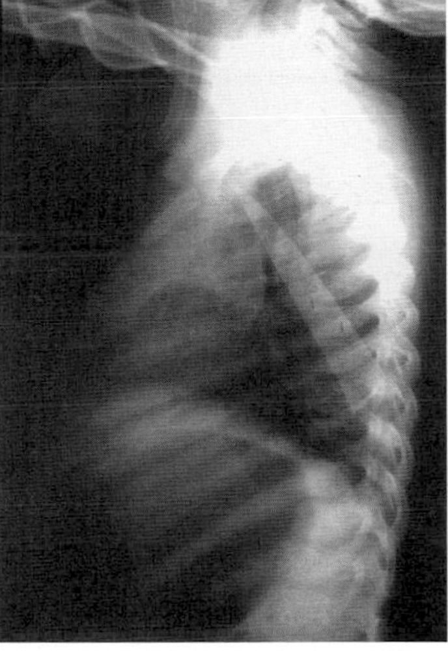
B

Fig. 14.4 ***A*** *AP and* ***B*** *lateral chest X-ray of a child dropped accidentally through a coffee table, which shattered. She was not shocked and was stable on arrival. Only a relatively small cut was seen on her back. It was only decided to take an X-ray as a precaution! The huge dagger of glass has passed upwards and laterally, missing the heart, the pulmonary artery and the aorta. Moral: a small cut can conceal a huge and potentially deadly foreign body. Also glass is opaque.*

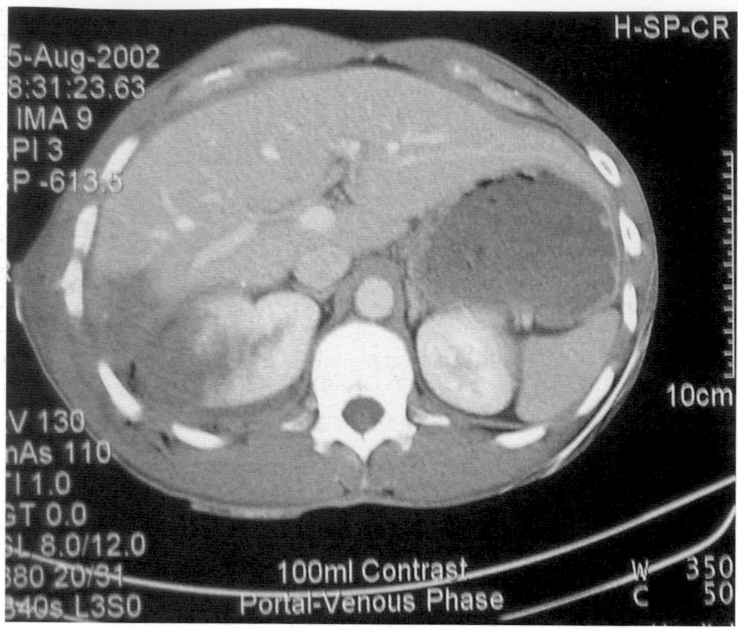

Fig. 14.5 *Gunshot wound to the abdomen – enhanced CT scan. The bullet has smashed through the liver, the lateral aspect of the right kidney and out of the back. Note: a patient with such major devastating trauma is often best sent directly to CT as soon as stabilized. In some parts of the world the majority of acute abdomens are gunshot wounds.*

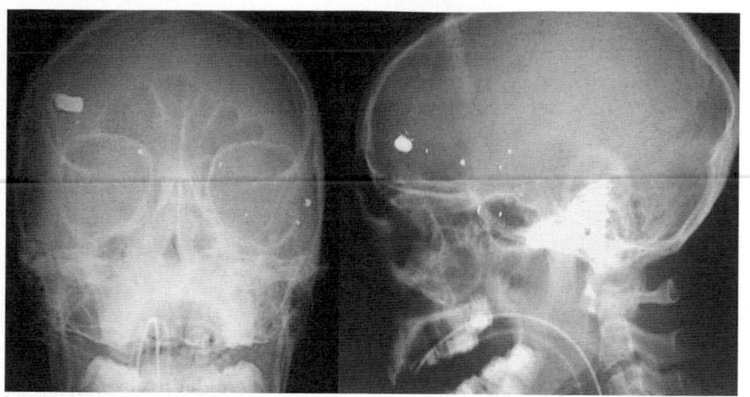

Fig. 14.6 **A** *AP and* **B** *lateral skull showing fatal gunshot wound to the head. Note the trail of debris. The entry point was behind the angle of the mandible. The patient did not survive long enough to reach CT.*

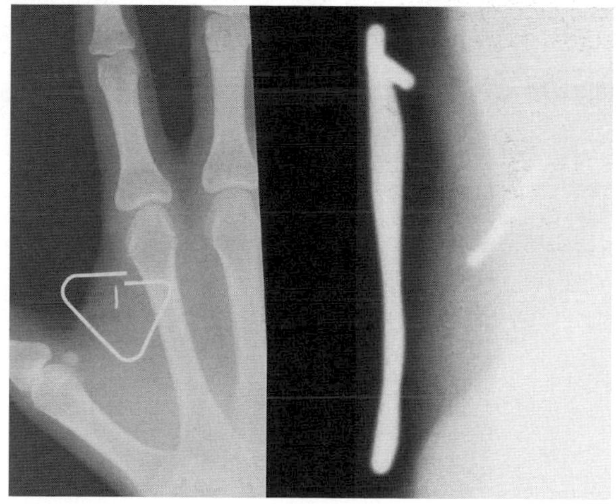

Fig. 14.7 **A** *Triangulating a wound over a foreign body with an unfolded paper clip. A metal detector will then actually help you to home in on it.* **B** *Magnified lateral view.*

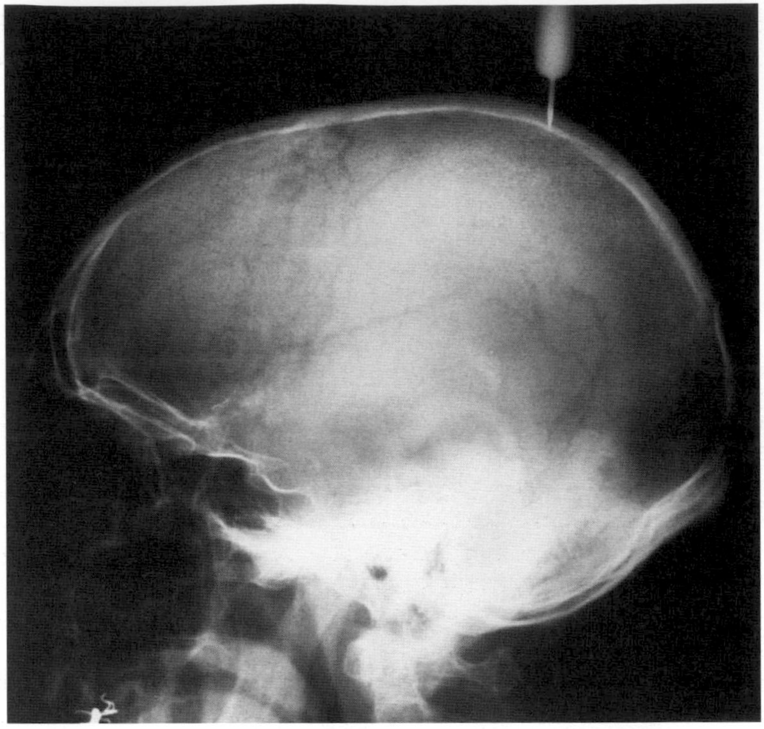

Fig. 14.8 *'I think he got the point.' Patient hit by a dart at a football match. Potential complications include: bleeding, tetanus, scalp cellulitis, osteomyelitis of the skull, septicaemia, meningitis, cerebral abscess, venous sinus thrombosis.*

Chapter 15

Non-accidental injury

Background: 'Shaken and stirred'

Whenever a baby or very young child (< 2 years) is brought in with trauma, there is the possibility of non-accidental injury (NAI). You can imagine how frightening it is for parents who have not harmed their baby to bring him or her in with a genuine injury. They will inevitably feel that people think they are guilty, just as we all do when a police car sits on our tail, and those who really have harmed their child will deny it – so the whole area is incredibly fraught. Be particularly wary of a history which does not fit the injuries, or if the history changes.

Really cunning child abusers can thump infants through a cushion to diffuse the effects of the blows; or they may dangle them by their ankles – causing less obvious injuries than when dangling them by the wrists.

Certain clinical signs like cigarette burns or a ruptured frenulum (detaching the lower lip from the gum) may be pathognomonic, but the tell-tale skeletal X-ray signs are bone injuries of different ages at particular sites.

Specifics to look out for include:

- *'Corner fractures'* at the metaphyses.
- *'Bucket-handle tears'* (Fig. 15.1) at the distal metaphyses of the long bones, which are basically more extensive 'corner fractures'.
- *Rib fractures* (Fig. 15.2) – may be due to shaking or squeezing the chest and present as little (or large) callus balls along the arcs of the ribs, particularly suspicious if bilateral and of different ages.
- *Periosteal reaction* (Fig. 15.3) of a long bone (e.g. the ulna) may indicate a response to trauma – but do not forget it may also indicate osteomyelitis in a

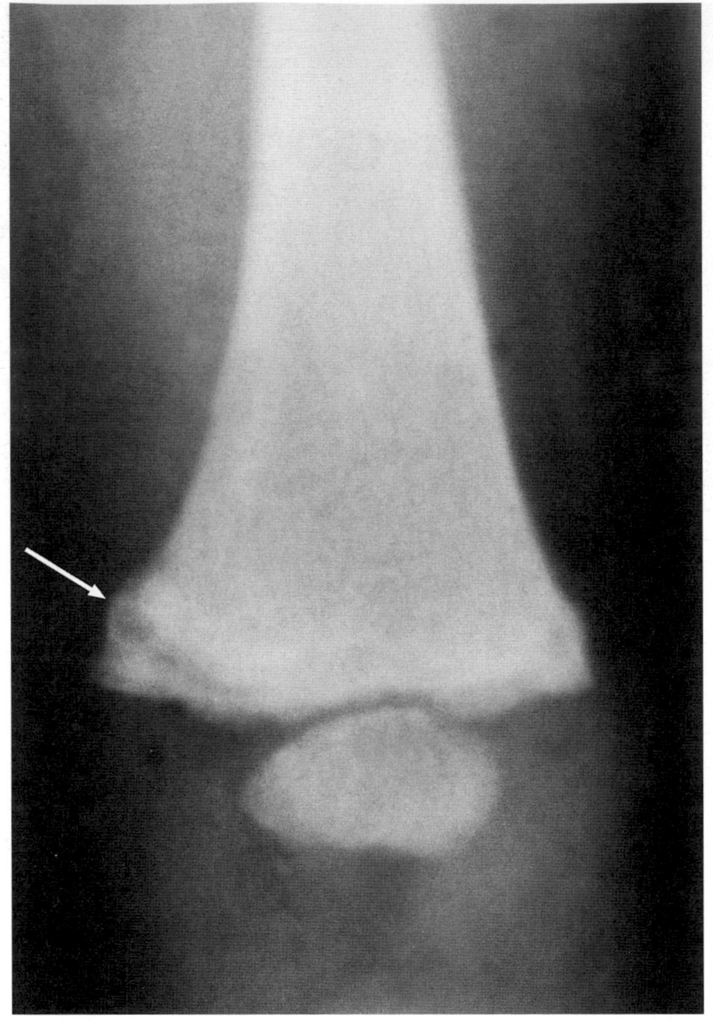

Fig. 15.1 *Bucket-handle fracture.*

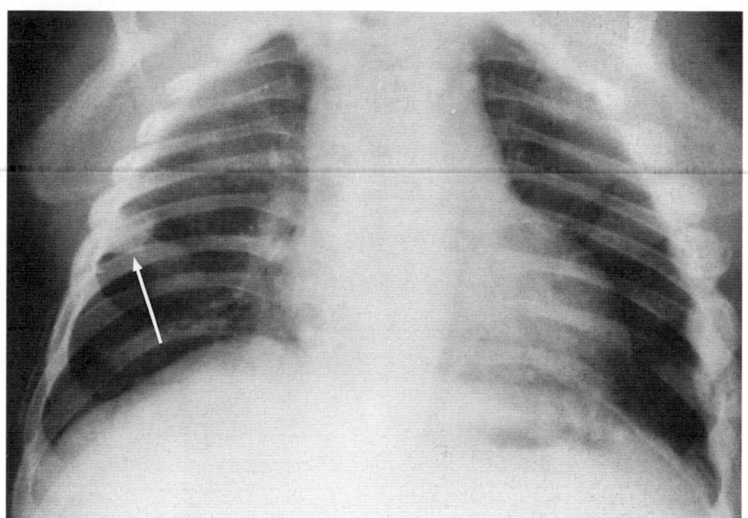

Fig. 15.2 *Multiple rib fractures in an infant. There are multiple callus balls down the left side from the 3rd rib and an isolated fracture of the right 5th rib anteriorly (arrow).*

child who is, for example, 'not using his arm, Doctor' And it does not have to be due to a fall – 'wringing' the soft tissues could just as easily do it – and this would be due to abuse.

- *Skull fracture* of course may indicate more severe trauma, e.g. smashing the head against a wall (Fig. 2.16).

What to do?

- Check the affect of the child – ? withdrawn.
- Be discreet and proceed with caution before making accusations.
- Has this child been in before?
- Check the at-risk register. Is this child on it?

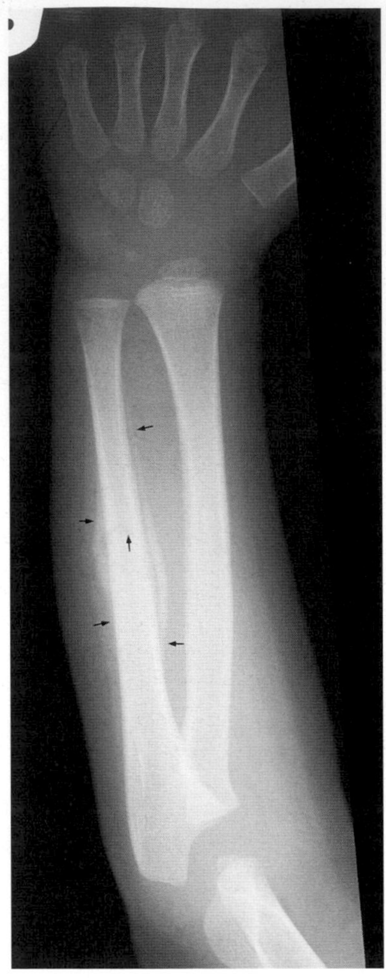

Fig. 15.3 *Periosteal reaction (arrows) on the ulna due to non-accidental injury. Note that osteomyelitis could generate an identical appearance and must always be kept in mind, for example when a child will not move a limb.*

- Get more experienced advice early – from a senior clinical colleague, the paediatricians, and if necessary, social services.

However:

- Maintain a high index of suspicion for and decide whether it is safe to let the child go home.
- **NB** Some experts regard rib fractures as an indication for a head scan (CT or MRI), and MRI has been mooted as the first examination of choice as it may confirm intracranial haematomas of different ages.

Gold medal points

- Instead of healing, skull fractures in young children can grow to produce *traumatic encephalocoeles* or *growing skull fractures*.
- *Necklace calcification* may be seen in the neck due to fat necrosis after attempted strangulation.
- *Ultrasound* may sometimes detect fractures in children sooner than X-rays.

NB Don't forget osteogenesis imperfecta. This may produce fractures with florid periosteal reactions, and it must be emphasized that many of the skeletal injuries described above may also occur in this condition, so are **not invariably pathognomonic of child abuse**. Check therefore for deafness, blue sclerae and wormian bones. Other rare skeletal dysplasias may also, on occasion, require to be entertained in the differential diagnosis.

Hints

- **Treat the patient, not the X-ray!**
- The head of the radius is at the elbow, not the wrist.
- Don't mix up metacarpals with metatarsals on request forms.
- Make sure you know your anatomy.
- Don't mix up the glenoid with the acetabulum. The glenoid is at the shoulder; the acetabulum is at the hip.
- Look right round the edge of every bone. It's laborious but you must force yourself to do it.
- It's not the skull fracture that matters but the damage underneath it.
- Make sure you do a thorough clinical examination before requesting X-rays.
- The most important part of a stethoscope is the bit between the ears.
- Tell the radiographer what you want to *see*, rather than requesting views you may not fully understand.
- Make sure you view the scalp with a bright light for air, glass, other foreign bodies and bumps.
- Not all foreign bodies under the skin are opaque, but ultrasound might show them.
- If you ask for a 'right foot' make sure it is a 'right foot' that comes back.
- Don't mistake normal epiphyses for fractures, or fractures for epiphyses.
- Two views at right angles is the minimum requirement.
- There will always be a 'helper' at your elbow to say 'That looks a bit funny' but you must make up your own mind on every film.

- Beware of the drunk. He is harder to assess clinically and the X-rays are likely to be degraded by obliquity and movement.
- Beware of artefacts and misleading images. There is nothing patients can't come up with to fox you or catch you out.
- Remember pathological fractures and pre-existing disease, even in the context of acute trauma, and especially in the context of sudden spontaneous pain.
- The 'retrospectoscope' is a cruel instrument.
- Keep good notes.
- Don't take any chances with the neck.
- 50% of the marks are for putting the films up the right way round.
- Find out if she is pregnant before you X-ray her pelvis, not after.
- Don't fall for a poorly inspired chest film.
- Each lobe collapses in its own way.
- X-rays won't show every fracture.
- Some fractures take weeks to appear.
- Some patients will walk on an impacted neck of femur, and let you move it around.
- Patients may only complain of their most severe pain thus masking other injuries.
- Oblique views will underestimate angulation.
- The bright light is your secret weapon.
- Don't let other people put the films up for you. 'Five'll get you ten' they'll put them up the wrong way round!
- Get someone else's opinion on the films you already have before exposing patients to more radiation.
- 'Seldom right but never in doubt' is not a good working aphorism.
- Never underestimate the value of previous films.

- 'A three-legged dog is still a dog', patients will not always present with all the symptoms and signs of disease.
- We are all looking for the signs that stop us thinking.
- Always be on the lookout for a second or third subtle finding, and the unexpected.
- If using conventional films, make sure you've taken all the films out of the packet. Not realizing that an axial view has been taken is a great way to miss a posterior dislocation of the shoulder!
- Listen to what the patient is saying to you. He's telling you what's wrong with him.
- A second film can add enormously to the diagnostic value of the first.
- Aim for the confidence of absolute knowledge.
- 'Bones are not full of red marrow but black ingratitude'. Miss a fracture and you'll find out what this means.
- And finally,

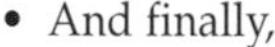

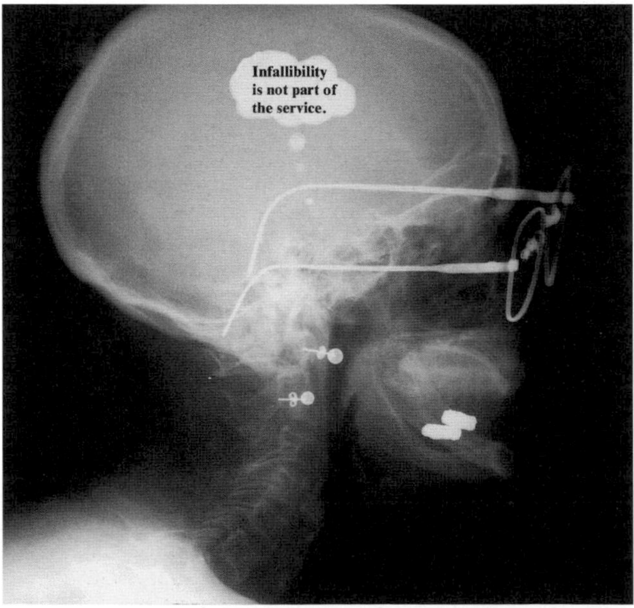

Index

Page numbers in bold print refer to illustrations and their captions.